Family Planning

A GLOBAL HANDBOOK FOR PROVIDERS

Evidence-based guidance developed
through worldwide collaboration

Updated 3rd edition
2018

World Health Organization
Department of
Reproductive Health and Research

Johns Hopkins
Bloomberg School of Public Health
Center for Communication Programs
Knowledge for Health Project

United States Agency for International Development
Bureau for Global Health
Office of Population and Reproductive Health

How to Obtain More Copies

The Knowledge for Health Project at Johns Hopkins Center for Communication Programs offers copies of *Family Planning: A Global Handbook for Providers* free of charge to readers in developing countries. All others, please contact the Knowledge for Health Project for more information.

To order by e-mail, write orders@jhuccp.org and include your name, complete mailing address, and telephone number.

To order via the Web, visit http://www.fphandbook.org/order-form.

The website http://www.fphandbook.org also offers downloads of printable files and files for e-readers in various languages of the Global Handbook and the updated wall chart, Do You Know Your Family Planning Choices?. The updates have been prepared in English. As they are translated into other languages, the translations will appear on the website.

ISBN 13: 978-0-9992037-0-5

Suggested citation: World Health Organization Department of Reproductive Health and Research (WHO/RHR) and Johns Hopkins Bloomberg School of Public Health/Center for Communication Programs (CCP), Knowledge for Health Project. Family Planning: A Global Handbook for Providers (2018 update). Baltimore and Geneva: CCP and WHO, 2018.

Published with support from the United States Agency for International Development, Global, GH/SPBO/OPS, under the terms of Grant No. AID-OAA-A-13-00068. Opinions expressed herein are those of the authors and do not necessarily reflect the views of USAID, The Johns Hopkins University, or the World Health Organization.

Family Planning

A GLOBAL HANDBOOK FOR PROVIDERS

Contents

BACK MATTER

Searchable online at www.fphandbook.org

JOB AIDS AND TOOLS

From the World Health Organization

Access to high-quality, affordable sexual and reproductive health services and information, including a full range of contraceptive methods, is fundamental to realizing the rights and well-being of women and girls, men and boys. Universal access to effective contraception ensures that all adults and adolescents can avoid the adverse health and socioeconomic consequences of unintended pregnancy and have a satisfying sexual life. Key global initiatives, including the Sustainable Development Goals and the Global Strategy for Women's, Children's and Adolescents' Health, call for universal access to family planning services as a right of women and girls and crucial to a healthy life.

However, reducing the vast unmet need for family planning remains a massive challenge to countries and the global health community. Services are still poor-quality or unavailable in many settings, while service delivery and social constraints persist.

Family planning providers are at the core of health system responses to these challenges. The Global Handbook offers clear, up-to-date information and advice to help providers meet clients' needs and inform their choice and use of contraception. The Handbook is also an excellent resource for training and can help to reinforce supervision.

The 2018 edition of the Handbook includes new WHO recommendations that expand contraceptive choices. For example, WHO now recommends that breastfeeding women can start progestogen-only pills or contraceptive implants any time after childbirth. More contraceptive options are now included: ulipristal acetate for emergency contraception; sub-cutaneous injection of DMPA; and the progesterone-releasing vaginal ring. Also, guidance on starting ongoing contraception following emergency contraception is provided. An important message throughout is WHO's recommendation that adolescent girls and young women are medically eligible to use any contraceptive method. In addition, the Handbook highlights opportunities for task sharing among providers to make contraceptive methods more available. This edition also includes the latest WHO guidance on hormonal contraception and HIV and advice for counselling clients at risk of HIV infection on their contraceptive choices.

WHO encourages all national health systems and other organizations providing family planning to consider this new edition of the Global Handbook a key document to help ensure the quality and safety of family planning services.

WHO appreciates the contributions of the many people, named in the Acknowledgements, who supported the updating and expanding this edition of the Handbook. Also, WHO thanks the Johns Hopkins Bloomberg School of Public Health/Center for Communication Programs for management and the United States Agency for International Development for financial and technical support of the Handbook.

Ian Askew, PhD
Director, Department of Reproductive Health and Research
World Health Organization

From the United States Agency for International Development

Access to voluntary family planning and reproductive health services for everyone, inclusive of women, men, couples, and adolescents, supports the health and well-being of individuals and can have positive economic, environmental, and social benefits for families and communities.

This handbook provides updated accurate and practical guidance to support program managers and providers in delivering high-quality family planning counseling, services and care. Prior editions were widely used to support strong programs: Over 500,000 copies have been distributed through USAID to governments and their partners. We anticipate this 2018 edition will continue to help family planning providers across the globe provide high-quality counseling and services.

Since the 2011 edition, many contraceptive methods have become more available in a range of markets. This edition updates information about these methods and covers new methods, including the LNG-IUD and implants, two long-acting reversible methods; subcutaneous depot medroxyprogesterone acetate (DMPA-SC), with the potential for self-injection; and the new progesterone-releasing vaginal ring for breastfeeding women. This update confirms that all women can safely use almost any method and that providing most methods is typically not complicated. Indeed, most methods can be provided even where resources are limited.

This handbook provides basic information that providers need to assist women and couples to choose, use, and change family planning methods as they move through their lives. As always, program managers and providers play a central role in supporting clients to make voluntary and informed choices from a range of safe and available methods. The client–provider relationship, grounded in evidence-based and skillful counseling, can help inform the client's understanding of family planning benefits in general and of the chosen method in particular. New clients may have a method already in mind, but they may not be aware of other options; continuing clients may have concerns with their current method, and knowledgeable counseling can help prevent discontinuation or help clients switch methods effectively. With the information in this book and the right resources, providers can ensure that a client's reproductive intentions, life situation, and preferences govern family planning decisions.

This update was developed in collaboration with the World Health Organization and experts from many organizations. USAID is proud to support its publication. We look forward to continuing the work with our many partners to empower women, men, couples, and adolescents to plan their families and their future.

Ellen H. Starbird
Director, Office of Population and Reproductive Health
Bureau for Global Health
United States Agency for International Development

Acknowledgements

Family Planning: A Global Handbook for Providers first appeared in 2007. It was updated in 2011 and now again in 2018. All 3 editions have benefited from the contributions of many people in many different organizations. The publishers wish to thank all these contributors. Without the collaboration and commitment of all involved, this book would not be possible.

First edition, 2007
Vera Zlidar, Ushma Upadhyay, and Robert Lande of the INFO Project, Center for Communication Programs at Johns Hopkins Bloomberg School of Public Health were the principal technical writers and led the handbook development process, together with Ward Rinehart from the INFO Project and Sarah Johnson of the World Health Organization, who also served as editors. Other contributors to the research and writing from the INFO Project include Fonda Kingsley, Sarah O'Hara, Hilary Schwandt, Ruwaida Salem, Vidya Setty, Deepa Ramchandran, Catherine Richey, Mahua Mandal, and Indu Adhikary.

Key technical advisors throughout the development of the book included Robert Hatcher, Roy Jacobstein, Enriquito Lu, Herbert Peterson, James Shelton, and Irina Yacobson. Kathryn Curtis, Anna Glasier, Robert Hatcher, Roy Jacobstein, Herbert Peterson, James Shelton, Paul Van Look, and Marcel Vekemans conducted final technical review of this book.

The following people provided their expertise during expert meetings in Baltimore in October 2004, Geneva in June 2005, or both: Yasmin Ahmed, Marcos Arevalo, Luis Bahamondes, Miriam Chipimo, Maria del Carmen Cravioto, Kathryn Curtis, Juan Diaz, Soledad Diaz, Mohammad Eslami, Anna Glasier, John Guillebaud, Ezzeldin Othman Hassan, Robert Hatcher, Mihai Horga, Douglas Huber, Carlos Huezo, Roy Jacobstein, Enriquito Lu, Pisake Lumbiganon, Pamela Lynam, Trent MacKay, Olav Meirik, Isaiah Ndong, Herbert Peterson, John Pile, Robert Rice, Roberto Rivera, Lois Schaefer, Markku Seppala, James Shelton, Bulbul Sood, Markus Steiner, James Trussell, Marcel Vekemans, and Wu Shangchun.

The key contributors to this handbook, who are listed above, declared no conflicts of interest.

The following organizations made extraordinary technical contributions to the creation of this handbook: The Centre for Development and Population Activities, EngenderHealth, Family Health International (now FHI360), Georgetown University Institute for Reproductive Health, Jhpiego, Management Sciences for Health, the Population Council, and the United States Agency for International Development.

Many others also contributed their expertise on specific topics and participated in the development of consensus on technical content. Contributors include Christopher Armstrong, Mark Barone, Mags Beksinska, Yemane Berhane, Ann Blouse, Julia Bluestone, Paul Blumenthal, Annette Bongiovanni, Débora Bossemeyer, Nathalie Broutet, Ward Cates, Venkatraman Chandra-Mouli, Kathryn Church, Samuel Clark, Carmela Cordero, Vanessa Cullins, Kelly Culwell, Johannes van Dam, Catherine d'Arcangues, Barbara Kinzie Deller, Sibongile Dludlu, Mary Drake, Paul Feldblum, Ron Frezieres, Claudia Garcia-Moreno, Kamlesh Giri, Patricia Gómez, Pio Iván Gómez Sánchez, Vera Halpern, Robert Hamilton, Theresa Hatzell, Helena von Hertzen, John Howson, Carol Joanis, Robert Johnson, Adrienne Kols, Deborah Kowal, Jan Kumar, Anne MacGregor, Luann Martin, Matthews Mathai, Noel McIntosh, Manisha Mehta, Kavita Nanda, Ruchira Tabassum Naved, Francis Ndowa, Nuriye Ortayli, Elizabeth Raymond, Heidi Reynolds, Mandy Rose, Sharon Rudy, Joseph Ruminjo, Dana Samu, Julia Samuelson, Harshad Sanghvi, George Schmid, Judith Senderowitz, Jacqueline Sherris, Nono Simelela, Irving Sivin, Jenni Smit, David Sokal, Jeff Spieler, Kay Stone, Maryanne Stone-Jimenez, Fatiha Terki, Kathleen Vickery, Lee Warner, Mary Nell Wegner, Peter Weis, and Tim Williams.

Family planning providers in Bangladesh, Brazil, China, Ghana, India, Indonesia, Kenya, Pakistan, the Philippines, and Zambia offered comments on draft covers and chapters of the book in sessions organized by Yasmin Ahmed, Ekta Chandra, Miriam Chipimo, Sharmila Das, Juan Diaz, Carlos Huezo, Enriquito Lu, Isaiah Ndong, Samson Radeny, Mary Segall, Sarbani Sen, Nina Shalita, Bulbul Sood, and Wu Shangchun.

John Fiege, Linda Sadler, and Rafael Avila created the layout of the book. Mark Beisser created the cover and initial design along with Linda Sadler, the staff at Prographics, and John Fiege. Rafael Avila managed the photographs and illustrations. Ushma Upadhyay, Vera Zlidar, and Robert Jacoby managed the book's production. Heather Johnson managed printing and distribution of the handbook along with Mandy Liberto, Tre Turner, Roslyn Suite-Parham, and Quan Wynder.

Second edition, 2011

The 2011 update incorporated all guidance from the WHO expert Working Group meeting in April 2008 for the *Medical Eligibility Criteria* and the *Selected Practice Recommendations,* and two Technical Consultations related to these guidelines in October 2008 and January 2010. It also incorporated guidance from an expert Working Group meeting on HIV and infant feeding in October 2009 and a Technical Consultation on community-based provision of injectable contraceptives in June 2009.

Selected members of the expert Working Group that met in 2005, experts who contributed to the handbook, and WHO staff contributed to and reviewed the update. They included Mario Festin, Mary Lyn Gaffield, Lucy Harber, Douglas Huber, Roy Jacobstein, Kirsten Krueger, Enriquito Lu, James Shelton, Jeff Spieler, and Irina Yacobson. Ward Rinehart and Sarah Johnson of Jura Editorial Services managed and edited the 2011 update.

Third edition, 2018

This update of the *Global Handbook* has involved a complete review of the contents of the 2011 edition and updating as needed. All chapters reflect the latest relevant WHO guidance. Thus, this update includes the recommendations of the fifth edition of the *Medical Eligibility Criteria for Contraceptive Use*, published in 2016, and of the third edition of the *Selected Practice Recommendations for Contraceptive Use*, published in 2016. (The bibliography on p. 422 lists WHO guidance documents.)

The following people contributed to this edition of the Global Handbook: Afeefa Abdur-Rahman, Moazzam Ali, Avni Amin, Ian Askew, Michal Avni, Rachel Baggaley, Beth Balderston, Pritha Biswas, Nathalie Broutet, Levent Cagatay, Heather Clark, Carmela Cordero, Jane Cover, Margaret D'Adamo, Hugo de Vuyst, Juan Diaz, Jennifer Drake, Jill Edwardson, Mohammed Eslami, Mario Festin, Melissa Freeman, Mary Lyn Gaffield, Victoria Graham, Metin Gulmezoglu, Denise Harrison, Roy Jacobstein, James Kiarie, Maggie Kilbourne-Brook, Robert Lande, Catherine Lane, Candace Lew, Enriquito (Ricky) Lu, Patricia MacDonald, Baker Maggwa, Shawn Malarcher, Judy Manning, Rachel Marcus, Jennifer Mason, Ruth Merkatz, Maureen Norton, Stephen Nurse-Findlay, Sarah Onyango, Kevin Peine, Rabab Petit, Kate Rademacher, Andrea Roe, Nigel Rollins, Vicky Samantha Rossi, Frans Roumen, Abdulmumin Saad, James Shelton, Jacqueline Sherris, Katherine Simmons, Regine Sitruk-Ware, Shelley Snyder, Jeff Spieler, Markus Steiner, Petrus Steyn, Melanie Taylor, Caitlin Thistle, Sara Tifft, John Townsend, James Trussell, Sheryl van der Poel, Elizabeth Westley, Teodora Wi, and Irina Yacobson. Sarah Johnson and Ward Rinehart of Jura Editorial Services managed and edited the 2018 update.

Several groups contributed new content to this edition. Beth Balderston, Jane Cover, Jenifer Drake, and Sara Tifft at PATH contributed the sections on giving subcutaneous injections in Chapter 4, Progestin-only Injectables. Heather Clark at the Population Council prepared Chapter 8, Progesterone-Releasing Vaginal Ring. Roy Jacobstein at Intrah and Markus Steiner at FHI 360 developed the section on counseling about effectiveness in Chapter 25, Family Planning Provision. John Stanback, Irina Yacobson, and Lucy Harber at FHI 360 created the job aids and text in the section on ruling out pregnancy (pages 439–440).

The Knowledge for Health Project at the Johns Hopkins Bloomberg School of Public Health, Center for Communication Programs, manages the production of the handbook and its distribution, with support from the United States Agency for International Development. Tara Sullivan is Project Director. As Operations Manager, Heather Finn oversaw development of this update. Susan Krenn directs the Center for Communication Programs.

WHO's Family Planning Guidance

The World Health Organization (WHO) develops guidance through a process that begins with systematic review and assessment of research evidence on key public health questions. Then, WHO convenes working groups of experts from around the world. The working groups assess the implications of the evidence and make recommendations for health care services and practice. Policy-makers and program managers can use these recommendations to write or update national guidelines and program policies.

Using this process, the Department of Reproductive Health and Research issues guidance on specific issues as important questions arise. It also maintains 2 sets of guidance that are updated and expanded periodically:

- The *Medical Eligibility Criteria for Contraceptive Use* provides guidance on whether people with certain medical conditions can safely and effectively use specific contraceptive methods.
- The *Selected Practice Recommendations for Contraceptive Use* answers questions about how to use various contraceptive methods.

This book, *Family Planning: A Global Handbook for Providers*, offers technical information to help health care providers deliver family planning methods appropriately and effectively. It incorporates and reflects the Medical Eligibility Criteria and the Selected Practice Recommendations as well as other WHO guidance. This third edition brings the Global Handbook up to date with current WHO guidance on all topics covered. A thorough reference guide, the handbook provides specific and practical guidance on 21 family planning methods. It also covers health issues that may arise in the context of family planning services. The intended primary audience for this handbook is health care providers who offer family planning in resource-limited settings around the world. Health care managers, supervisors, and policy-makers also may find this book helpful.

The *Decision-Making Tool for Family Planning Clients and Providers* incorporates WHO guidance into a tool that helps family planning providers and clients to discuss family planning choices and helps clients make informed decisions. This flipchart tool leads provider and client through a structured yet tailored process that facilitates choosing and using a family planning method. The tool also helps to guide return visits by family planning clients.

Together, these 4 publications—the Medical Eligibility Criteria, the Selected Practice Recommendations, the Global Handbook, and the Decision-Making Tool—are known as the 4 Cornerstones of WHO's family planning guidance.

On the Internet:

- Medical Eligibility Criteria: www.who.int/reproductivehealth/publications/family_planning/MEC-5/en/
- Selected Practice Recommendations: www.who.int/reproductivehealth/publications/family_planning/SPR-3/en/
- Family Planning: A Global Handbook for Providers: www.fphandbook.org
- Decision-Making Tool for Family Planning Clients and Providers: www.who.int/reproductivehealth/publications/family_planning/9241593229index/en/

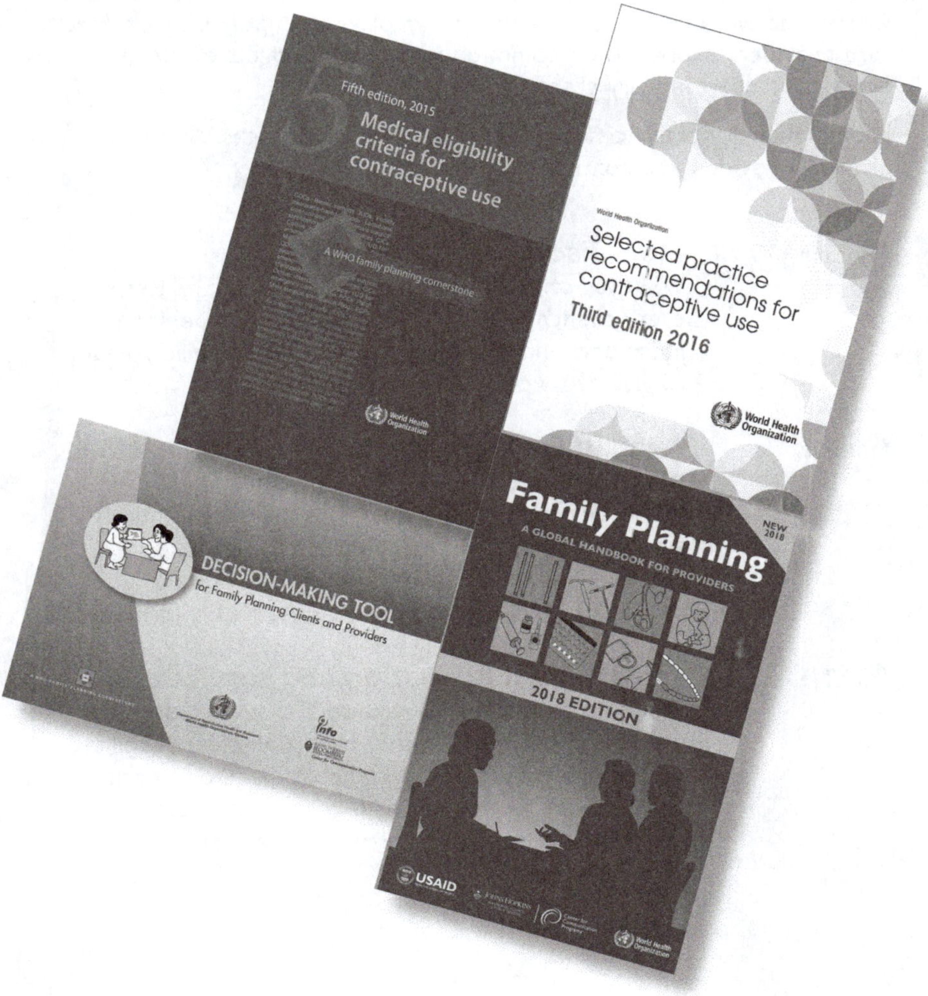

Human Rights: Family Planning Providers' Contribution

All people deserve the right to determine, as best they can, the course of their own lives. Whether and when to have children, how many, and with whom are important parts of this right. Family planning providers have the privilege and responsibility to help people to make and carry out these decisions. Furthermore, programs that honor their clients' human rights contribute to positive sexual health outcomes.

Thus, high-quality family planning services and the people who deliver them respect, protect, and fulfill the human rights of all their clients. Everyone working at every level of the health system plays an important part. Health care providers express their commitment to human rights every day in every contact with every client.

Nine human rights principles guide family planning services. As a family planning provider, you contribute to all of them.

Principle **1**

Non-discrimination
What you can do: Welcome all clients equally. Respect every client's needs and wishes. Set aside personal judgments and any negative opinions. Promise yourself to give every client the best care you can.

Principle **2**

Availability of contraceptive information and services
What you can do: Know the family planning methods available and how to provide them. Help make sure that supplies stay in stock. Do not rule out any method for a client, and do not hold back information.

Principle **3**

Accessible information and services
What you can do: Help make sure that everyone can use your facility, even if they have a physical disability. Participate in outreach, when possible. Do not ask clients, even young clients, to get someone else's permission to use family planning or a certain family planning method.

Principle **4** **Acceptable information and services**

What you can do: Be friendly and welcoming, and help make your facility that way. Put yourself in the client's shoes. Think what is important to the clients—what they want and how they want it provided.

Principle **5** **Quality**

What you can do: Keep your knowledge and skills up-to-date. Use good communication skills. Check that contraceptives you provide are not out-of-date.

Principle **6** **Informed decision-making**

What you can do: Explain family planning methods clearly, including how to use them, how effective they are, and what side effects they may have, if any. Help clients consider what is important to them in a family planning method.

Principle **7** **Privacy and confidentiality**

What you can do: Do not discuss your clients with others except with permission and as needed for their care. When talking with clients, find a place where others cannot hear. Do not tell others what your clients have said. Promptly put away clients' records.

Principle **8** **Participation**

What you can do: Ask clients what they think about family planning services. Act on what they say to improve care.

Principle **9** **Accountability**

What you can do: Hold yourself accountable for the care that you give clients and for their rights.

These human rights principles guide WHO's work and serve as the framework for WHO's guidance on contraceptive methods. The full statement of these principles can be found in *Ensuring human rights in the provision of contraceptive information and services: Guidance and recommendations*; 2014 (http://www.who.int/reproductivehealth/publications/family_planning/human-rights-contraception/en/).

Collaborating and Supporting Organizations

Abt Associates

African Population and Health Research Center (APHRC)

Afrihealth Optonet Association (CSOs Network), Nigeria

Al-Mustafa Welfare Association (CSOs Network), Sindh

Amref Health Africa

Ansul-India Health & Management Services (AIHMS)

Asesorías Internacionales en Salud Integral y Desarrollo (ASID), Costa Rica

Asociación Hondureña de Planificación de Familia (ASHONPLAFA)

Asociación Pro Bienestar de la Familia de Guatemala (APROFAM)

Asociación TAN UX'IL, Guatemala

Associação Moçambicana de Obstetras e Ginecologistas (AMOG)

Association Burkinabè pour le bien être familal (ABBEF) du Burkina Faso

Association for the Well-Being of the Colombian Family (Profamilia)

Association of Reproductive Health Professionals (ARHP)

Association for Reproductive and Family Health

Balanced Stewardship Development Association

Bill & Melinda Gates Institute for Population and Reproductive Health

Bixby Center for Global Reproductive Health, University of California, San Francisco

Bridges of Hope Training

CARE International

CARE USA

Carolina Population Center, University of North Carolina at Chapel Hill

Centre for the Development of People (CEDEP), Ghana

Centro de Investigación y Promoción para América Central de Derechos Humanos – CIPAC, Costa Rica

Chemonics

CILSIDA, Togo

Civil Society for Family Planning in Nigeria (CiSFP)

Concept Foundation

Consortium of Reproductive Health Associations (CORHA).

CORE Group

Croatian Society for Reproductive Medicine and Gynecologic Endocrinology of Croatian Medical Association

Cultural Practice, LLC

East European Institute for Reproductive Health

EngenderHealth

Equilibres & Populations

Family Guidance Association of Ethiopia

Family Planning Association of Swaziland

Federation of Obstetric & Gynecological Societies of India

Female Health Company

FHI 360

Foundation for Integrated Rural Development (FIRD), Uganda

FP2020

FUSA AC, Argentina

Georgetown University, Institute for Reproductive Health

Grameen Foundation USA (GF USA)

Guttmacher Institute

Health NGOs Network (HENNET)

Health, Development and Performance (HDP), Rwanda

Hesperian Health Guides

Hindustan Latex Family Planning Promotion Trust (HLFPPT)

Implementing Best Practices (IBP) Consortium

Initiative Supporting Adolescents & Youths in Education and Sexual Health (ISAYES), Nigeria

Institute of Health Management, Pachod (IHMP)

Institute of Tropical Medicine, Antwerp, Belgium

Instituto Nacional de Ciencias Médicas y Nutrición Salvador Zubirán.

Intensive Rescue Foundation International (IRFI)

International Community of Women Living with HIV

International Community of Women Living with HIV – Eastern Africa (ICWEA)

International Confederation of Midwives

International Consortium for Emergency Contraception (ICEC)

International Federation of Gynecology and Obstetrics (FIGO)

International Islamic Center for Population Studies and Research (IICPSR) – Al Azhar University.

International Medical Corps

International Planned Parenthood Federation (IPPF)

International Planned Parenthood Federation/Western Hemisphere Region (IPPF/WHR)

IntraHealth International, Inc.

Investigación en Salud y Demografía, S.C. (INSAD)

Ipas Africa Alliance

Jhpiego

John Snow, Inc (JSI)

Johns Hopkins Bloomberg School of Public Health

Kwa-Zulu Natal Maternal Women, Child and Nutrition Directorate

Last Mile Health and Development Association, Nigeria

LiveWell Initiative LWI, Nigeria

Management Sciences for Health (MSH)

Marie Stopes International

Ministry of Health and Medical Services, Solomon Islands

Ministry of Health Belize

Ministry of Health of the Republic of Zambia

Mozambican Association for Family Development (AMODEFA)

Muslim Family Counselling Services

National Population and Family Planning Board, Indonesia

Network of People Living with HIV/AIDS in Nigeria (NEPHWAN)

NGALAKERI

Options Consultancy Services

Overseas Strategic Consulting, Ltd

Palladium

Pan African Positive Women's Coalition, Zimbabwe

Pan American Health Organization, Latin American Center for Perinatology, Women and Reproductive Health (CLAP/WR-PAHO/WHO)

PATH

Pathfinder International

PLAFAM, Asociación Civil de Planificación Familiar

Plan International

Planned Parenthood Association of Ghana (PPAG)

Planned Parenthood Association of Zambia (PPAZ)

Planned Parenthood Global

Population Council

Population Foundation of India (PFI)

Population Media Center (PMC)

Population Reference Bureau

Population Services International (PSI)

Princeton University, Office of Population Research

PT Tunggal Idaman Abdi

Public Health Informatics Foundation (PHIF)

Public Health Institute (PHI)

Real Agency for Community Development (RACD), Uganda

Reproductive Health Supplies Coalition (RHSC)

Reproductive Health Uganda (RHU)

Réseau Siggil Jigéen Sénégal

Romanian Family Planning Network

Rotarian Action Group for Population & Development (RFPD)

Salud y Famila

Save the Children

SOCOBA Inc. (Society for Children Orphaned by AIDS)

Trust Women Foundation

Tulane University School of Public Health and Tropical Medicine

Uganda Youth Alliance for Family Planning and Adolescent Health (UYAFPAH)

United Nations Population Fund

University of Gadjah Mada (UGM), Indonesia

University of North Carolina Gillings School of Global Public Health

University of the Witwatersrand, Reproductive Health and HIV Institute

University Research Co., LLC

Venture Strategies for Health and Development

We Care Solar

Wellbeing Foundation Africa

West African Health Organization (WAHO)

WINGS/ALAS Guatemala

YLabs

Zimbabwe National Family Planning Council (ZNFPC)

Combined Oral Contraceptives

Key Points for Providers and Clients

- **Take one pill every day.** For greatest effectiveness a woman must take pills daily and start each new pack of pills on time.
- **Take any missed pill as soon as possible.** Missing pills risks pregnancy and may make some side effects worse.
- **Bleeding changes are common but not harmful.** Typically, there is irregular bleeding for the first few months and then lighter and more regular bleeding.
- **Can be given to a woman at any time to start now or later.**

What Are Combined Oral Contraceptives?

- Pills that contain low doses of 2 hormones—a progestin and an estrogen—like the natural hormones progesterone and estrogen in a woman's body.
- Combined oral contraceptives (COCs) are also called "the Pill," low-dose combined pills, OCPs, and OCs.
- Work primarily by preventing the release of eggs from the ovaries (ovulation).

How Effective?

Effectiveness depends on the user: Risk of pregnancy is greatest when a woman starts a new pill pack 3 or more days late, or misses 3 or more pills near the beginning or end of a pill pack.

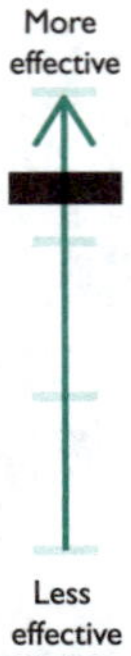

- As commonly used, about 7 pregnancies per 100 women using COCs over the first year. This means that 93 of every 100 women using COCs will not become pregnant.
- When no pill-taking mistakes are made, less than 1 pregnancy per 100 women using COCs over the first year (3 per 1,000 women).

Return of fertility after COCs are stopped: No delay

Protection against sexually transmitted infections (STIs): None

Why Some Women Say They Like Combined Oral Contraceptives

- Are controlled by the woman
- Can be stopped at any time without a provider's help
- Do not interfere with sex
- Are easy to use
- Easy to obtain, for example, in drug shops or pharmacies

Side Effects, Health Benefits, and Health Risks

Side Effects (see also Managing Any Problems, p. 20)

Some users report the following:

- Changes in bleeding patterns,[†] including:
  - Lighter bleeding and fewer days of bleeding
  - Irregular bleeding
  - Infrequent bleeding
  - No monthly bleeding
- Headaches
- Dizziness
- Nausea
- Breast tenderness
- Weight change (see Question 6, p. 25)
- Mood changes
- Acne (can improve or worsen, but usually improves)

> Bleeding changes are normal and not harmful. If a woman finds them bothersome, counseling and support can help.

Other possible physical changes:

- Blood pressure increases a few points (mm Hg). When increase is due to COCs, blood pressure declines quickly after use of COCs stops.

† *For definitions of bleeding patterns, see "vaginal bleeding," page 407.*

Known Health Benefits

Help protect against:

- Risks of pregnancy
- Cancer of the lining of the uterus (endometrial cancer)
- Cancer of the ovary
- Symptomatic pelvic inflammatory disease

May help protect against:

- Ovarian cysts
- Iron-deficiency anemia

Reduce:

- Menstrual cramps
- Menstrual bleeding problems
- Ovulation pain
- Excess hair on face or body
- Symptoms of polycystic ovarian syndrome (irregular bleeding, acne, excess hair on face or body)
- Symptoms of endometriosis (pelvic pain, irregular bleeding)

Known Health Risks

Very rare:

- Blood clot in deep veins of legs or lungs (deep vein thrombosis or pulmonary embolism)

Extremely rare:

- Stroke
- Heart attack

See also Facts About Combined Oral Contraceptives and Cancer, p. 4.

Correcting Misunderstandings (see also Questions and Answers, p. 25)

Combined oral contraceptives:

- Do not build up hormones in a woman's body. Women do not need a "rest" from taking COCs.
- Must be taken every day, whether or not a woman has sex that day.
- Do not make women infertile after they stop taking COCs.
- Do not cause birth defects or multiple births.
- Do not change women's sexual behavior.
- Do not collect in the stomach. Instead, the pill dissolves each day.
- Do not disrupt an existing pregnancy.

Facts About Combined Oral Contraceptives and Cancer

Overall risk of developing cancer over a lifetime is similar among women who have used COCs and women who have not used COCs. COC users may have small increases in risk of some types of cancer, but they also have long-term reductions in other types of cancer.

Ovarian and endometrial cancer

- Use of COCs helps *protect* users from 2 important kinds of cancer—cancer of the ovaries and cancer of the lining of the uterus (endometrial cancer).
- This protection continues for 15 years or more after stopping use of COCs.

Breast cancer

- Research findings about COCs and breast cancer are difficult to interpret:
  - Studies find that women who used COCs more than 10 years ago face the same risk of breast cancer as similar women who have never used COCs. In contrast, some studies find that current users of COCs and women who have used COCs within the past 10 years are slightly more likely to be diagnosed with breast cancer. On balance, there may be little difference in lifetime risk. It is unclear whether these findings are explained by earlier detection of existing breast cancers among COC users or by a biologic effect of COCs on breast cancer.
  - Previous use of COCs does not increase the risk of breast cancer later in life, when breast cancer is more common.
  - When a current or former COC user is diagnosed with breast cancer, the cancers generally are less advanced than cancers diagnosed in other women.
  - COC use does not increase risk of breast cancer for women whose relatives have had breast cancer.

Cervical cancer

- Cervical cancer is caused by certain types of human papillomavirus (HPV). HPV is a common sexually transmitted infection that usually clears on its own without treatment, but sometimes it persists and sometimes leads to cervical cancer. A vaccine can help to prevent cervical cancer. (See Cervical Cancer, p. 340.) If cervical screening is available, providers can advise all women to be screened every 3 years (or as national guidelines recommend).
- Use of COCs for 5 years or more appears to increase slightly the risk of cervical cancer. After a woman stops using COCs, this risk decreases. By 10 years after stopping COCs, a former COC user has the same risk of cervical cancer as a woman who has never used COCs. The number of cervical cancers associated with COC use is small.

Other cancers

- Use of COCs may decrease the risk of colorectal cancer.
- There is no clear evidence that COC use either decreases or increases the risk of any other type of cancer.

Who Can and Cannot Use Combined Oral Contraceptives

Safe and Suitable for Nearly All Women

Nearly all women can use COCs safely and effectively, including women who:

- Have or have not had children
- Are married or are not married
- Are of any age, including adolescents and women over 40 years old
- After childbirth and during breastfeeding, after a period of time
- Have just had an abortion, miscarriage, or ectopic pregnancy
- Smoke cigarettes—if under 35 years old
- Have anemia now or had in the past
- Have varicose veins
- Are living with HIV, whether or not on antiretroviral therapy

Avoid Unnecessary Procedures

(see Importance of Procedures, p. 368)

Women can begin using COCs:

- Without a pelvic examination
- Without any blood tests or other routine laboratory tests
- Without cervical cancer screening
- Without a breast examination
- Without a pregnancy test. A woman can begin using COCs at any time, even when she is not having monthly bleeding at the time, if it is reasonably certain she is not pregnant (see Pregnancy Checklist, inside back cover).

> Blood pressure measurement is desirable before starting a hormonal method. However, where the risks of pregnancy are high and few methods are available, a woman should not be denied a hormonal method simply because her blood pressure cannot be measured. If possible, she can have her blood pressure measured later at a time and place convenient for her.

Medical Eligibility Criteria for

Combined Oral Contraceptives

Ask the client the questions below about known medical conditions. Examinations and tests are not necessary. If she answers "no" to all of the questions, then she can start COCs if she wants. If she answers "yes" to a question, follow the instructions. In some cases she can still start COCs. These questions also apply for the combined patch (see p. 117) and the combined vaginal ring (see p. 123).

1. Are you breastfeeding a baby less than 6 months old?

❑ NO ❑ **YES**

- If fully or nearly fully breastfeeding: Give her COCs and tell her to start taking them 6 months after giving birth or when breast milk is no longer the baby's main food—whichever comes first (see Fully or nearly fully breastfeeding, p. 11).
- If partially breastfeeding: She can start COCs as soon as 6 weeks after childbirth (see Partially breastfeeding, p. 12).

2. Have you had a baby in the last 3 weeks and you are not breastfeeding?

❑ NO ❑ **YES** Give her COCs now and tell her to start taking them 3 weeks after childbirth. (If there is an additional risk that she might develop a blood clot in a deep vein (deep vein thrombosis, or VTE), then she should not start COCs at 3 weeks after childbirth, but start at 6 weeks instead. These additional risk factors include previous VTE, thrombophilia, caesarean delivery, blood transfusion at delivery, postpartum hemorrhage, pre-eclampsia, obesity ($\geq$30 kg/m^2), smoking, and being bedridden for a prolonged time.)

3. Do you smoke cigarettes?

❑ NO ❑ **YES** If she is 35 years of age or older and smokes, do not provide COCs. Urge her to stop smoking and help her choose another method, but not patch or ring if she smokes fewer than 15 cigarettes a day, and also not monthly injectables if more than 15 cigarettes a day.

4. Do you have cirrhosis of the liver, a liver infection, or liver tumor? Have you ever had jaundice when using COCs?

❑ NO ❑ **YES** If she reports serious liver disease (such as severe cirrhosis or liver tumor), acute or flare of viral hepatitis, or ever had jaundice while using COCs, do not provide COCs. Help her choose a method without hormones. (She can use monthly injectables if she has had jaundice only with past COC use.)

5. Do you have high blood pressure?

❑ NO ❑ **YES** If you cannot check blood pressure and she reports a history of high blood pressure, or if she is being treated for high blood pressure, do not provide COCs. Refer her for a blood pressure check if possible or help her choose a method without estrogen.

Check blood pressure if possible:

- If her blood pressure is below 140/90 mm Hg, provide COCs. No need to retest before starting COCs.
- If blood pressure is 160/100 mm Hg or higher, do not provide COCs. Help her choose a method without estrogen, but not a progestin-only injectable.
- If blood pressure is 140–159/90–99 mm Hg, one measurement is not enough to diagnose high blood pressure. Give her a backup method* to use until she can return for another blood pressure measurement, or help her choose another method.
  - If her next blood pressure measurement is below 140/90 mm Hg, she can start COCs.
  - However, if her next blood pressure measurement is 140/90 mm Hg or higher, do not provide COCs. Help her choose a method without estrogen, but not a progestin-only injectable if systolic blood pressure is 160 or higher or diastolic pressure is 100 or higher.

(See also Question 18, p. 28.)

(Continued on next page)

* *Backup methods include abstinence, male and female condoms, spermicides, and withdrawal. Tell her that spermicides and withdrawal are the least effective contraceptive methods. If possible, give her condoms.*

6. Have you had diabetes for more than 20 years or damage to your arteries, vision, kidneys, or nervous system caused by diabetes?

❑ NO ❑ **YES** Do not provide COCs. Help her choose a method without estrogen but not progestin-only injectables.

7. Do you have gallbladder disease now or take medication for gallbladder disease?

❑ NO ❑ **YES** Do not provide COCs. Help her choose another method but not the combined patch or combined vaginal ring.

8. Have you ever had a stroke, blood clot in your leg or lungs, heart attack, or other serious heart problems?

❑ NO ❑ **YES** If she reports heart attack, heart disease due to blocked or narrowed arteries, or stroke, do not provide COCs. Help her choose a method without estrogen but not progestin-only injectables. If she reports a current blood clot in the deep veins of the legs (not superficial clots) or lungs, help her choose a method without hormones.

9. Do you have or have you ever had breast cancer?

❑ NO ❑ **YES** Do not provide COCs. Help her choose a method without hormones.

10. Do you sometimes see a bright area of lost vision in the eye before a very bad headache (migraine aura)? Do you get throbbing, severe head pain, often on one side of the head, that can last from a few hours to several days and can cause nausea or vomiting (migraine headaches)? Such headaches are often made worse by light, noise, or moving about.

❑ NO ❑ **YES** If she has migraine aura at any age, do not provide COCs. If she has migraine headaches *without* aura *and* is age 35 or older, do not provide COCs. Help these women choose a method without estrogen. If she is under 35 and has migraine headaches without aura, she can use COCs (see Identifying Migraine Headaches and Auras, p. 436).

11. Are you taking medications for seizures? Are you taking rifampicin or rifabutin for tuberculosis or other illness?

❑ NO ❑ **YES** If she is taking barbiturates, carbamazepine, lamotrigine, oxcarbazepine, phenytoin, primidone, topiramate, rifampicin, or rifabutin, do not provide COCs. They can make COCs less effective. Help her choose another method but not progestin-only pills, patch, or combined ring. If she is taking lamotrigine, help her choose a method without estrogen.

12. Are you planning major surgery that will keep you from walking for one week or more?

❑ NO ❑ **YES** If so, she can start COCs 2 weeks after she can move about again. Until she can start COCs, she should use a backup method.

13. Do you have several conditions that could increase your chances of heart disease (coronary artery disease) or stroke, such as older age, smoking, high blood pressure, or diabetes?

❑ NO ❑ **YES** Do not provide COCs. Help her choose a method without estrogen but not progestin-only injectables.

Also, women should not use COCs if they report having thrombogenic mutations or lupus with positive (or unknown) antiphospholipid antibodies. For complete classifications, see Medical Eligibility Criteria for Contraceptive Use, p. 388.

Be sure to explain the health benefits and risks and the side effects of the method that the client will use. Also, point out any conditions that would make the method inadvisable, when relevant to the client.

Combined Oral Contraceptives for Women With HIV

- Women living with HIV or on antiretroviral therapy can safely use COCs.
- Urge these women to use condoms along with COCs. Used consistently and correctly, condoms help prevent transmission of HIV and other STIs.

Using Clinical Judgment in Special Cases

Usually, a woman with any of the conditions listed below should not use COCs. In special circumstances, however, when other, more appropriate methods are not available or acceptable to her, a qualified provider who can carefully assess a specific woman's condition and situation may decide that she can use COCs. The provider needs to consider the severity of her condition and, for most conditions, whether she will have access to follow-up.

- Not breastfeeding and less than 3 weeks since giving birth, without additional risk that she might develop a blood clot in a deep vein (VTE)
- Not breastfeeding and between 3 and 6 weeks postpartum with additional risk that she might develop VTE
- Primarily breastfeeding between 6 weeks and 6 months since giving birth
- Age 35 or older and smokes fewer than 15 cigarettes a day
- High blood pressure (systolic blood pressure between 140 and 159 mm Hg or diastolic blood pressure between 90 and 99 mm Hg)
- Controlled high blood pressure, where continuing evaluation is possible
- History of high blood pressure, where blood pressure cannot be taken (including pregnancy-related high blood pressure)
- History of jaundice while using COCs in the past
- Gallbladder disease (current or medically treated)
- Age 35 or older and has migraine headaches without aura
- Younger than age 35 and has migraine headaches without aura that have developed or have gotten worse while using COCs
- Had breast cancer more than 5 years ago, and it has not returned
- Diabetes for more than 20 years or damage to arteries, vision, kidneys, or nervous system caused by diabetes
- Multiple risk factors for arterial cardiovascular disease such as older age, smoking, diabetes, and high blood pressure
- Taking barbiturates, carbamazepine, oxcarbazepine, phenytoin, primidone, topiramate, rifampicin, or rifabutin. A backup contraceptive method should also be used because these medications reduce the effectiveness of COCs.
- Taking lamotrigine. Combined hormonal methods may make lamotrigine less effective.

Providing Combined Oral Contraceptives

When to Start

IMPORTANT: A woman can start using COCs any time she wants if it is reasonably certain she is not pregnant. To be reasonably certain she is not pregnant, use the Pregnancy Checklist (see inside back cover). Also, a woman can be given COCs at any time and told when to start taking them.

Woman's situation	When to start
Having menstrual cycles or switching from a nonhormonal method	**Any time of the month** • If she is starting within 5 days after the start of her monthly bleeding, no need for a backup method. • If it is more than 5 days after the start of her monthly bleeding, she can start COCs any time it is reasonably certain she is not pregnant. She will need a backup method* for the first 7 days of taking pills. (If you cannot be reasonably certain, see How and When to Use the Pregnancy Checklist and Pregnancy Tests, p. 440.) • If she is switching from an IUD, she can start COCs immediately (see Copper-Bearing IUD, Switching From an IUD to Another Method, p. 172).
Switching from a hormonal method	• Immediately, if she has been using the hormonal method consistently and correctly or if it is otherwise reasonably certain she is not pregnant. No need to wait for her next monthly bleeding. No need for a backup method. • If she is switching from injectables, she can begin taking COCs when the repeat injection would have been given. No need for a backup method.
Fully or nearly fully breastfeeding	
Less than 6 months after giving birth	• Give her COCs and tell her to start taking them 6 months after giving birth or when breast milk is no longer the baby's main food—whichever comes first.

* *Backup methods include abstinence, male and female condoms, spermicides, and withdrawal. Tell her that spermicides and withdrawal are the least effective contraceptive methods. If possible, give her condoms.*

Woman's situation	When to start
Fully or nearly fully breastfeeding (continued)	
More than 6 months after giving birth	• If her monthly bleeding has not returned, she can start COCs any time it is reasonably certain she is not pregnant. She will need a backup method for the first 7 days of taking pills. (If you cannot be reasonably certain, see How and When to Use the Pregnancy Checklist and Pregnancy Tests, p. 440.) • If her monthly bleeding has returned, she can start COCs as advised for women having menstrual cycles (see previous page).
Partially breastfeeding	
Less than 6 weeks after giving birth	• Give her COCs and tell her to start taking them 6 weeks after giving birth. • Also give her a backup method to use until 6 weeks since giving birth if her monthly bleeding returns before this time.
More than 6 weeks after giving birth	• If her monthly bleeding has not returned, she can start COCs any time it is reasonably certain she is not pregnant.† She will need a backup method for the first 7 days of taking pills. (If you cannot be reasonably certain, see How and When to Use the Pregnancy Checklist and Pregnancy Tests, p. 440.) • If her monthly bleeding has returned, she can start COCs as advised for women having menstrual cycles (see previous page).

† *Where a visit 6 weeks after childbirth is routinely recommended and other opportunities to obtain contraception are limited, some providers and programs may give COCs at the 6-week visit, without further evidence that the woman is not pregnant, if her monthly bleeding has not yet returned.*

Woman's situation	When to start
Not breastfeeding	
Less than 4 weeks after giving birth	• She can start COCs at any time on days 21–28 after giving birth. Give her pills any time to start during these 7 days. No need for a backup method. (If additional risk for VTE, wait until 6 weeks. See Question 2, p. 6.)
More than 4 weeks after giving birth	• If her monthly bleeding has not returned, she can start COCs any time it is reasonably certain she is not pregnant.† She will need a backup method for the first 7 days of taking pills. (If you cannot be reasonably certain, see How and When to Use the Pregnancy Checklist and Pregnancy Tests, p. 440.) • If her monthly bleeding has returned, she can start COCs as advised for women having menstrual cycles (see p. 11).
No monthly bleeding (not related to childbirth or breastfeeding)	• She can start COCs any time it is reasonably certain she is not pregnant. She will need a backup method for the first 7 days of taking pills.
After miscarriage or abortion	• Immediately. If she is starting within 7 days after first- or second-trimester miscarriage or abortion, no need for a backup method. • If it is more than 7 days after first- or second-trimester miscarriage or abortion, she can start COCs any time it is reasonably certain she is not pregnant. She will need a backup method for the first 7 days of taking pills. (If you cannot be reasonably certain, see How and When to Use the Pregnancy Checklist and Pregnancy Tests, p. 440.)

Woman's situation	When to start
After taking emergency contraceptive pills (ECPs)	**After taking progestin-only or combined ECPs:** • She can start or restart COCs immediately after she takes the ECPs. *No need to wait for her next monthly bleeding.* – A continuing user who needed ECPs due to pill-taking errors can continue where she left off with her current pack. • If she does not start immediately but returns for COCs, she can start at any time if it is reasonably certain she is not pregnant. • All women will need to use a backup method for the first 7 days of taking pills. **After taking ulipristal acetate (UPA) ECPs:** • She can start or restart COCs on the 6th day after taking UPA-ECPs. *No need to wait for her next monthly bleeding.* COCs and UPA interact. If COCs are started sooner, and thus both are present in the body, one or both may be less effective. • Give her a supply of pills and tell her to start them on the 6th day after taking the UPA-ECPs. • She will need to use a backup method from the time she takes the UPA-ECPs until she has been taking COCs for 7 days. • If she does not start on the 6th day but returns later for COCs, she may start at any time if it is reasonably certain she is not pregnant.

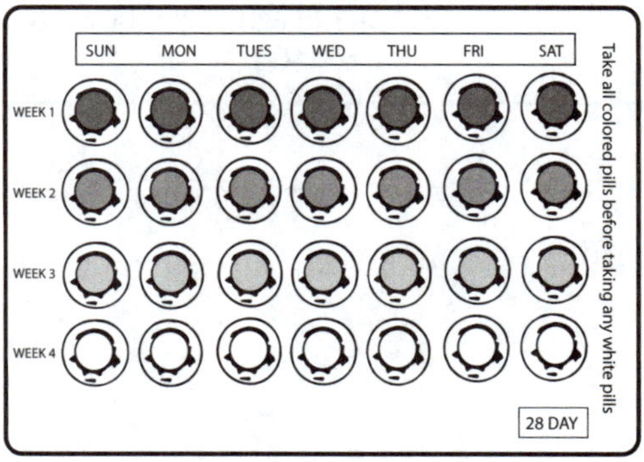

Giving Advice on Side Effects

IMPORTANT: Thorough counseling about bleeding changes and other side effects is an important part of providing the method. Counseling about bleeding changes may be the most important help a woman needs to keep using the method without concern.

Describe the most common side effects	• In the first few months, bleeding at unexpected times (irregular bleeding). Then lighter, shorter, and more regular monthly bleeding. • Headaches, breast tenderness, weight change, and possibly other side effects.
Explain about these side effects	• Side effects are not signs of illness. • Most side effects usually become less or stop within the first few months of using COCs. • Common, but some women do not have them.
Explain what to do in case of side effects	• Keep taking COCs. Skipping pills risks pregnancy and can make some side effects worse. • Take each pill at the same time every day to help reduce irregular bleeding and also help with remembering. • Take pills with food or at bedtime to help avoid nausea. • The client can come back for help if side effects bother her or if she has other concerns.

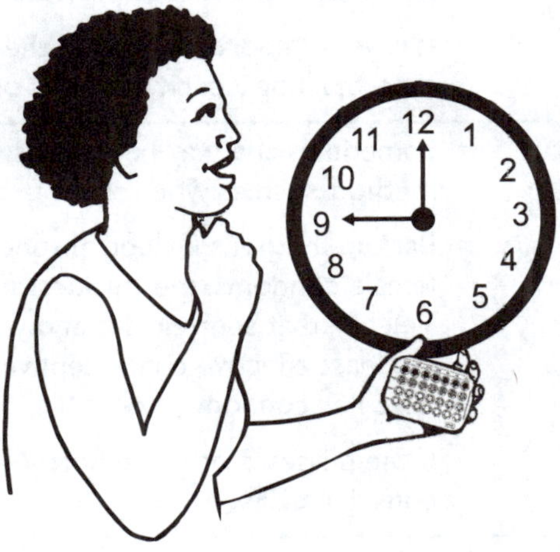

Explaining How to Use

1. Give pills	• Give up to 1 year's supply (13 packs) depending on the woman's preference and planned use.
2. Explain pill pack	• Show which kind of pack—21 pills or 28 pills. With 28-pill packs, point out that the last 7 pills are a different color and do not contain hormones (some brands may differ). • Show how to take the first pill from the pack and then how to follow the directions or arrows on the pack to take the rest of the pills.
3. Give key instruction	• **Take one pill each day**—until the pack is empty. • Discuss cues for taking a pill every day. Linking pill-taking to a daily activity—such as cleaning her teeth—may help her remember. • Taking pills at the same time each day helps to remember them. It also may help reduce some side effects.
4. Explain starting next pack	• 28-pill packs: When she finishes one pack, she should take the first pill from the next pack on the very next day. • 21-pill packs: After she takes the last pill from one pack, she should wait 7 days—no more—and then take the first pill from the next pack. • It is very important to start the next pack on time. Starting a pack late risks pregnancy.
5. Provide backup method and explain use	• Sometimes she may need to use a backup method, such as when she misses pills. • Backup methods include abstinence, male or female condoms, spermicides, and withdrawal. Tell her that spermicides and withdrawal are the least effective contraceptive methods. Give her condoms, if possible. • If she misses 3 or more hormonal pills, she can consider ECPs.

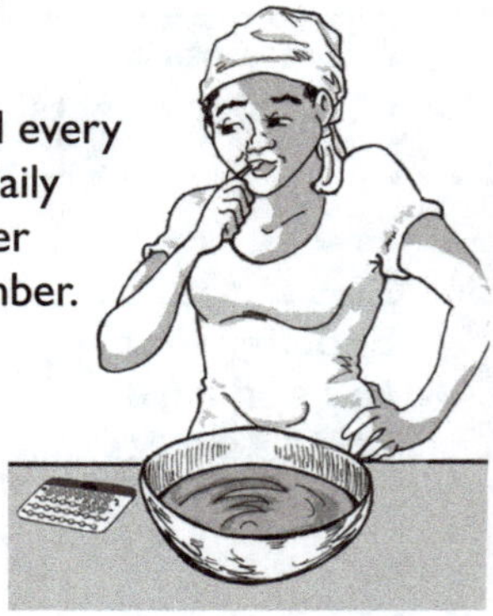

Supporting the User

Managing Missed Pills

It is easy to forget a pill or to be late in taking it. Adolescents are more likely to forget pills and so may need extra support and guidance.

COC users should know what to do if they forget to take pills. **If a woman misses one or more pills, she should follow the instructions below.** Use the tool on p. 431 to help explain these instructions to the client.

Making Up Missed Pills With 30–35 µg Estrogen‡

Key message	• **Take a missed hormonal pill as soon as possible.** • Keep taking pills as usual, one each day. (She may take 2 pills at the same time or on the same day.)
Missed 1 or 2 pills? Started new pack 1 or 2 days late?	• Take a hormonal pill as soon as possible. • Little or no risk of pregnancy.
Missed pills 3 or more days in a row in the first or second week? Started new pack 3 or more days late?	• Take a hormonal pill as soon as possible. • Use a backup method for the next 7 days. • Also, if she had sex in the past 5 days, she can consider ECPs (see Emergency Contraceptive Pills, p. 49).
Missed 3 or more pills in the third week?	• Take a hormonal pill as soon as possible. • Finish all hormonal pills in the pack. Throw away the 7 nonhormonal pills in a 28-pill pack. • Start a new pack the next day. • Use a backup method for the next 7 days. • Also, if she had sex in the past 5 days, she can consider ECPs (see Emergency Contraceptive Pills, p. 49).

(Continued on next page)

‡ *For pills with 20 µg of estrogen or less, women missing one pill should follow the same guidance as for missing one or two 30–35 µg pills. Women missing 2 or more pills should follow the same guidance as for missing 3 or more 30–35 µg pills.*

Missed any non-hormonal pills? (last 7 pills in 28-pill pack)	• Discard the missed nonhormonal pill(s). • Keep taking COCs, one each day. Start the new pack as usual.
Severe vomiting or diarrhea	• If she vomits within 2 hours after taking a pill, she should take another pill from her pack as soon as possible, then keep taking pills as usual. • If she has vomiting or diarrhea for more than 2 days, follow instructions for 3 or more missed pills, above.

How Can a Partner Help?

The client's partner is welcome to participate in counseling and learn about the method and what support he can give to his partner. A male partner can:

- Support a woman's choice of COCs
- Help her to remember to take a pill each day and to start a new pack on time
- Show understanding and support if she has side effects
- Help her to make sure that she has a new pill pack on hand to start on time
- Help to make sure she has ECPs on hand in case she misses pills or starts a new pill pack late
- Use condoms consistently in addition to COCs if he has an STI/HIV or thinks he may be at risk of an STI/HIV

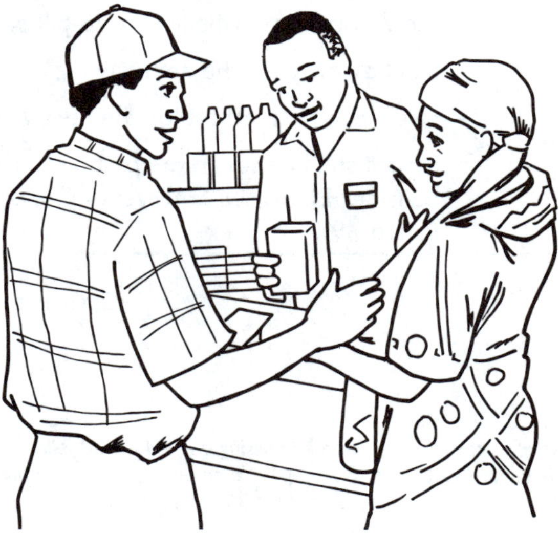

"Come Back Any Time": Reasons to Return

Assure every client that she is welcome to come back any time—for example, if she has problems, questions, or wants another method; she has any major change in health status; or she thinks she might be pregnant. Also if:

- She needs more pills.
- She wants ECPs because she started a new pack 3 or more days late or missed 3 or more hormonal pills or, if she is using pills with 20 µg of estrogen or less, because she started a new pack 2 or more days late or missed 2 or more hormonal pills.

General health advice: Anyone who suddenly feels that something is seriously wrong with her health should immediately seek medical care from a nurse or doctor. Her contraceptive method is most likely not the cause of the condition, but she should tell the nurse or doctor what method she is using.

Planning the Next Visit

1. Encourage her to come back for more pills before she uses up her supply of pills.
2. An annual visit is recommended.
3. Some women can benefit from contact after 3 months of COC use. This offers an opportunity to answer any questions, help with any problems, and check on correct use.

Helping Continuing Users

1. Ask how the client is doing with the method and whether she is satisfied. Ask if she has any questions or anything to discuss.
2. Ask especially if she is concerned about bleeding changes. Give her any information or help that she needs (see Managing Any Problems, next page).
3. Ask if she often has problems remembering to take a pill every day. If so, discuss ways to remember, making up missed pills, and ECPs, or choosing another method. Adolescents may need extra support.
4. Give her more pill packs—a full year's supply (13 packs), if possible. Plan her next resupply visit before she will need more pills.
5. Every year or so, check blood pressure if possible (see Medical Eligibility Criteria, Question 5, p. 7).
6. Ask a long-term client if she has had any new health problems since her last visit. Address problems as appropriate. For new health problems that may require switching methods, see p. 22.
7. Ask a long-term client about major life changes that may affect her needs—particularly plans for having children and STI/HIV risk. Follow up as needed.

Managing Any Problems

Problems Reported as Side Effects or Problems With Use

May or may not be due to the method.

- Problems with side effects affect women's satisfaction and use of COCs. They deserve the provider's attention. If the client reports side effects or problems, listen to her concerns, give her advice, and support, and, if appropriate, treat. Make sure she understands the advice and agrees.
- Encourage her to keep taking a pill every day even if she has side effects. Missing pills can risk pregnancy and may make some side effects worse.
- Many side effects will subside after a few months of use. For a woman whose side effects persist, give her a different COC formulation, if available, for at least 3 months.
- Offer to help the client choose another method—now, if she wishes, or if problems cannot be overcome.

Missed pills

- See Managing Missed Pills, p. 17.

Irregular bleeding (bleeding at unexpected times that bothers the client)

- Reassure her that many women using COCs experience irregular bleeding. It is not harmful and usually becomes less or stops after the first few months of use.
- Other possible causes of irregular bleeding include:
  - Missed pills
  - Taking pills at different times each day
  - Vomiting or diarrhea
  - Taking anticonvulsants, rifampicin, or rifabutin (see Starting treatment with anticonvulsants, rifampicin or rifabutin, p. 23)
- To reduce irregular bleeding:
  - Urge her to take a pill each day and at the same time each day.
  - Teach her to make up for missed pills properly, including after vomiting or diarrhea (see Managing Missed Pills, p. 17).
  - For modest short-term relief, she can try 800 mg ibuprofen 3 times daily after meals for 5 days or other nonsteroidal anti-inflammatory drug (NSAID), beginning when irregular bleeding starts. NSAIDs provide some relief of irregular bleeding for implants, progestin-only injectables, and IUDs, and they may also help for COCs.
  - If she has been taking the pills for more than a few months and NSAIDs do not help, give her a different COC formulation, if available. Ask her to try the new pills for at least 3 months.

- If irregular bleeding continues or starts after several months of normal or no monthly bleeding, or you suspect that something may be wrong for other reasons, consider underlying conditions unrelated to method use (see Unexplained vaginal bleeding, next page).

No monthly bleeding

- Ask if she is having any bleeding at all. (She may have just a small stain on her underclothing and not recognize it as monthly bleeding.) If she is, reassure her.
- Reassure her that some women using COCs stop having monthly bleeding, and this is not harmful. There is no need to lose blood every month. It is similar to not having monthly bleeding during pregnancy. She is not pregnant or infertile. Blood is not building up inside her. (Some women are happy to be free from monthly bleeding, and for some women this may help prevent anemia.)
- Ask if she has been taking a pill every day. If so, reassure her that she is not likely to be pregnant. She can continue taking her COCs as before.
- Did she skip the 7-day break between packs (21-day packs) or skip the 7 nonhormonal pills (28-day pack)? If so, reassure her that she is not pregnant. She can continue using COCs.
- If she has missed hormonal pills or started a new pack late:
  - She can continue using COCs.
  - Tell a woman who has missed 3 or more pills or started a new pack 3 or more days late to return if she has signs and symptoms of early pregnancy.
  - See p. 17 for instructions on how to make up for missed pills.

Ordinary headaches (nonmigrainous)

- Try the following (one at a time):
  - Suggest aspirin (325–650 mg), ibuprofen (200–400 mg), paracetamol (325–1000 mg), or other pain reliever.
  - Some women get headaches during the hormone-free week (the 7 days a woman does not take hormonal pills). Consider extended use (see Extended and Continuous Use of Combined Oral Contraceptives, p. 24).
- Any headaches that get worse or occur more often during COC use should be evaluated.

Nausea or dizziness

- For nausea, suggest taking COCs at bedtime or with food.

If symptoms continue:

- Consider locally available remedies.
- Consider extended use if her nausea comes after she starts a new pill pack (see Extended and Continuous Use of Combined Oral Contraceptives, p. 24).

Breast tenderness

- Recommend that she wear a supportive bra (including during strenuous activity and sleep).
- Try hot or cold compresses.
- Suggest aspirin (325–650 mg), ibuprofen (200–400 mg), paracetamol (325–1000 mg), or other pain reliever.
- Consider locally available remedies.

Weight change

- Review diet and counsel as needed.

Mood changes or changes in sex drive

- Some women have changes in mood during the hormone-free week (the 7 days when a woman does not take hormonal pills). Consider extended use (see Extended and Continuous Use of Combined Oral Contraceptives, p. 24).
- Ask about changes in her life that could affect her mood or sex drive, including changes in her relationship with her partner. Give her support as appropriate.
- Clients who have serious mood changes such as major depression should be referred for care.
- Consider locally available remedies.

Acne

- Acne usually improves with COC use. It may worsen for a few women.
- If she has been taking pills for more than a few months and acne persists, give her a different COC formulation, if available. Ask her to try the new pills for at least 3 months.
- Consider locally available remedies.

New Problems That May Require Switching Methods

May or may not be due to the method.

Unexplained vaginal bleeding (that suggests a medical condition not related to the method) or heavy or prolonged bleeding

- Refer or evaluate by history and pelvic examination. Diagnose and treat as appropriate.
- She can continue using COCs while her condition is being evaluated.
- If bleeding is caused by sexually transmitted infection or pelvic inflammatory disease, she can continue using COCs during treatment.

Starting treatment with anticonvulsants, rifampicin, or rifabutin

- Barbiturates, carbamazepine, oxcarbazepine, phenytoin, primidone, topiramate, rifampicin, and rifabutin may make COCs, patch, and combined vaginal ring less effective. Combined hormonal methods, including combined pills and monthly injectables, may make lamotrigine less effective. If using these medications long-term, she may want a different method, such as a progestin-only injectable, implant, a copper-bearing IUD, or an LNG-IUD.
- If using these medications short-term, she can use a backup method along with COCs for greater protection from pregnancy.

Migraine headaches (see Identifying Migraine Headaches and Auras, p. 436)

- Regardless of her age, a woman who develops migraine headaches, with or without aura, or whose migraine headaches become worse while using COCs should stop using COCs.
- Help her choose a method without estrogen.

Circumstances that will keep her from walking for one week or more

- If she is having major surgery, or her leg is in a cast, or for other reasons she will be unable to move about for several weeks, she should:
  - Tell her doctors that she is using COCs.
  - Stop taking COCs and use a backup method during this period.
  - Restart COCs 2 weeks after she can move about again.

Certain serious health conditions (suspected heart or serious liver disease, high blood pressure, blood clots in deep veins of legs or lungs, stroke, breast cancer, damage to arteries, vision, kidneys, or nervous system caused by diabetes, or gallbladder disease). See Signs and Symptoms of Serious Health Conditions, p. 384.

- Tell her to stop taking COCs.
- Give her a backup method to use until the condition is evaluated.
- Refer for diagnosis and care if not already under care.

Suspected pregnancy

- Assess for pregnancy.
- Tell her to stop taking COCs if pregnancy is confirmed.
- There are no known risks to a fetus conceived while a woman is taking COCs (see Question 5, p. 25).

Extended and Continuous Use of Combined Oral Contraceptives

Some COC users do not follow the usual cycle of 3 weeks taking hormonal pills followed by one week without hormones. Some women take hormonal pills for 12 weeks without a break, followed by one week of nonhormonal pills (or no pills). This is extended use. Other women take hormonal pills without any breaks at all. This is continuous use. Monophasic pills are recommended for such use (see Question 16, p. 27).

Women easily manage taking COCs in different ways when properly advised how to do so. Many women value controlling when they have monthly bleeding—if any—and tailoring pill use as they wish.

Benefits of Extended and Continuous Use

- Women have vaginal bleeding only 4 times a year or not at all.
- Reduces how often some women suffer headaches, premenstrual syndrome, mood changes, and heavy or painful bleeding during the week without hormonal pills.

Disadvantages of Extended and Continuous Use

- Irregular bleeding may last as long as the first 6 months of use—especially among women who have never before used COCs.
- More supplies needed—15 to 17 packs every year instead of 13.

Extended Use Instructions

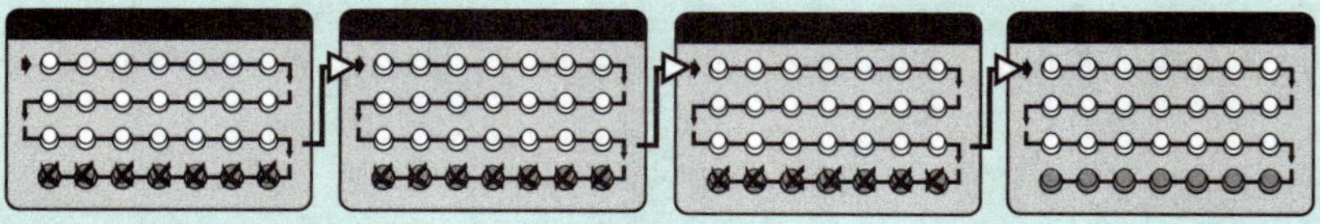

- Take 84 hormonal pills in a row, one each day. (These are the hormonal pills in 4 monthly packs.) Users of 28-pill packs do not take the non-hormonal pills.
- After 84 hormonal pills, wait 7 days and start the next pack of pills on the 8th day. (Users of 28-pill packs can take the nonhormonal pills in the 4th pack if they wish and start the hormonal pills the day after the last nonhormonal pill.) Expect some bleeding during this week of not taking the hormonal pills.

Continuous Use Instructions

A woman should take one hormonal pill every day for as long as she wishes to use COCs. If bothersome irregular bleeding occurs, she can stop taking pills for 3 or 4 days and then start taking hormonal pills continuously again.

Questions and Answers About Combined Oral Contraceptives

1. Should a woman take a "rest" from COCs after taking them for a time?

No. There is no evidence that taking a "rest" is helpful. In fact, taking a "rest" from COCs can lead to unintended pregnancy. COCs can safely be used for many years without having to stop taking them periodically.

2. If a woman has been taking COCs for a long time, will she still be protected from pregnancy after she stops taking COCs?

No. A woman is protected only as long as she takes her pills regularly.

3. How long does it take to become pregnant after stopping COCs?

Women who stop using COCs can become pregnant as quickly as women who stop nonhormonal methods. COCs do not delay the return of a woman's fertility after she stops taking them. The bleeding pattern a woman had before she used COCs generally returns after she stops taking them. Some women may have to wait a few months before their usual bleeding pattern returns.

4. Do COCs cause abortion?

No. Research on COCs finds that they do not disrupt an existing pregnancy. They should not be used to try to cause an abortion. They will not do so.

5. Do COCs cause birth defects? Will the fetus be harmed if a woman accidentally takes COCs while she is pregnant?

No. Good evidence shows that COCs will not cause birth defects and will not otherwise harm the fetus if a woman becomes pregnant while taking COCs or accidentally starts to take COCs when she is already pregnant.

6. Do COCs cause women to gain or lose a lot of weight?

No. Most women do not gain or lose weight due to COCs. Weight changes naturally as life circumstances change and as people age. Because these changes in weight are so common, many women think that COCs cause these gains or losses in weight. Studies find, however, that, on average, COCs do not affect weight. A few women experience sudden changes in weight when using COCs. These changes reverse after they stop taking COCs. It is not known why these women respond to COCs in this way.

7. Do COCs lower women's mood or sex drive?

Generally, no. Some women using COCs report these complaints. The great majority of COC users do not report any such changes, however, and some report that both mood and sex drive improve. It is difficult to tell whether such changes are due to the COCs or to other reasons. Providers can help a client with these problems (see Mood changes or changes in sex drive, p. 22). There is no evidence that COCs affect women's sexual behavior.

8. What can a provider say to a client asking about COCs and breast cancer?

The provider can point out that both COC users and women who do not use COCs can have breast cancer. In scientific studies breast cancer was slightly more common among women using COCs and those who had used COCs in the past 10 years than among other women. Scientists do not know whether or not COCs actually caused the slight increase in breast cancers. It is possible that the cancers were already there before COC use but were found sooner in COC users (see Facts About Combined Oral Contraceptives and Cancer, p. 4).

9. Can COCs be used as a pregnancy test?

No. A woman may experience some vaginal bleeding (a "withdrawal bleed") as a result of taking several COCs or one full cycle of COCs, but studies suggest that this practice does not accurately identify who is or is not pregnant. Thus, giving a woman COCs to see if she has bleeding later is not recommended as a way to tell if she is pregnant. COCs should not be given to women as a pregnancy test of sorts because they do not produce accurate results.

10. Must a woman have a pelvic examination before she can start COCs or at follow-up visits?

No. A pelvic examination to check for pregnancy is not necessary. Instead, asking the right questions usually can help to make reasonably certain that a woman is not pregnant (see Pregnancy Checklist, inside back cover). No other condition that could be detected by a pelvic examination rules out COC use.

11. Can women with varicose veins use COCs?

Yes. COCs are safe for women with varicose veins. Varicose veins are enlarged blood vessels close to the surface of the skin. They are not dangerous. They are not blood clots, nor are these veins the deep veins in the legs where a blood clot can be dangerous (deep vein thrombosis). A woman who has or has had deep vein thrombosis should not use COCs.

12. Can a woman safely take COCs throughout her life?

Yes. There is no minimum or maximum age for COC use. COCs can be an appropriate method for most women from onset of monthly bleeding (menarche) to menopause (see Women Near Menopause, p. 325).

COCs can be an appropriate method for adolescents. Adolescents may need extra support and encouragement to use COCs consistently and effectively.

13. Can women who smoke use COCs safely?

Women younger than age 35 who smoke can use COCs. Women age 35 and older who smoke should choose a method without estrogen or, if they smoke fewer than 15 cigarettes a day, monthly injectables. Older women who smoke can take the progestin-only pill if they prefer pills. All women who smoke should be urged to stop smoking.

14. What if a client wants to use COCs but it is not reasonably certain that she is not pregnant after using the pregnancy checklist?

A woman who answers "No" to all 6 questions on the Pregnancy Checklist (see inside back cover) can still start taking COCs. Ask her to come back for a pregnancy test if her next monthly bleeding is late. See Ruling Out Pregnancy, p. 439.

15. Can COCs be used as emergency contraceptive pills (ECPs) after unprotected sex?

Yes. As soon as possible, but no more than 5 days after unprotected sex, a woman can take COCs as ECPs (see Pill Formulations and Dosing for Emergency Contraception, p. 55). Progestin-only pills, however, are more effective and cause fewer side effects such as nausea and stomach upset.

16. What are the differences among monophasic, biphasic, and triphasic pills?

Monophasic pills provide the same amount of estrogen and progestin in every hormonal pill. Biphasic and triphasic pills change the amount of estrogen and progestin at different points of the pill-taking cycle. For biphasic pills, the first 10 pills have one dosage, and then the next 11 pills have another level of estrogen and progestin. For triphasic pills, the first 7 or so pills have one dosage, the next 7 pills have another dosage, and the last 7 hormonal pills have yet another dosage. All prevent pregnancy in the same way. Differences in side effects, effectiveness, and continuation appear to be slight.

17. Is it important for a woman to take her COCs at the same time each day?

A woman can take her COCs at different times of day, and they will still be effective. However, taking them at the same time each day can be helpful for 2 reasons. Some side effects may be reduced by taking the pill at the same time each day. Also, taking a pill at the same time each day can help women remember to take their pills more consistently. Linking pill taking with a daily activity also helps women remember to take their pills.

18. Should women who choose COCs and certain other hormonal contraceptives be routinely tested for high blood pressure?

It is desirable for all women to have blood pressure measurements taken routinely before starting a hormonal method of contraception. However, in some settings blood pressure measurements are unavailable. In many of these settings, pregnancy-related morbidity and mortality risks are high, and these methods are among the few methods that are widely available. In such settings women should not be denied use of these methods simply because their blood pressure cannot be measured.

Women with high blood pressure or very high blood pressure should not use combined hormonal methods—COCs, monthly injectables, patch, or combined ring. Where blood pressure cannot be measured, women with a history of high blood pressure should not use these methods. Women with very high blood pressure should not use progestin-only injectables. Women can use progestin-only pills (POPs), implants, and LNG-IUDs even if they have high or very high blood pressure readings or a history of high or very high blood pressure.

High blood pressure is defined as systolic pressure 140 mm Hg or higher or diastolic pressure 90 mm Hg or higher. Very high blood pressure is defined as systolic pressure 160 mm Hg or higher or diastolic pressure 100 mm Hg or higher.

For more guidance concerning blood pressure, see the Medical Eligibility Criteria checklists in the chapters on COCs (p. 6), progestin-only injectables (p. 72), and monthly injectables (p. 101).

CHAPTER 2

Progestin-Only Pills

This chapter on progestin-only pills focuses on breastfeeding women. Women who are not breastfeeding also can use progestin-only pills. Guidance that differs for women who are not breastfeeding is noted.

Key Points for Providers and Clients

- **Take one pill every day.** No breaks between packs.
- **Safe for breastfeeding women and their babies.** Progestin-only pills do not affect milk production.
- **Add to the contraceptive effect of breastfeeding.** Together, they provide effective pregnancy protection.
- **Bleeding changes are common but not harmful.** Typically, pills lengthen how long breastfeeding women have no monthly bleeding. For women having monthly bleeding, frequent or irregular bleeding is common.
- **Can be given to a woman at any time to start now or later.**

What Are Progestin-Only Pills?

- Pills that contain very low doses of a progestin like the natural hormone progesterone in a woman's body.
- Do not contain estrogen, and so can be used throughout breastfeeding and by women who cannot use methods with estrogen.
- Progestin-only pills (POPs) are also called "minipills" and progestin-only oral contraceptives.
- Work primarily by:
  - Thickening cervical mucus (this blocks sperm from meeting an egg)
  - Disrupting the menstrual cycle, including preventing the release of eggs from the ovaries (ovulation)

How Effective?

Effectiveness depends on the user: For women who have monthly bleeding, risk of pregnancy is greatest if pills are taken late or missed completely.

Breastfeeding women:

- As commonly used, about 1 pregnancy per 100 women using POPs over the first year. This means that 99 of every 100 women will not become pregnant.
- When pills are taken every day, less than 1 pregnancy per 100 women using POPs over the first year (3 per 1,000 women).

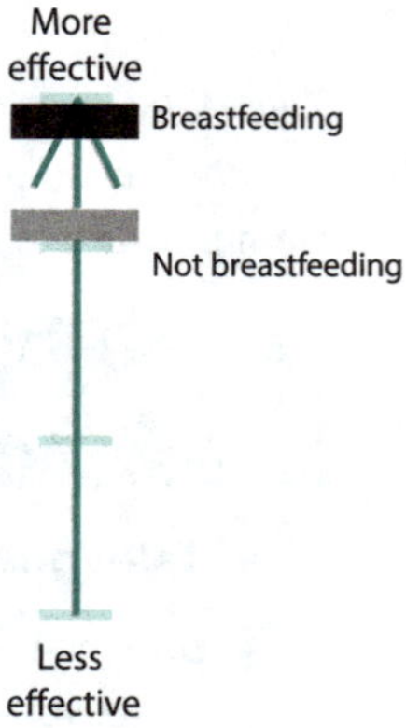

Less effective for women not breastfeeding:

- As commonly used, about 7 pregnancies per 100 women using POPs over the first year. This means that 93 of every 100 women will not become pregnant.
- When pills are taken every day at the same time, less than 1 pregnancy per 100 women using POPs over the first year (3 per 1,000 women).

Return of fertility after POPs are stopped: No delay

Protection against sexually transmitted infections (STIs): None

Why Some Women Say They Like Progestin-Only Pills

- Can be used while breastfeeding
- Can be stopped at any time without a provider's help
- Do not interfere with sex
- Are controlled by the woman

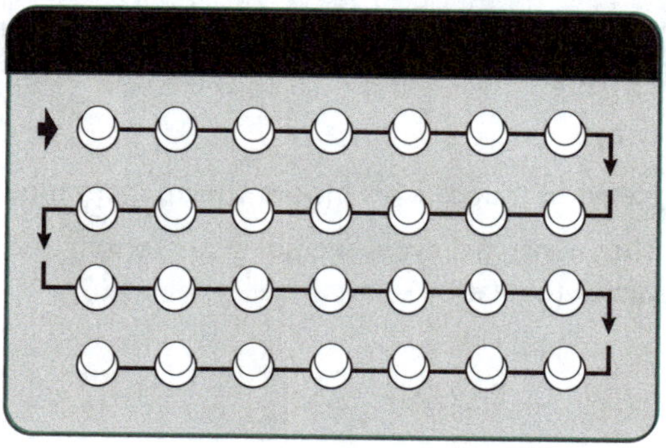

Side Effects, Health Benefits, and Health Risks

Side Effects (see also Managing Any Problems, p. 42)

Some users report the following:

- Changes in bleeding patterns,† including:
  - For breastfeeding women, longer delay in return of monthly bleeding after childbirth (lengthened postpartum amenorrhea)
  - Frequent bleeding
  - Irregular bleeding
  - Infrequent bleeding
  - Prolonged bleeding
  - No monthly bleeding

  Breastfeeding also affects a woman's bleeding patterns.

> Bleeding changes are normal and not harmful. If a woman finds them bothersome, counseling and support can help.

- Headaches
- Dizziness
- Mood changes
- Breast tenderness
- Abdominal pain
- Nausea

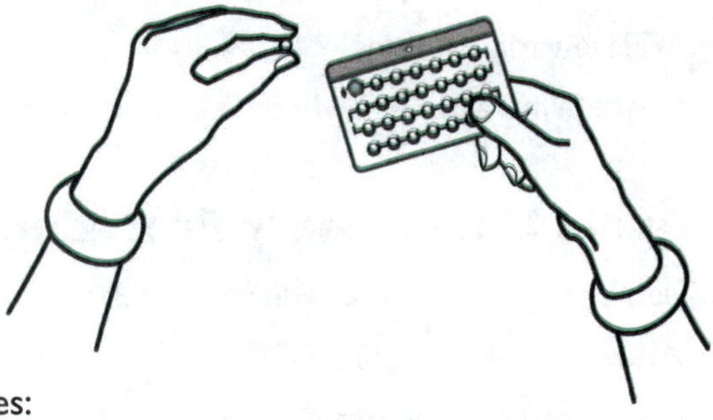

Other possible physical changes:

- For women not breastfeeding, enlarged ovarian follicles

Known Health Benefits

Help protect against:

- Risks of pregnancy

Known Health Risks

None

Correcting Misunderstandings (see also Questions and Answers, p. 46)

Progestin-only pills:

- Do not cause a breastfeeding woman's milk to dry up
- Must be taken every day, whether or not a woman has sex that day
- Do not make women infertile
- Do not cause diarrhea in breastfeeding babies
- Reduce the risk of ectopic pregnancy

† *For definitions of bleeding patterns, see "vaginal bleeding," p. 407.*

Who Can and Cannot Use Progestin-Only Pills

Safe and Suitable for Nearly All Women

Nearly all women can use POPs safely and effectively, including women who:

- Are breastfeeding (she can start immediately after childbirth)
- Have or have not had children
- Are married or are not married
- Are of any age, including adolescents and women over 40 years old
- Have just had an abortion, miscarriage, or ectopic pregnancy
- Smoke cigarettes, regardless of woman's age or number of cigarettes smoked
- Have anemia now or had in the past
- Have varicose veins
- Are living with HIV, whether or not on antiretroviral therapy

Avoid Unnecessary Procedures

(see Importance of Procedures, p. 368)

Women can begin using POPs:

- Without a pelvic examination
- Without any blood tests or other routine laboratory tests
- Without cervical cancer screening
- Without a breast examination
- Without a pregnancy test. A woman can begin using POPs at any time, even when she is not having monthly bleeding at the time, if it is reasonably certain she is not pregnant (see Pregnancy Checklist, inside back cover).

> Blood pressure measurement is desirable before starting a hormonal method. However, where the risks of pregnancy are high and few methods are available, a woman should not be denied a hormonal method simply because her blood pressure cannot be measured. If possible, she can have her blood pressure measured later at a time and place convenient for her.

Medical Eligibility Criteria for

Progestin-Only Pills

Ask the client the questions below about known medical conditions. Examinations and tests are not necessary. If she answers "no" to all of the questions, then she can start POPs if she wants. If she answers "yes" to a question, follow the instructions. In some cases she can still start POPs.

1. Do you have severe cirrhosis of the liver or severe tumor?

❑ NO ❑ **YES** If she severe cirrhosis or severe liver tumor, such as liver cancer), do not provide POPs. Help her choose a method without hormones.

2. Do you have a serious problem now with a blood clot in your leg or lungs?

❑ NO ❑ **YES** If she reports a current blood clot in a leg (affecting deep veins, not superficial veins) or in a lung, and she is not on anticoagulant therapy, do not provide POPs. Help her choose a method without hormones.

3. Are you taking medication for seizures? Are you taking rifampicin or rifabutin for tuberculosis or other illness?

❑ NO ❑ **YES** If she is taking barbiturates, carbamazepine, oxcarbazepine, phenytoin, primidone, topiramate, rifampicin, or rifabutin, do not provide POPs. They can make POPs less effective. Help her choose another method but not combined oral contraceptives.

4. Do you have or have you ever had breast cancer?

❑ NO ❑ **YES** Do not provide POPs. Help her choose a method without hormones.

Also, women should not use POPs if they report having thrombogenic mutations or lupus with positive (or unknown) antiphospholipid antibodies. For complete classifications, see Medical Eligibility Criteria for Contraceptive Use, p. 388.

Be sure to explain the health benefits and risks and the side effects of the method that the client will use. Also, point out any conditions that would make the method inadvisable, when relevant to the client.

Using Clinical Judgment in Special Cases

Usually, a woman with any of the conditions listed below should not use POPs. In special circumstances, however, when other, more appropriate methods are not available or acceptable to her, a qualified provider who can carefully assess a specific woman's condition and situation may decide that she can use POPs. The provider needs to consider the severity of her condition and, for most conditions, whether she will have access to follow-up.

- Acute blood clot in deep veins of legs or lungs
- Had breast cancer more than 5 years ago, and it has not returned
- Severe cirrhosis or severe liver tumor
- Systemic lupus erythematosus with positive (or unknown) antiphospholipid antibodies
- Taking barbiturates, carbamazepine, oxcarbazepine, phenytoin, primidone, topiramate, rifampicin, or rifabutin. A backup contraceptive method should also be used because these medications reduce the effectiveness of POPs.

Progestin-Only Pills for Women With HIV

- Women living with HIV or on antiretroviral therapy can safely use POPs.
- Urge these women to use condoms along with POPs. Used consistently and correctly, condoms help prevent transmission of HIV and other STIs.
- For appropriate breastfeeding practices for women with HIV, see Maternal and Newborn Health, Preventing Mother-to-Child Transmission of HIV, p. 352.

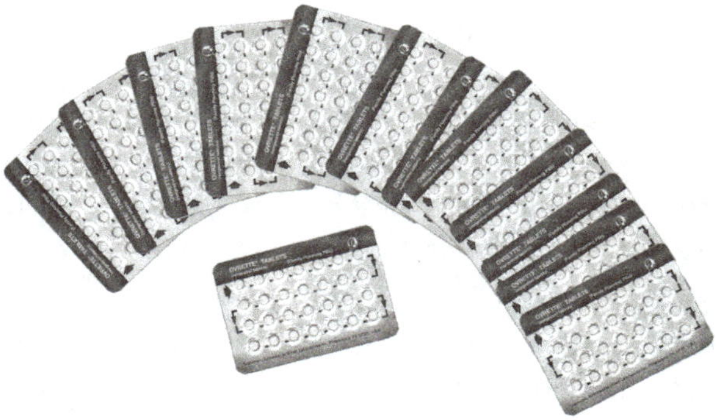

Providing Progestin-Only Pills

When to Start

IMPORTANT: A woman can start using POPs any time she wants if it is reasonably certain she is not pregnant. To be reasonably certain she is not pregnant, use the Pregnancy Checklist (see inside back cover). Also, a woman can be given POPs at any time and told when to start taking them.

Woman's situation	When to start
Fully or nearly fully breastfeeding	
Less than 6 months after giving birth	• If her monthly bleeding has not returned, she can start POPs any time between giving birth and 6 months. No need for a backup method. • If her monthly bleeding has returned, she can start POPs as advised for women having menstrual cycles (see next page).
More than 6 months after giving birth	• If her monthly bleeding has not returned, she can start POPs any time it is reasonably certain she is not pregnant. She will need a backup method* for the first 2 days of taking pills. (If you cannot be reasonably certain, see How and When to Use the Pregnancy Checklist and Pregnancy Tests, p. 440.) • If her monthly bleeding has returned, she can start POPs as advised for women having menstrual cycles (see next page).
Partially breastfeeding	
If her monthly bleeding has not returned	• She can start POPs any time it is reasonably certain she is not pregnant.† She will need a backup method for the first 2 days of taking pills. (If you cannot be reasonably certain, see How and When to Use the Pregnancy Checklist and Pregnancy Tests, p. 440.)
If her monthly bleeding has returned	• She can start POPs as advised for women having menstrual cycles (see next page).

* *Backup methods include abstinence, male and female condoms, spermicides, and withdrawal. Tell her that spermicides and withdrawal are the least effective contraceptive methods. If possible, give her condoms.*

† *Where a visit 6 weeks after childbirth is routinely recommended and other opportunities to obtain contraception are limited, some providers and programs may allow a woman to start POPs at the 6-week visit, without further evidence that the woman is not pregnant, if her monthly bleeding has not yet returned.*

Woman's situation	When to start
Not breastfeeding	
Less than 4 weeks after giving birth	• She can start POPs at any time. No need for a backup method.
More than 4 weeks after giving birth	• If her monthly bleeding has not returned, she can start POPs any time it is reasonably certain she is not pregnant.[†] She will need a backup method for the first 2 days of taking pills. (If you cannot be reasonably certain, see How and When to Use the Pregnancy Checklist and Pregnancy Tests, p. 440.) • If her monthly bleeding has returned, she can start POPs as advised for women having menstrual cycles (see below).
Switching from a hormonal method	• Immediately, if she has been using the hormonal method consistently and correctly or if it is otherwise reasonably certain she is not pregnant. No need to wait for her next monthly bleeding. No need for a backup method. • If she is switching from injectables, she can begin taking POPs when the repeat injection would have been given. No need for a backup method.
Having menstrual cycles or switching from a nonhormonal method	**Any time of the month** • If she is starting within 5 days after the start of her monthly bleeding, no need for a backup method. • If it is more than 5 days after the start of her monthly bleeding, she can start POPs any time it is reasonably certain she is not pregnant. She will need a backup method for the first 2 days of taking pills. (If you cannot be reasonably certain, see How and When to Use the Pregnancy Checklist and Pregnancy Tests, p. 440.) • If she is switching from an IUD, she can start POPs immediately (see Copper-Bearing IUD, Switching From an IUD to Another Method, p. 172).

[†] *Where a visit 6 weeks after childbirth is routinely recommended and other opportunities to obtain contraception are limited, some providers and programs may allow a woman to start POPs at the 6-week visit, without further evidence that the woman is not pregnant, if her monthly bleeding has not yet returned.*

Woman's situation	When to start
No monthly bleeding (not related to childbirth or breastfeeding)	• She can start POPs any time it is reasonably certain she is not pregnant. She will need a backup method for the first 2 days of taking pills.
After miscarriage or abortion	• Immediately. If she is starting within 7 days after first- or second-trimester miscarriage or abortion, no need for a backup method. • If it is more than 7 days after first- or second-trimester miscarriage or abortion, she can start POPs any time it is reasonably certain she is not pregnant. She will need a backup method for the first 2 days of taking pills. (If you cannot be reasonably certain, see How and When to Use the Pregnancy Checklist and Pregnancy Tests, p. 440.)
After taking emergency contraceptive pills (ECPs)	**After taking progestin-only or combined ECPs:** • She can start or restart POPs immediately after she takes the ECPs. *No need to wait for her next monthly bleeding.* – A continuing user who needed ECPs due to pill-taking errors can continue where she left off with her current pack. • If she does not start immediately, but returns for POPs, she can start at any time if it is reasonably certain she is not pregnant. • All women will need to use a backup method for the first 2 days of taking pills. **After taking ulipristal acetate (UPA) ECPs:** • She can start or restart POPs on the 6th day after taking UPA-ECPs. *No need to wait for her next monthly bleeding.* POPs and UPA interact. If POPs are started sooner, and thus both are present in the body, one or both may be less effective. • Give her a supply of pills and tell her to start them on the 6th day after taking the UPA-ECPs. • She will need to use a backup method from the time she takes UPA-ECPs until she has been taking POPs for 2 days. • If she does not start on the 6th day but returns later for POPs, she may start at any time if it is reasonably certain she is not pregnant.

Giving Advice on Side Effects

IMPORTANT: Thorough counseling about bleeding changes and other side effects is an important part of providing the method. Counseling about bleeding changes may be the most important help a woman needs to keep using the method without concern.

Describe the most common side effects	• Breastfeeding women normally do not have monthly bleeding for several months after giving birth. POPs lengthen this period of time. • Women who are not breastfeeding may have frequent or irregular bleeding for the first several months, followed by regular bleeding or continued irregular bleeding. • Headaches, dizziness, breast tenderness, and possibly other side effects.
Explain about these side effects	• Side effects are not signs of illness. Lack of bleeding does not mean pregnancy. • Usually become less or stop within the first few months of using POPs. Bleeding changes, however, usually persist. • Common, but some women do not have them.
Explain what to do in case of side effects	• Keep taking POPs. Skipping pills risks pregnancy. • Try taking pills with food or at bedtime to help avoid nausea. • The client can come back for help if side effects bother her or if she has other concerns.

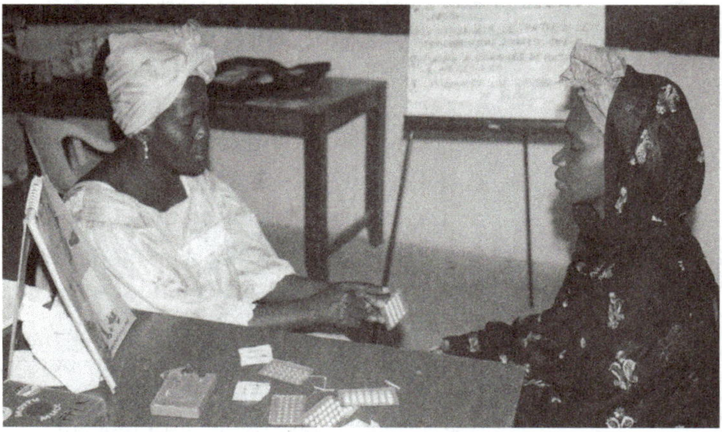

Explaining How to Use

1. Give pills	• Give as many packs as possible—even as much as a year's supply (11 packs of 35 pills each or 13 packs of 28 pills each).
2. Explain pill pack	• Show which kind of pack—28 pills or 35 pills. • Explain that all pills in POP packs are the same color and all are active pills, containing a hormone that prevents pregnancy. • Show how to take the first pill from the pack and then how to follow the directions or arrows on the pack to take the rest of the pills.
3. Give key instruction	• **Take one pill each day**—until the pack is empty. • Women who are not breastfeeding should take a pill at the same time each day. Taking a pill more than 3 hours late makes it less effective. • Discuss cues for taking a pill every day. Linking pill-taking to a daily activity—such as cleaning her teeth—may help her remember.
4. Explain starting next pack	• When she finishes one pack, she should take the first pill from the next pack on the very next day. • It is very important to start the next pack on time. Starting a pack late risks pregnancy.
5. Provide backup method and explain use	• Sometimes she may need to use a backup method, such as when she misses pills or is late taking a pill. • Backup methods include abstinence, male or female condoms, spermicides, and withdrawal. Tell her that spermicides and withdrawal are the least effective contraceptive methods. Give her condoms, if possible.
6. Explain that effectiveness decreases when breastfeeding stops	• Without the additional protection of breastfeeding itself, POPs are not as effective as most other hormonal methods. • When she stops breastfeeding, she can continue taking POPs if she is satisfied with the method, or she is welcome to come back for another method.

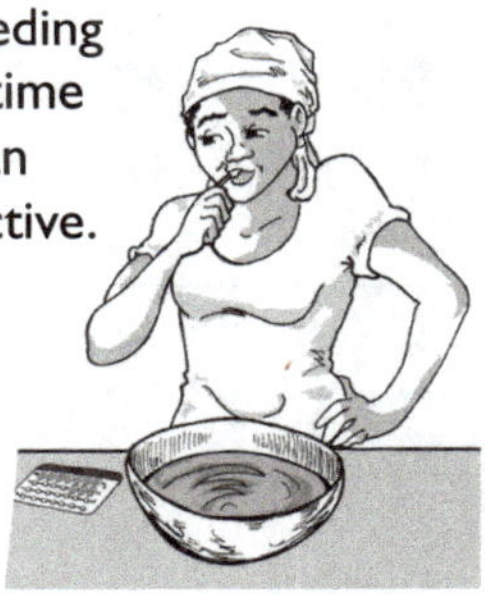

Supporting the User

Managing Missed Pills

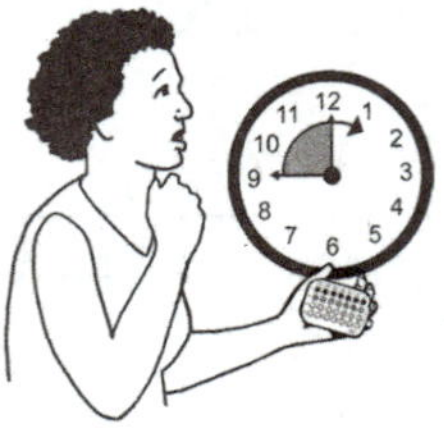

It is easy to forget a pill or to be late in taking it. Adolescents are more likely to forget pills and so may need extra support and guidance.

POP users should know what to do if they forget to take pills. **If a woman is 3 or more hours late taking a pill (12 or more hours late taking a POP containing desogestrel 75 mg), or if she misses a pill completely, she should follow the instructions below.** For breastfeeding women, whether missing a pill places her at risk of pregnancy depends on whether or not her monthly bleeding has returned.

Making Up Missed Progestin-Only Pills

Key message	• **Take a missed pill as soon as possible.** • Keep taking pills as usual, one each day. (She may take 2 pills at the same time or on the same day.)
Do you have monthly bleeding regularly?	• If yes, she also should use a backup method for the next 2 days. • Also, if she had sex in the past 5 days, she can consider taking ECPs (see Emergency Contraceptive Pills, p. 49).
Severe vomiting or diarrhea	• If she vomits within 2 hours after taking a pill, she should take another pill from her pack as soon as possible, and keep taking pills as usual.

How Can a Partner Help?

The client's partner is welcome to participate in counseling and learn about the method and what support he can give to his partner. A male partner can:

- Support a woman's choice of POPs
- Help her to remember to take a pill at about the same time each day
- Show understanding and support if she has side effects
- Help her to make sure that she has a new pill pack on hand to start on time
- Help to make sure she has ECPs on hand in case she misses pills or starts a new pill pack late
- Use condoms consistently in addition to POPs if he has an STI/HIV or thinks he may be at risk of an STI/HIV

"Come Back Any Time": Reasons to Return

Assure every client that she is welcome to come back any time—for example, if she has problems, questions, or wants another method; she has a major change in health status; or she thinks she might be pregnant. Also if:

- She has stopped breastfeeding and wants to switch to another method.
- For a woman who has monthly bleeding: If she took a pill more than 3 hours late or missed one completely, and also had sex during the last 5 days, she may wish to consider ECPs (see Emergency Contraceptive Pills, p. 49).

General health advice: Anyone who suddenly feels that something is seriously wrong with her health should immediately seek medical care from a nurse or doctor. Her contraceptive method is most likely not the cause of the condition, but she should tell the nurse or doctor what method she is using.

Planning the Next Visit

1. Encourage her to come back for more pills before she uses up her supply of pills.
2. Contacting women after the first 3 months of POP use is recommended. This offers an opportunity to answer any questions, help with any problems, and check on correct use.

Helping Continuing Users

1. Ask how the client is doing with the method and whether she is satisfied. Ask if she has any questions or anything to discuss.
2. Ask especially if she is concerned about bleeding changes. Give her any information or help that she needs (see Managing Any Problems, p. 42).
3. Ask if she often has problems remembering to take a pill every day. If so, discuss ways to remember, making up for missed pills, and ECPs, or choosing another method. Adolescents may need extra support.
4. Give her more pill packs—as much as a full year's supply (11 or 13 packs), if possible. Plan her next resupply visit before she will need more pills.
5. Ask a long-term client if she has had any new health problems since her last visit. Address problems as appropriate. For new health problems that may require switching methods, see p. 45.
6. Ask a long-term client about major life changes that may affect her needs—particularly plans for having children and STI/HIV risk. Follow up as needed.

Managing Any Problems

Problems Reported as Side Effects or Problems With Use

May or may not be due to the method.

- Problems with side effects affect women's satisfaction and use of POPs. They deserve the provider's attention. If the client reports side effects or problems, listen to her concerns, give her advice and support, and, if appropriate, treat. Make sure she understands the advice and agrees.
- Encourage her to keep taking a pill every day even if she has side effects. Missing pills can risk pregnancy.
- Many side effects will subside after a few months of use. For a woman whose side effects persist, give her a different POP formulation, if available, for at least 3 months.
- Offer to help the client choose another method—now, if she wishes, or if problems cannot be overcome.

No monthly bleeding

- Breastfeeding women:
  - Reassure her that this is normal during breastfeeding. It is not harmful.
- Women not breastfeeding:
  - Reassure her that some women using POPs stop having monthly bleeding, and this is not harmful. There is no need to lose blood every month. It is similar to not having monthly bleeding during pregnancy. She is not pregnant or infertile. Blood is not building up inside her. (Some women are happy to be free from monthly bleeding.)

Irregular bleeding (bleeding at unexpected times that bothers the client)

- Reassure her that many women using POPs experience irregular bleeding—whether breastfeeding or not. (Breastfeeding itself also can cause irregular bleeding.) It is not harmful and sometimes becomes less or stops after the first several months of use. Some women have irregular bleeding the entire time they are taking POPs, however.
- Other possible causes of irregular bleeding include:
  - Vomiting or diarrhea
  - Taking anticonvulsants or rifampicin (see Starting treatment with anticonvulsants, rifampicin, or rifabutin, p. 45)
- To reduce irregular bleeding:
  - Teach her to make up for missed pills properly, including after vomiting or diarrhea (see Managing Missed Pills, p. 40).
  - For modest short-term relief she can try 800 mg ibuprofen 3 times daily after meals for 5 days, or other nonsteroidal anti-inflammatory drug (NSAID), beginning when irregular bleeding starts. NSAIDs

provide some relief of irregular bleeding for implants, progestin-only injectables, and IUDs, and they may also help POP users.

- If she has been taking the pills for more than a few months and NSAIDs do not help, give her a different POP formulation, if available. Ask her to try the new pills for at least 3 months.

- If irregular bleeding continues or starts after several months of normal or no monthly bleeding, or you suspect that something may be wrong for other reasons, consider underlying conditions unrelated to method use (see Unexplained vaginal bleeding, p. 45).

Heavy or prolonged bleeding (twice as much as usual or longer than 8 days)

- Reassure her that some women using POPs experience heavy or prolonged bleeding. It is generally not harmful and usually becomes less or stops after a few months.
- For modest short-term relief she can try NSAIDs, beginning when heavy bleeding starts. Try the same treatments as for irregular bleeding (see previous page).
- To help prevent anemia, suggest she take iron tablets and tell her it is important to eat foods containing iron, such as meat and poultry (especially beef and chicken liver), fish, green leafy vegetables, and legumes (beans, bean curd, lentils, and peas).
- If heavy or prolonged bleeding continues or starts after several months of normal or no monthly bleeding, or you suspect that something may be wrong for other reasons, consider underlying conditions unrelated to method use (see Unexplained vaginal bleeding, p. 45).

Missed pills

- See Managing Missed Pills, p. 40.

Ordinary headaches (nonmigrainous)

- Suggest aspirin (325–650 mg), ibuprofen (200–400 mg), paracetamol (325–1000 mg), or other pain reliever.
- Any headaches that get worse or occur more often during POP use should be evaluated.

Mood changes or changes in sex drive

- Ask about changes in her life that could affect her mood or sex drive, including changes in her relationship with her partner. Give her support as appropriate.
- Some women experience depression in the year after giving birth. This is not related to POPs. Clients who have serious mood changes such as major depression should be referred for care.
- Consider locally available remedies.

Breast tenderness

- Breastfeeding women:
  - See Maternal and Newborn Health, Sore Breasts, p. 356.
- Women not breastfeeding:
  - Recommend that she wear a supportive bra (including during strenuous activity and sleep).
  - Try hot or cold compresses.
  - Suggest aspirin (325–650 mg), ibuprofen (200–400 mg), paracetamol (325–1000 mg), or other pain reliever.
  - Consider locally available remedies.

Severe pain in lower abdomen

- Abdominal pain may be due to various problems, such as enlarged ovarian follicles or cysts.
  - A woman can continue to use POPs during evaluation and treatment.
  - There is no need to treat enlarged ovarian follicles or cysts unless they grow abnormally large, twist, or burst. Reassure the client that they usually disappear on their own. To be sure the problem is resolving, see the client again in 6 weeks, if possible.
- With severe abdominal pain, be particularly alert for additional signs or symptoms of ectopic pregnancy, which is rare and not caused by POPs, but it can be life-threatening (see Question 13, p. 48).
- In the early stages of ectopic pregnancy, symptoms may be absent or mild, but eventually they will become severe. A combination of these signs or symptoms should increase suspicion of ectopic pregnancy:
  - Unusual abdominal pain or tenderness
  - Abnormal vaginal bleeding or no monthly bleeding—especially if this is a change from her usual bleeding pattern
  - Light-headedness or dizziness
  - Fainting
- If ectopic pregnancy or other serious health condition is suspected, refer at once for immediate diagnosis and care. (See Female Sterilization, Managing Ectopic Pregnancy, p. 227, for more on ectopic pregnancies.)

Nausea or dizziness

- For nausea, suggest taking POPs at bedtime or with food.
- If symptoms continue, consider locally available remedies.

New Problems That May Require Switching Methods

May or may not be due to the method.

Unexplained vaginal bleeding (that suggests a medical condition not related to the method)

- Refer or evaluate by history and pelvic examination. Diagnose and treat as appropriate.
- She can continue using POPs while her condition is being evaluated.
- If bleeding is caused by a sexually transmitted infection or pelvic inflammatory disease, she can continue using POPs during treatment.

Starting treatment with anticonvulsants, rifampicin, or rifabutin

- Barbiturates, carbamazepine, oxcarbazepine, phenytoin, primidone, topiramate, rifampicin, rifabutin, and ritonavir may make POPs less effective. If using these medications long-term, she may want a different method, such as progestin-only injectables or a copper-bearing IUD or LNG-IUD.
- If using these medications short-term, she can use a backup method along with POPs.

Migraine headaches (see Identifying Migraine Headaches and Auras, p. 436)

- A woman who has migraine headaches with or without aura can safely start POPs.
- If she develops migraine headaches without aura while taking POPs, she can continue to use POPs if she wishes.
- If she develops migraine aura while using POPs, stop POPs. Help her choose a method without hormones.

Certain serious health conditions (suspected blood clots in deep veins of legs or lungs, liver disease, or breast cancer). See Signs and Symptoms of Serious Health Conditions, p. 384.

- Tell her to stop taking POPs.
- Give her a backup method to use until the condition is evaluated.
- Refer for diagnosis and care if not already under care.

Heart disease due to blocked or narrowed arteries (ischemic heart disease) **or stroke**

- A woman who has one of these conditions can safely start POPs. If, however, the condition develops after she starts using POPs, she should stop. Help her choose a method without hormones.
- Refer for diagnosis and care if not already under care.

Suspected pregnancy

- Assess for pregnancy, including ectopic pregnancy.
- Tell her to stop taking POPs if pregnancy is confirmed.
- There are no known risks to a fetus conceived while a woman is taking POPs (see Question 4, p. 46).

Questions and Answers About Progestin-Only Pills

1. **Can a woman who is breastfeeding safely use POPs?**

   In 2016 WHO considered this question and updated its guidance to allow a woman to use progestin-only pills after childbirth regardless of how recently she gave birth. She does not need to wait until 6 weeks postpartum. POPs are safe for both the mother and the baby and do not affect milk production.

2. **What should a woman do when she stops breastfeeding her baby? Can she continue taking POPs?**

   A woman who is satisfied with using POPs can continue using them when she has stopped breastfeeding. She is less protected from pregnancy than when breastfeeding, however. She can switch to another method if she wishes.

3. **Can a woman take POPs at any age?**

   Yes. There is no minimum or maximum age for POP use.

   POPs can be an appropriate method for adolescents. Adolescents who are breastfeeding have the same need for an effective way to space births as older women. They may need extra support and encouragement to use POPs consistently and effectively.

4. **Do POPs cause birth defects? Will the fetus be harmed if a woman accidentally takes POPs while she is pregnant?**

   No. Good evidence shows that POPs will not cause birth defects and will not otherwise harm the fetus if a woman becomes pregnant while taking POPs or accidentally takes POPs when she is already pregnant.

5. **How long does it take to become pregnant after stopping POPs?**

   Women who stop using POPs can become pregnant as quickly as women who stop nonhormonal methods. POPs do not delay the return of a woman's fertility after she stops taking them. The bleeding pattern a woman had before she used POPs generally returns after she stops taking them. Some women may have to wait a few months before their usual bleeding pattern returns.

6. If a woman does not have monthly bleeding while taking POPs, does this mean that she is pregnant?

Probably not, especially if she is breastfeeding. If she has been taking her pills every day, she is probably not pregnant and can keep taking her pills. If she is still worried after being reassured, she can be offered a pregnancy test, if available, or referred for one. If not having monthly bleeding bothers her, switching to another method may help—but not to another progestin-only method. These methods sometimes stop monthly bleeding.

7. Must the POP be taken every day?

Yes. All of the pills in the POP package contain the hormone that prevents pregnancy. If a woman does not take a pill every day—especially a woman who is not breastfeeding—she could become pregnant. (In contrast, the last 7 pills in a 28-pill pack of combined oral contraceptives are not active. They contain no hormones.)

8. Is it important for a woman to take her POPs at the same time each day?

Yes, for 2 reasons. POPs contain very little hormone, and taking a pill more than 3 hours late (more than 12 hours late with POPs containing desogestrel 75 mg) could reduce their effectiveness for women who are not breastfeeding. (Breastfeeding women have the additional protection from pregnancy that breastfeeding provides, and so taking pills late is not as risky.) Also, taking a pill at the same time each day can help women remember to take their pills more consistently. Linking pill taking with a daily activity also helps women remember to take their pills.

9. Do POPs cause cancer?

No. Few large studies exist on POPs and cancer, but smaller studies of POPs are reassuring. Larger studies of implants have not shown any increased risk of cancer. Implants contain hormones similar to those used in POPs, and, during the first few years of implant use, at about twice the dosage.

10. Can POPs be used as emergency contraceptive pills (ECPs) after unprotected sex?

Yes. As soon as possible, but no more than 5 days after unprotected sex, a woman can take POPs as ECPs (see Pill Formulations and Dosing for Emergency Contraception, p. 55). Depending on the type of POP, she will have to take 40 to 50 pills. This is many pills, but it is safe because there is very little hormone in each pill.

11. Do POPs lower women's mood or sex drive?

Generally, no. Some women using POPs report these complaints. The great majority of POP users do not report any such changes, however, and some report that both mood and sex drive improve. It is difficult to tell whether such changes are due to the POPs or to other reasons. Providers can help a client with these problems (see Mood changes or changes in sex drive, p. 43). There is no evidence that POPs affect women's sexual behavior.

12. What should be done if a POP user has an ovarian cyst?

The great majority of cysts are not true cysts but actually fluid-filled structures in the ovary (follicles) that continue to grow beyond the usual size in a normal menstrual cycle. They may cause some mild abdominal pain, but they require treatment only if they grow abnormally large, twist, or burst. These follicles usually go away without treatment (see Severe pain in lower abdomen, p. 44).

13. Do POPs increase the risk of ectopic pregnancy?

No. On the contrary, POPs reduce the risk of ectopic pregnancy. Ectopic pregnancies are rare among POP users. The rate of ectopic pregnancy among women using POPs is 48 per 10,000 women per year. The rate of ectopic pregnancy among women in the United States using no contraceptive method is 65 per 10,000 women per year.

On the uncommon occasions that POPs fail and pregnancy occurs, 5 to 10 of every 100 of these pregnancies are ectopic. Thus, the great majority of pregnancies after POPs fail are not ectopic. Still, ectopic pregnancy can be life-threatening, and so a provider should be aware that ectopic pregnancy is possible if POPs fail.

CHAPTER 3

Emergency Contraceptive Pills

Key Points for Providers and Clients

- **Emergency contraceptive pills (ECPs) help a woman avoid pregnancy after she has sex without contraception.**
- **ECPs help to prevent pregnancy when taken up to 5 days after unprotected sex.** The sooner they are taken, the better.
- **Do not disrupt an existing pregnancy.**
- **Safe for all women**—even women who cannot use ongoing hormonal contraceptive methods.
- **Provide an opportunity for women to start using an ongoing family planning method.**
- **Several options can be used as emergency contraceptive pills.** Dedicated products, progestin-only pills, and combined oral contraceptives all can act as emergency contraceptives.

What Are Emergency Contraceptive Pills?

- ECPs are sometimes called "morning after" pills or postcoital contraceptives.
- Work by preventing or delaying the release of eggs from the ovaries (ovulation). They do not work if a woman is already pregnant.

(The copper-bearing IUD also can be used for emergency contraception. See p. 166.)

What Pills Can Be Used as Emergency Contraceptive Pills?

- A special ECP product with levonorgestrel only, or ulipristal acetate (UPA)
- Progestin-only pills with levonorgestrel or norgestrel
- Combined oral contraceptives with estrogen and a progestin—levonorgestrel, norgestrel, or norethindrone (also called norethisterone)

When to Take Them?

- *As soon as possible* after unprotected sex. The sooner ECPs are taken after unprotected sex, the better they prevent pregnancy.
- Can help to prevent pregnancy when taken any time up to 5 days after unprotected sex.

How Effective?

- If 100 women each had sex once during the second or third week of the menstrual cycle without using contraception, 8 women would likely become pregnant.
- If all 100 women used ulipristal acetate ECPs, fewer than one woman would likely become pregnant.
- If all 100 women used progestin-only ECPs, one woman would likely become pregnant.
- If all 100 women used combined estrogen and progestin ECPs, 2 women would likely become pregnant.

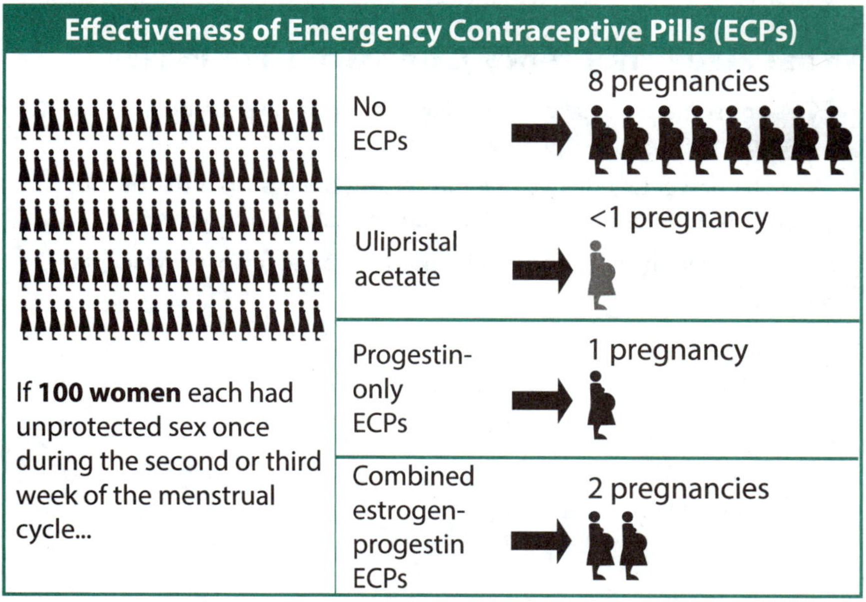

Return of fertility after taking ECPs: No delay. A woman can become pregnant immediately after taking ECPs. Taking ECPs prevents pregnancy only from acts of sex that took place in the 5 days before. They will not protect a woman from pregnancy from acts of sex more than 24 hours after she takes ECPs. To stay protected from pregnancy, women must begin to use another contraceptive method (see Planning Ongoing Contraception, p. 61).

Protection against sexually transmitted infections (STIs): None

Side Effects, Health Benefits, and Health Risks

Side Effects (see also Managing Any Problems, p. 61)

Some users report the following:

- Changes in bleeding patterns, including:
  - Slight irregular bleeding for 1–2 days after taking ECPs
  - Monthly bleeding that starts earlier or later than expected

In the first several days after taking ECPs:

- Nausea‡
- Abdominal pain
- Fatigue
- Headaches
- Breast tenderness
- Dizziness
- Vomiting‡

Known Health Benefits

Help protect against:

- Risks of pregnancy

Known Health Risks

None

Correcting Misunderstandings (see also Questions and Answers, p. 62)

Emergency contraceptive pills:

- Can be used by women of any age, including adolescents
- Do not cause abortion
- Do not prevent or affect implantation
- Do not cause birth defects if pregnancy occurs
- Are not dangerous to a woman's health

(Continued on next page)

‡ *Women using progestin-only or ulipristal acetate ECP formulations are much less likely to experience nausea and vomiting than women using estrogen and progestin ECP formulations.*

- Do not increase risky sexual behavior
- Do not make women infertile
- Can be used more than once in a woman's cycle

Avoid Unnecessary Procedures

- A woman can take ECPs when needed without first seeing a health care provider.
- No procedures or tests are needed before takings ECPs. The exception is that a woman who missed her last menses should have a pregnancy test before taking UPA-ECPs.

Why Some Women Say They Like Emergency Contraceptive Pills

- Can be used as needed
- Offer a second chance at preventing unwanted pregnancy
- Enable a woman to avoid pregnancy if sex was forced or she was prevented from using contraception
- Are controlled by the woman
- Reduce the need for abortion in the case of contraceptive errors or if contraception is not used
- Can have on hand in case the need arises

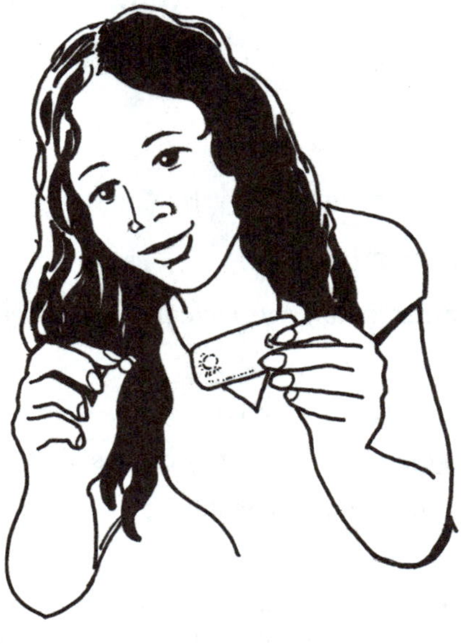

Who Can Use Emergency Contraceptive Pills

Safe and Suitable for All Women

Tests and examinations are not necessary for using ECPs.

Medical Eligibility Criteria for

Emergency Contraceptive Pills

All women can use ECPs safely and effectively, including women who cannot use ongoing hormonal contraceptive methods. Because of the short-term nature of their use, there are no medical conditions that make ECPs unsafe for any woman.

Providing Emergency Contraceptive Pills

ECPs may be needed in many different situations. Many women do not know about them, however. Women who use contraceptive methods that depend on the user, such as pills and condoms, particularly benefit from learning about ECPs.

If possible, give all women who may need ECPs a supply in advance. If giving an advance supply is not possible, an advance prescription may be given in some settings or a woman can be told where to obtain them locally.

An advance supply is helpful because a woman can keep them in case she needs them. Women are more likely to use ECPs if they already have them when needed. Also, having them on hand enables women to take them as soon as possible after unprotected sex, when they will be most effective.

When to Use

- Any time within 5 days after unprotected sex. The sooner after unprotected sex that ECPs are taken, the more effective they are.

ECPs Appropriate in Many Situations

ECPs can be used any time a woman is worried that she might become pregnant. For example, after:

- Sexual assault
- Any unprotected sex
- Mistakes using contraception, such as:
  - Condom was used incorrectly, slipped, or broke
  - Couple incorrectly used a fertility awareness method (for example, failed to abstain or to use another method during the fertile days)
  - Man failed to withdraw, as intended, before he ejaculated
  - Woman has had unprotected sex after she has missed 3 or more combined oral contraceptive pills or has started a new pack 3 or more days late
  - IUD has come out of place
  - Woman has had unprotected sex when she is more than 4 weeks late for her repeat injection of DMPA, more than 2 weeks late for her repeat injection of NET-EN, or more than 7 days late for her repeat monthly injection

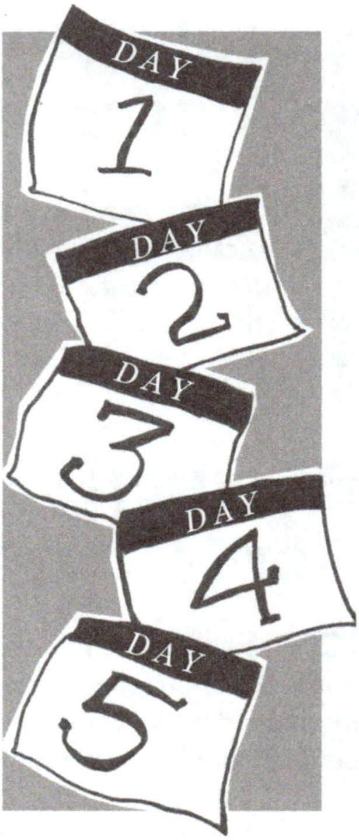

Pill Formulations and Dosing
for Emergency Contraception

Pill Type and Hormone	Formulation	Pills to Take: At First	Pills to Take: 12 Hours Later
Dedicated ECP Products			
Progestin-only	1.5 mg LNG	1	0
	0.75 mg LNG	2	0
Ulipristal acetate	30 mg ulipristal acetate	1	0
Oral Contraceptive Pills Used for Emergency Contraception			
Combined (estrogen-progestin) oral contraceptives	0.02 mg EE + 0.1 mg LNG	5	5
	0.03 mg EE + 0.15 mg LNG	4	4
	0.03 mg EE + 0.15 mg LNG	4	4
	0.03 mg EE + 0.125 mg LNG	4	4
	0.05 mg EE + 0.25 mg LNG	2	2
	0.03 mg EE + 0.3 mg norgestrel	4	4
	0.05 mg EE + 0.5 mg norgestrel	2	2
Progestin-only pills	0.03 mg LNG	50*	0
	0.0375 mg LNG	40*	0
	0.075 mg norgestrel	40*	0

* Many pills, but safe. See Question 8, p. 63.

LNG = levonorgestrel EE = ethinyl estradiol

For information on brands of ECPs and oral contraceptive pills, see: The Emergency Contraception Website (http:/ec.princeton.edu) and the International Consortium for Emergency Contraception (http:/www.cecinfo.org).

Giving Emergency Contraceptive Pills

1. Give pill (or pills)	• She can take the pill or pills immediately. • If she is using a 2-dose regimen, tell her to take the next dose in 12 hours.
2. Describe the most common side effects	• Nausea, abdominal pain, possibly others. • Slight bleeding or change in timing of monthly bleeding. • Side effects are not signs of illness and they do not last long. Most women have no side effects.
3. Explain what to do about side effects	• Nausea: – Routine use of anti-nausea medications is not recommended. – Women who have had nausea with previous ECP use or with the first dose of a 2-dose regimen can take anti-nausea medication such as 25–50 mg meclizine hydrochloride (such as Agyrax, Antivert, Bonine, Postafene) one-half to one hour before taking ECPs. • Vomiting: – If the woman vomits within 2 hours after taking progestin-only or combined ECPs, she should take another dose. If she vomits within 3 hours of taking ulipristal acetate ECPs, she should take another dose. (She can use anti-nausea medication with this repeat dose, as above.) If vomiting continues, she can take a repeat dose of progestin-only or combined ECPs by placing the pills high in her vagina. If vomiting occurs more than 2 hours after taking progestin-only or combined ECPs, or 3 hours after taking UPA-ECPs, then she does not need to take any extra pills.
4. Give more ECPs and help her start an ongoing method	• If possible, give her more ECPs to take home in case she needs them in the future. • See Planning Ongoing Contraception, p. 61.
5. Follow-up	• Encourage her to return for an early pregnancy test if her monthly bleeding is more than 7 days late.

"Come Back Any Time": Reasons to Return

No routine return visit is required. Assure every client that she is welcome to come back any time, however, and also if:

- She thinks she might be pregnant, especially if she has no monthly bleeding or her next monthly bleeding is delayed by more than 7 days.
- She did not start a continuing method immediately and now wants one.

How Can a Partner Help?

The client's partner is welcome to participate in counseling and learn about the method and what support he can give to his partner. A male partner can:

- Support a woman's decision to use ECPs
- Understand and support her need to choose and use a continuing method
- Help to make sure she has ECPs on hand in case she needs them again
- If she needed ECPs because of a mistake with a method, understand and support correct use of the method or discuss using a different method

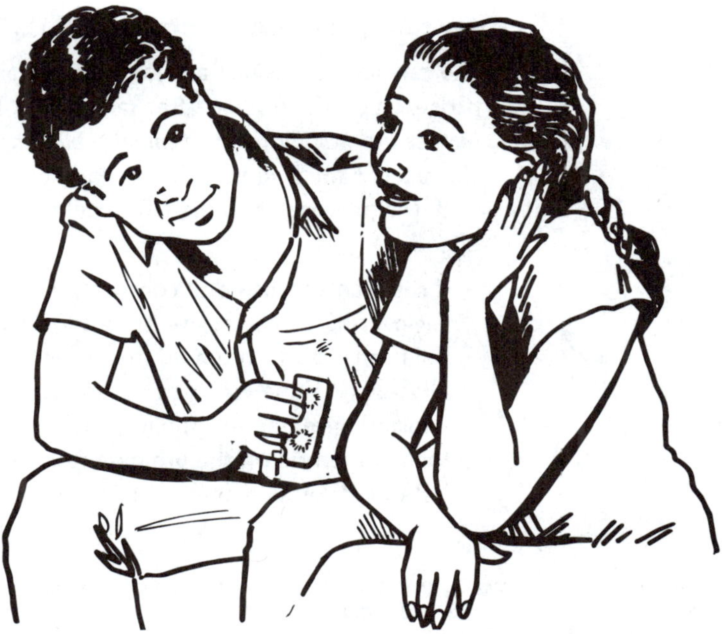

When to Start or Restart Contraception After ECP Use

Method	When to start or restart
Hormonal methods (combined oral contraceptives, progestin-only pills, progestin-only injectables, monthly injectables, implants, combined patch, combined vaginal ring)	**After taking progestin-only or combined ECPs:** • Can start or restart any method immediately after she takes the ECPs. *No need to wait for her next monthly bleeding.* – The continuing user of oral contraceptive pills who needed ECPs due to error can resume use as before. She does not need to start a new pack. – Patch users should begin a new patch. – Ring users should follow the instructions for late replacement or removal on page 126. • All women need to abstain from sex or use a backup method* for the first 7 days of using their method. • If she does not start immediately, but instead returns for a method, she can start any method at any time if it is reasonably certain she is not pregnant. **After taking ulipristal acetate (UPA) ECPs:** • She can start or restart any method containing progestin on the 6th day after taking UPA-ECPs. *No need to wait for her next monthly bleeding.* (If she starts a method containing progestin earlier, both the progestin and the UPA could be less effective.) – If she wants to use oral contraceptive pills, vaginal ring, or patch, give her a supply and tell her to start on the 6th day after taking UPA-ECPs. If she wants to use injectables or implants, give her an appointment to return for the method on the 6th day after taking UPA-ECPs or as soon as possible after that.

* *Backup methods include abstinence, male and female condoms, spermicides, and withdrawal. Tell her that spermicides and withdrawal are the least effective contraceptive methods. If possible, give her condoms.*

Method	When to start or restart
	– All women need to use a backup method from the time they take UPA-ECPs until they have been using a hormonal method for 7 days (or 2 days for progestin-only pills). • If she does not start on the 6th day, but instead returns later for a method, she may start any method at any time if it is reasonably certain she is not pregnant.
Levonorgestrel intrauterine device	**After taking progestin-only or combined ECPs:** • She can have the LNG-IUD inserted *at any time it can be determined that she is not pregnant* (see Ruling Out Pregnancy, p. 439). • She should use a backup method* for the first 7 days after LNG-IUD insertion. **After taking UPA-ECPs:** • She can have the LNG-IUD inserted on the 6th day after taking UPA-ECPs *if it can be determined that she is not pregnant.* – If she wants to use the LNG-IUD, give her an appointment to return to have it inserted on the 6th day after taking UPA-ECPs or as soon as possible after that. • She will need to use a backup method from the time she takes UPA-ECPs until 7 days after the LNG-IUD is inserted. • If she does not have the LNG-IUD inserted on the 6th day, but instead returns later, she can have it inserted at any time if it can be determined she is not pregnant.
Copper-bearing intrauterine device	**After taking progestin-only, combined, or UPA-ECPs:** • If she decides to use a copper-bearing IUD after taking ECPs, she can have it inserted on the same day she takes the ECPs. No need for a backup method.

3 Emergency Contraceptive Pills

Method	When to start or restart
Copper-bearing intrauterine device (continued)	• If she does not have it inserted immediately, but instead returns for the method, she can have the copper-bearing IUD inserted any time if it can be determined that she is not pregnant. Note: The copper-bearing IUD can be used for emergency contraception. A woman who wants to use the IUD for regular contraception can have it inserted for emergency contraception within the first 5 days after unprotected sex and then continue using it (see Copper-Bearing IUD, p. 155).
Female sterilization	**After taking progestin-only, combined, or UPA-ECPs:** • The sterilization procedure can be done within 7 days after the start of her next monthly bleeding or any other time if it is reasonably certain she is not pregnant. Give her a backup method to use until she can have the procedure.
Male and female condoms, spermicides, diaphragms, cervical caps, withdrawal	**After taking progestin-only, combined, or UPA-ECPs:** • Immediately.
Fertility awareness methods	**After taking progestin-only, combined, or UPA-ECPs:** • Standard Days Method: With the start of her next monthly bleeding. • Symptoms-based methods: Once normal secretions have returned. • Give her a backup method to use until she can begin the method of her choice.

Helping Users

Planning Ongoing Contraception

1. Explain that ECPs will not protect her from pregnancy from acts of sex more than 24 hours after she takes them. Discuss the need for and choice of ongoing pregnancy prevention and, if at risk, protection from STIs including HIV (see Sexually Transmitted Infections, Including HIV, p. 329).
2. If she does not want to start a contraceptive method now, give her condoms or a cycle of oral contraceptives and ask her to use them if she changes her mind. Give instructions on use. Invite her to come back any time if she wants another method or has any questions or problems.
3. If possible, give her more ECPs to use in the future in case of unprotected sex. She may need them if she has unprotected sex again as soon as 24 hours after taking the previous ECPs.

Managing Any Problems

Problems Reported as Side Effects

May or may not be due to the method.

Slight irregular bleeding

- Irregular bleeding due to ECPs will stop without treatment.
- Assure the woman that this is not a sign of illness or pregnancy.

Change in timing of next monthly bleeding or suspected pregnancy

- Monthly bleeding may start a few days earlier or later than expected. This is not a sign of illness or pregnancy.
- If her next monthly bleeding is more than 7 days later than expected after she takes ECPs, assess for pregnancy. There are no known risks to a fetus conceived if ECPs fail to prevent pregnancy (see Question 3, next page).

Questions and Answers About Emergency Contraceptive Pills

1. How do ECPs work?

ECPs prevent the release of an egg from the ovary or delay its release by 5 to 7 days. By then, any sperm in the woman's reproductive tract will have died, since sperm can survive there for only about 5 days. If ovulation has occurred and the egg was fertilized, ECPs do not prevent implantation or disrupt an already established pregnancy.

2. Do ECPs disrupt an existing pregnancy?

No. ECPs do not work if a woman is already pregnant.

3. Will ECPs harm the fetus if a woman accidentally takes them while she is pregnant?

No. Evidence does not show that ECPs will cause birth defects or otherwise harm the fetus if a woman is already pregnant when she takes ECPs or if ECPs fail to prevent pregnancy.

4. How long do ECPs protect a woman from pregnancy?

Women who take ECPs should understand that they could become pregnant the next time they have sex unless they begin to use another method of contraception at once. Because ECPs delay ovulation in some women, *she may be most fertile soon after taking ECPs.* If she wants ongoing protection from pregnancy, she must start using another contraceptive method by the next day, including a backup method if starting her continuing method requires it. In particular, a woman who has taken UPA-ECPs should wait until the 6th day to start a hormonal contraceptive. She should use a backup method during this period.

5. Can ECPs be used more than once?

Yes. If needed, ECPs can be taken again, even in the same cycle. A woman who needs ECPs often may want to consider a longer-acting and more effective family planning method.

6. Should women use ECPs as a continuing method of contraception?

A woman can use ECPs whenever she needs them, even more than once in the same cycle. However, relying on ECPs as an ongoing method should not be advised. It is not certain that ECPs, taken every time after sex, would be as effective as regular, continuing methods of contraception. Also, women who often take ECPs may have more side effects. Repeated use of ECPs poses no known health risks. It may be helpful, however, to screen women who take ECPs often for health conditions that can limit use of hormonal contraceptives.

7. What oral contraceptive pills can be used as ECPs?

Many combined (estrogen-progestin) oral contraceptives and progestin-only pills can be used as ECPs. Any pills containing the hormones used for emergency contraception—levonorgestrel, norgestrel, norethindrone, and any of these progestins together with estrogen (ethinyl estradiol)—can be used.

8. Is it safe to take 40 or 50 progestin-only pills as ECPs?

Yes. Progestin-only pills contain very small amounts of hormone. Thus, it is necessary to take many pills in order to receive the total ECP dose needed. In contrast, the ECP dosage with combined (estrogen-progestin) oral contraceptives is generally only 2 to 5 pills in each of 2 doses 12 hours apart. Women should not take 40 or 50 combined (estrogen-progestin) oral contraceptive pills as ECPs.

For women who have been continuing users of POPs, this may be the method of emergency contraception most convenient for her, or the only method available in time.

9. What is ulipristal acetate (UPA)?

UPA is an anti-progestin—that is, it modifies the activity of the natural hormone progesterone in a woman's monthly cycle. Thus, like other ECPs, UPA-ECPs probably work by blocking or delaying release of an egg from the ovary (ovulation). All ECPs should be taken as soon as possible for greatest effectiveness. UPA-ECPs may be more effective than other ECPs between 72 hours and 120 hours after unprotected sex. UPA-ECPs have been available in Europe since 2009 and received approval from the United States Food and Drug Administration in 2010 for use as an emergency contraceptive. They are now available in more than 50 countries. UPA-ECPs are not intended for use as a continuing oral contraceptive.

10. Are ECPs safe for women living with HIV? Can women on antiretroviral therapy safely use ECPs?

Yes. Women living with HIV and those on antiretroviral therapy can safely use ECPs.

11. Are ECPs appropriate for adolescents?

Yes. A study of ECP use among girls 13 to 16 years old found it safe. Furthermore, all of the study participants were able to use ECPs correctly. Also, access to ECPs does not influence sexual behavior.

Adolescents might particularly need ECPs because of high rates of forced sex, stigma about obtaining contraceptives, limited ability to plan for sex, and errors in using contraceptives.

12. Can a woman who cannot use combined (estrogen-progestin) oral contraceptives or progestin-only pills as an ongoing method still safely use ECPs?

Yes. This is because ECP treatment is very brief and the dose is small.

13. If ECPs failed to prevent pregnancy, does a woman have a greater chance of that pregnancy being an ectopic pregnancy?

No evidence suggests that ECPs increase the risk of ectopic pregnancy. Worldwide studies of progestin-only ECPs, including a US Food and Drug Administration review, have not found higher rates of ectopic pregnancy after ECPs failed than are found among pregnancies generally.

14. Why give women ECPs before they need them? Won't that discourage or otherwise affect contraceptive use?

No. Studies of women given ECPs in advance report these findings:

- Women who had ECPs on hand took them sooner after having unprotected sex than women who had to seek out ECPs. Progestin-only ECPs are more likely to be effective when taken sooner.
- Women given ECPs ahead of time were more likely to use them when needed than women who had to go to a provider to get ECPs.
- Women continued to use other contraceptive methods as they did before obtaining ECPs in advance.
- Women did not have unprotected sex more often.

If ECPs require a prescription and cannot be given in advance, give a prescription that can be use as needed.

15. If a woman buys ECPs over the counter, can she use them correctly?

Yes. Taking ECPs is simple, and medical supervision is not needed. Studies show that both young and adult women find the label and instructions easy to understand. In some countries ECPs are approved for over-the-counter sales or nonprescription use. These countries include Canada, China, India, the United States, and many others around the world.

CHAPTER 4

Progestin-Only Injectables

Key Points for Providers and Clients

- **Bleeding changes are common but not harmful.** Typically, irregular bleeding for the first several months and then no monthly bleeding.
- **Return for injections regularly.** Coming back every 3 months (13 weeks) for DMPA or every 2 months for NET-EN is important for greatest effectiveness.
- **Injection can be as much as 4 weeks late for DMPA or 2 weeks late for NET-EN.** Even if later, she may still be able to have the injection.
- **Gradual weight gain is common**, averaging 1–2 kg per year.
- **Return of fertility is often delayed.** It takes several months longer on average to become pregnant after stopping progestin-only injectables than after stopping other methods.

What Are Progestin-Only Injectables?

- The injectable contraceptives depot medroxyprogesterone acetate (DMPA) and norethisterone enanthate (NET-EN) each contain a progestin like the natural hormone progesterone in a woman's body. (In contrast, monthly injectables contain both estrogen and progestin. See Monthly Injectables, p. 97.)
- Do not contain estrogen, and so can be used throughout breastfeeding, starting 6 weeks after giving birth, and by women who cannot use methods with estrogen.
- Given by injection into the muscle (intramuscular injection) or, with a new formulation of DMPA, just under the skin (subcutaneous injection). The hormone is then released slowly into the bloodstream. (See DMPA for Subcutaneous Injection, p. 68.)

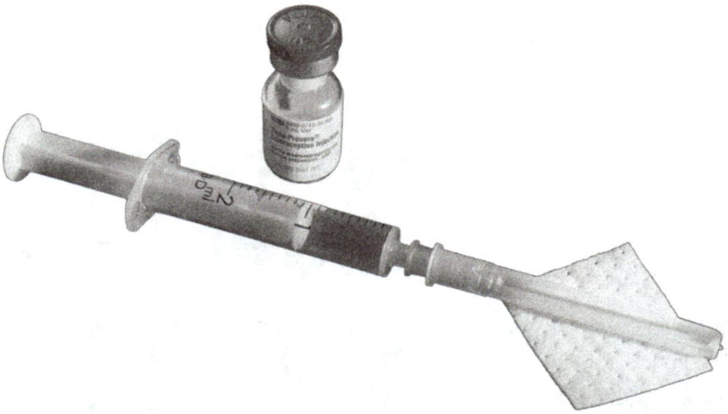

- DMPA, the most widely used progestin-only injectable, is also known in its intramuscular form as "the shot," "the jab," the injection, Depo, Depo-Provera, and Petogen. The subcutaneous version in the Uniject injection system is currently marketed under the name Sayana Press and in prefilled single-dose disposable hypodermic syringes as depo-subQ provera 104.
- NET-EN is also known as norethindrone enanthate, Noristerat, Norigest, and Syngestal. (See Comparing Injectables, p. 427, for differences between DMPA and NET-EN.)
- Work primarily by preventing the release of eggs from the ovaries (ovulation).

How Effective?

Effectiveness depends on getting injections regularly: Risk of pregnancy is greatest when a woman misses an injection.

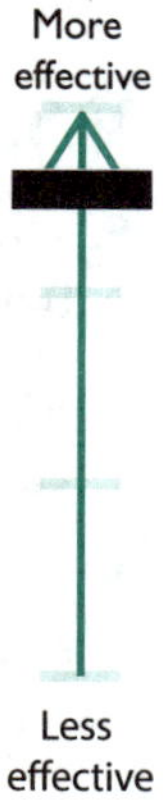

- As commonly used, about 4 pregnancies per 100 women using progestin-only injectables over the first year. This means that 96 of every 100 women using injectables will not become pregnant.
- When women have injections on time, less than 1 pregnancy per 100 women using progestin-only injectables over the first year (2 per 1,000 women).

Return of fertility after injections are stopped: An average of about 4 months longer for DMPA and 1 month longer for NET-EN than with most other methods (see Question 8, p. 94).

Protection against sexually transmitted infections (STIs): None

Side Effects, Health Benefits, and Health Risks

Side Effects (see also Managing Any Problems, p. 89)

> Bleeding changes are normal and not harmful. If a woman finds them bothersome, counseling and support can help.

Most users report some changes in monthly bleeding.†

- Typically, these include, with DMPA:

  First 3 months:

  – Irregular bleeding

  – Prolonged bleeding

  At one year:

  – No monthly bleeding

  – Infrequent bleeding

  – Irregular bleeding

- NET-EN affects bleeding patterns less than DMPA. NET-EN users have fewer days of bleeding in the first 6 months and are less likely than DMPA users to have no monthly bleeding after one year.

Some users report the following:

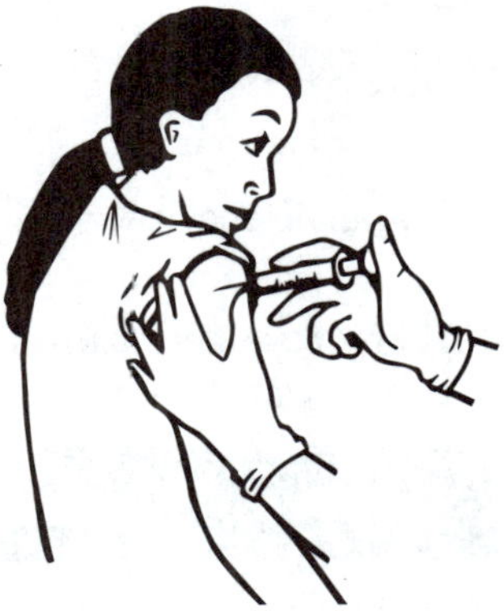

- Weight gain (see Question 5, p. 93)
- Headaches
- Dizziness
- Abdominal bloating and discomfort
- Mood changes
- Less sex drive

Other possible physical changes:

- Loss of bone density (see Question 11, p. 95)

Why Some Women Say They Like Progestin-Only Injectables

- Requires action only every 2 or 3 months. No daily pill-taking.
- Do not interfere with sex
- Are private: No one else can tell that a woman is using contraception
- Stop monthly bleeding (for many women)
- May help women to gain weight

† *For definitions of bleeding patterns, see "vaginal bleeding," p. 407.*

Known Health Benefits	*Known Health Risks*
DMPA	
Helps protect against: • Risks of pregnancy • Cancer of the lining of the uterus (endometrial cancer) • Uterine fibroids May help protect against: • Symptomatic pelvic inflammatory disease • Iron-deficiency anemia Reduces: • Sickle cell crises among women with sickle cell anemia • Symptoms of endometriosis (pelvic pain, irregular bleeding)	None
NET-EN	
Helps protect against: • Risks of pregnancy • Iron-deficiency anemia	None

NET-EN may offer many of the same health benefits as DMPA, but this list of benefits includes only those for which there is available research evidence.

DMPA for Subcutaneous Injection

DMPA is now available in a special formulation, called DMPA-SC, that is meant only for subcutaneous injection (just under the skin) and not for injection into muscle. Subcutaneous injection is easier to learn than intramuscular injection.

DMPA-SC is available in two injection systems—in the Uniject device and in prefilled, single-dose, conventional syringes. Both have short needles meant for injection just below the skin.

With the Uniject system, the user squeezes a flexible reservoir that pushes the fluid through the needle. DMPA-SC in the Uniject system is marketed under the brand name Sayana Press. This product may be particularly useful for community-based programs (see box, next page). Also, women can easily learn to give themselves subcutaneous injections with this system (see instructions on p. 84–85).

Correcting Misunderstandings (see also Questions and Answers, p. 92)

Progestin-only injectables:

- Can stop monthly bleeding, but this is not harmful and could help prevent anemia. It is similar to not having monthly bleeding during pregnancy. Blood is not building up inside the woman. Effectiveness is high regardless of the bleeding pattern.
- Do not disrupt an existing pregnancy.
- Do not make women infertile.

Delivering Injectable Contraception in the Community

Injectable contraceptives are popular with many women. This method can be more widely available when it is offered in the community as well as in clinics.

In 2012 WHO noted that using lay health workers to give injectable contraceptives may increase access to injectables and does not appear to raise safety concerns. WHO suggested that provision of injectables could be added to well-functioning programs that employ lay health workers.

These recommendations are part of a global movement known as task-sharing—empowering more types of health care workers to provide various health services. The goal of task-sharing is to serve more people, especially where there are few highly trained health care providers (see Who Provides Family Planning?, p. 372).

Lay health workers, auxiliary nurses, and other community-based providers of injectables should be trained and able to give injections safely. Also, they should be able to screen clients for pregnancy and for medical eligibility. They can inform women about delayed return of fertility and common side effects, including irregular bleeding, no monthly bleeding, and weight gain, and explain the importance of dual protection if a woman is at risk for sexually transmitted infections, including HIV. They also can inform women about the range of methods available, including methods available at the clinic. All providers of injectables need specific competency-based training and supportive supervision to carry out these tasks. WHO recommends specific monitoring and evaluation of the provision of injectables by lay health workers.

(Continued on next page)

Delivering Injectable Contraception in the Community *(continued)*

Prefilled syringes aid community-based programs

Prefilled single-dose, single-use injection devices make community and home delivery easier because providers do not have to draw a measured dose into the syringe from a vial. Also, these devices cannot be reused. DMPA is available in a number of prefilled single-dose injection systems: The older formulation for intramuscular injection (DMPA-IM) is available in auto-disable syringes. The newer subcutaneous formulation (DMPA-SC), which is suitable only for injection just under the skin, comes in the Uniject injection system under the brand name Sayana Press and in single-use conventional syringes (see DMPA for Subcutaneous Injection, p. 68).

The new subcutaneous formulation, particularly in the Uniject system, is likely to make delivery of DMPA injections in the community and the home easier. In fact, women can learn to inject themselves with this formulation (see p. 83).

Working together, in communities and clinics

For success, clinic-based providers and community-based providers need to work together closely. Programs vary, but these are some ways that clinic-based providers can support community-based providers:

- Managing side effects (see pp. 89–90)
- Using clinical judgment concerning medical eligibility in special cases (see p. 74)
- Ruling out pregnancy in women who are more than 4 weeks late for an injection of DMPA or 2 weeks late for NET-EN (see Managing Late Injections, p. 88)
- Responding to concerns of clients referred by the community-based providers

The clinic also can serve as "home" for the community-based providers, where they go for resupply, for supervision, training, and advice, and to turn in their records.

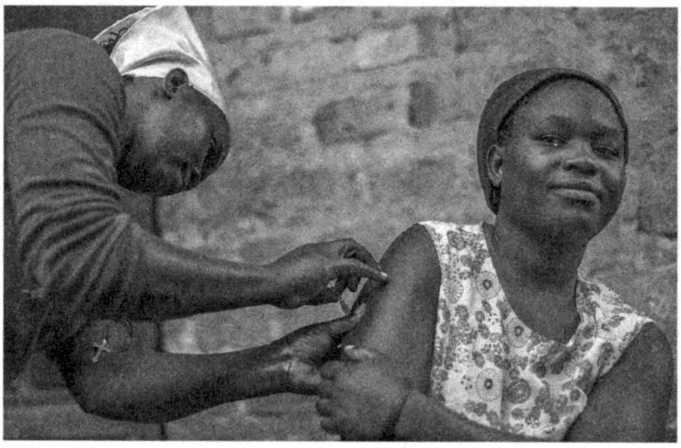

Who Can and Cannot Use Progestin-Only Injectables

Safe and Suitable for Nearly All Women

Nearly all women can use progestin-only injectables safely and effectively, including women who:

- Have or have not had children
- Are married or are not married
- Are of any age, including adolescents and women over 40 years old
- Have just had an abortion or miscarriage
- Smoke cigarettes, regardless of woman's age or number of cigarettes smoked
- Are breastfeeding, starting as soon as 6 weeks after childbirth
- Are living with HIV, whether or not on antiretroviral therapy (see Progestin-Only Injectables for Women With HIV, p. 74)

Avoid Unnecessary Procedures

(see Importance of Procedures, p. 368)

Women can begin using progestin-only injectables:

- Without a pelvic examination
- Without any blood tests or other routine laboratory tests
- Without cervical cancer screening
- Without a breast examination
- Without a pregnancy test. A woman can begin using a progestin-only injectable at any time, even when she is not having monthly bleeding at the time, if it is reasonably certain she is not pregnant (see Pregnancy Checklist, inside back cover).

> Blood pressure measurement is desirable before starting a hormonal method. However, where the risks of pregnancy are high and few methods are available, a woman should not be denied a hormonal method simply because her blood pressure cannot be measured. If possible, she can have her blood pressure measured later at a time and place convenient for her.

Medical Eligibility Criteria for

Progestin-Only Injectables

Ask the client the questions below about known medical conditions. Examinations and tests are not necessary. If she answers "no" to all of the questions, then she can start progestin-only injectables if she wants. If she answers "yes" to a question, follow the instructions. In some cases she can still start progestin-only injectables.

1. Are you breastfeeding a baby less than 6 weeks old?

❑ NO ❑ **YES** She can start using progestin-only injectables as soon as 6 weeks after childbirth (see Fully or nearly fully breastfeeding or Partially breastfeeding, p. 76).

2. Do you have severe cirrhosis of the liver or severe liver tumor?

❑ NO ❑ **YES** If she reports severe cirrhosis or severe liver tumor, such as liver cancer, do not provide progestin-only injectables. Help her choose a method without hormones.

3. Do you have high blood pressure?

❑ NO ❑ **YES**

Check her blood pressure if possible:

- If she is currently being treated for high blood pressure and it is adequately controlled, or her blood pressure is below 160/100 mm Hg, provide progestin-only injectables.
- If systolic blood pressure is 160 mm Hg or higher or diastolic blood pressure is 100 or higher, do not provide progestin-only injectables. Help her choose another method, one without estrogen.
- If she reports having high blood pressure in the past, and you cannot check blood pressure, provide progestin-only injectables.

4. Have you had diabetes for more than 20 years *or* damage to your arteries, vision, kidneys, or nervous system caused by diabetes?

❑ NO ❑ **YES** Do not provide progestin-only injectables. Help her choose another method, one without estrogen.

5. Have you ever had a stroke, blood clot in your leg or lungs, heart attack, or other serious heart problems?

❑ NO ❑ **YES** If she reports heart attack, heart disease due to blocked or narrowed arteries, or stroke, do not provide progestin-only injectables. Help her choose another method, one without estrogen. If she reports a current blood clot in legs (affecting deep veins, not superficial veins) or in a lung and she is not on anticoagulant therapy, help her choose a method without hormones.

6. Are you having vaginal bleeding that is unusual for you?

❑ NO ❑ **YES** If she has unexplained vaginal bleeding that suggests pregnancy or an underlying medical condition, progestin-only injectables could make diagnosis and monitoring of any treatment more difficult. Help her choose another method to use while being evaluated and treated (but not implants or a copper-bearing or hormonal IUD). After treatment, re-evaluate for use of progestin-only injectables.

7. Do you have or have you ever had breast cancer?

❑ NO ❑ **YES** Do not provide progestin-only injectables. Help her choose a method without hormones.

8. Do you have several conditions that could increase your chances of heart disease (coronary artery disease) or stroke, such as high blood pressure <u>and</u> diabetes?

❑ NO ❑ **YES** Do not provide progestin-only injectables. Help her choose another method, one without estrogen.

Also, women should not use progestin-only injectables if they report having lupus with positive (or unknown) antiphospholipid antibodies and not on immunosuppressive treatment, or severe thrombocytopenia. For complete classifications, see Medical Eligibility Criteria for Contraceptive Use, p. 388.

Be sure to explain the health benefits and risks and the side effects of the method that the client will use. Also, point out any conditions that would make the method inadvisable, when relevant to the client.

Using Clinical Judgment in Special Cases

Usually, a woman with any of the conditions listed below should not use progestin-only injectables. In special circumstances, however, when other, more appropriate methods are not available or acceptable to her, a qualified provider who can carefully assess a specific woman's condition and situation may decide that she can use progestin-only injectables. The provider needs to consider the severity of her condition and, for most conditions, whether she will have access to follow-up.

- Breastfeeding and less than 6 weeks since giving birth (considering the risks of another pregnancy and that a woman may have limited further access to injectables)
- Severe high blood pressure (systolic 160 mm Hg or higher or diastolic 100 mm Hg or higher)
- Acute blood clot in deep veins of legs or lungs
- History of heart disease or current heart disease due to blocked or narrowed arteries (ischemic heart disease)
- History of stroke
- Multiple risk factors for arterial cardiovascular disease such as diabetes and high blood pressure
- Unexplained vaginal bleeding before evaluation for possible serious underlying condition
- Had breast cancer more than 5 years ago, and it has not returned
- Diabetes for more than 20 years or damage to arteries, vision, kidneys, or nervous system caused by diabetes
- Severe cirrhosis or liver tumor
- Systemic lupus erythematosus with positive (or unknown) antiphospholipid antibodies and not on immunosuppressive treatment, or severe thrombocytopenia.

Progestin-Only Injectables for Women With HIV

- Women who are living with HIV or are on antiretroviral (ARV) therapy can safely use progestin-only injectables.
- The time between injections does not need to be shortened for women taking ARVs.
- Urge these women to use condoms as well. Used consistently and correctly, condoms help prevent transmission of HIV and other STIs.

Counseling Women Who Want a Progestin-Only Injectable Where HIV Risk Is High

Some research has found that women who use a progestin-only injectable and are exposed to HIV are more likely than other women to get HIV infection (see Question 2, p. 92). It is not clear whether this is due to the progestin-only injectable or to the way that the research was conducted.

In countries and programs where many family planning clients are at high risk of HIV, providers should discuss this finding with women interested in a progestin-only injectable. For counseling tips see Considering Progestin-Only Injectables Where HIV Risk Is High, p. 438. Women who are at high risk for HIV can still choose a progestin-only injectable if they wish (MEC Category 2).

Providing Progestin-Only Injectables

When to Start

IMPORTANT: A woman can start injectables any time she wants if it is reasonably certain she is not pregnant. To be reasonably certain she is not pregnant, use the Pregnancy Checklist (see inside back cover).

Woman's situation	When to start
Having menstrual cycles or switching from a nonhormonal method	**Any time of the month** • If she is starting within 7 days after the start of her monthly bleeding, no need for a backup method. • If it is more than 7 days after the start of her monthly bleeding, she can start injectables any time it is reasonably certain she is not pregnant. She will need a backup method* for the first 7 days after the injection. • If she is switching from an IUD, she can start injectables immediately (see Copper-Bearing IUD, Switching From an IUD to Another Method, p. 172).

* *Backup methods include abstinence, male and female condoms, spermicides, and withdrawal. Tell her that spermicides and withdrawal are the least effective contraceptive methods. If possible, give her condoms.*

Woman's situation	When to start
Switching from a hormonal method	• Immediately, if she has been using the hormonal method consistently and correctly or if it is otherwise reasonably certain she is not pregnant. No need to wait for her next monthly bleeding. No need for a backup method. • If she is switching from another injectable, she can have the new injectable when the repeat injection would have been given. No need for a backup method.
Fully or nearly fully breastfeeding	
Less than 6 months after giving birth	• If she gave birth less than 6 weeks ago, delay her first injection until at least 6 weeks after giving birth. • If her monthly bleeding has not returned, she can start injectables any time between 6 weeks and 6 months. No need for a backup method. • If her monthly bleeding has returned, she can start injectables as advised for women having menstrual cycles (see previous page).
More than 6 months after giving birth	• If her monthly bleeding has not returned, she can start injectables any time if it is reasonably certain she is not pregnant. She will need a backup method for the first 7 days after the injection. • If her monthly bleeding has returned, she can start injectables as advised for women having menstrual cycles (see previous page).
Partially breastfeeding	
Less than 6 weeks after giving birth	• Delay her first injection until at least 6 weeks after giving birth.

Woman's situation	When to start
Partially breastfeeding (continued)	
More than 6 weeks after giving birth	• If her monthly bleeding has not returned, she can start injectables any time if it is reasonably certain she is not pregnant.† She will need a backup method for the first 7 days after the injection. • If her monthly bleeding has returned, she can start injectables as advised for women having menstrual cycles (see p. 75).
Not breastfeeding	
Less than 4 weeks after giving birth	• She can start injectables at any time. No need for a backup method.
More than 4 weeks after giving birth	• If her monthly bleeding has not returned, she can start injectables any time if it is reasonably certain she is not pregnant.† She will need a backup method for the first 7 days after the injection. • If her monthly bleeding has returned, she can start injectables as advised for women having menstrual cycles (see p. 75).
No monthly bleeding (not related to childbirth or breastfeeding)	• She can start injectables any time if it is reasonably certain she is not pregnant. She will need a backup method for the first 7 days after the injection.
After miscarriage or abortion	• Immediately. If she is starting within 7 days after first- or second-trimester miscarriage or abortion, no need for a backup method. • If it is more than 7 days after first- or second-trimester miscarriage or abortion, she can start injectables any time if it is reasonably certain she is not pregnant. She will need a backup method for the first 7 days after the injection.

† *Where a visit 6 weeks after childbirth is routinely recommended and other opportunities to obtain contraception are limited, some providers and programs may give the first injection at the 6-week visit, without further evidence that the woman is not pregnant, if her monthly bleeding has not yet returned.*

Woman's situation	When to start
After taking emergency contraceptive pills (ECPs)	**After taking progestin-only or combined ECPs:** • She can start or restart injectables on the same day as taking the ECPs. *No need to wait for her next monthly bleeding to have the injection.* – She will need to use a backup method for the first 7 days after the injection. • If she does not start immediately but returns for injectables, she can start at any time if it is reasonably certain she is not pregnant. **After taking ulipristal acetate (UPA) ECPs:** • She can start or restart injectables on the 6th day after taking UPA-ECPs. *No need to wait for her next monthly bleeding to have the injection.* Injectables and UPA interact. If an injectable is started sooner, and thus both are present in the body, one or both may be less effective. • Make an appointment for her to return for the injection on the 6th day after taking UPA-ECPs, or as soon as possible after that. • She will need to use a backup method from the time she takes UPA-ECPs until 7 days after the injection. • If she does not start on the 6th day but returns later for injectables, she may start at any time if it is reasonably certain she is not pregnant.

Giving Advice on Side Effects

IMPORTANT: Thorough counseling about bleeding changes and other side effects must come before giving the injection. Counseling about bleeding changes may be the most important help a woman needs to keep using the method without concern.

Describe the most common side effects	• For the first several months, irregular bleeding, prolonged bleeding, frequent bleeding. Later, no monthly bleeding. • Weight gain (about 1–2 kg per year), headaches, dizziness, and possibly other side effects.
Explain about these side effects	• Side effects are not signs of illness. • Common, but some women do not have them. • The client can come back for help if side effects bother her.

Giving Intermuscular Injection with a Conventional Syringe

1. Obtain one dose of injectable, needle, and syringe

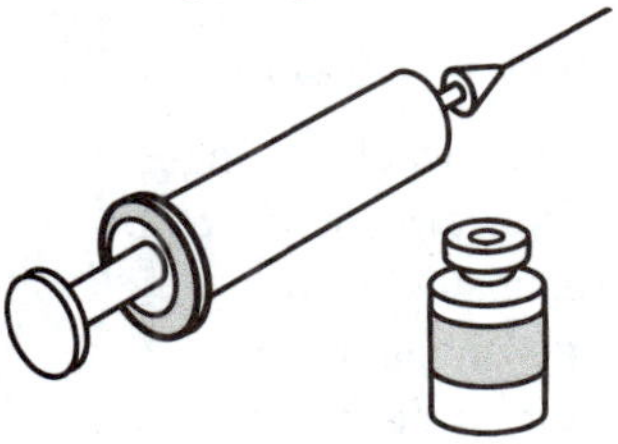

- DMPA: 150 mg for injections into the muscle (intramuscular injection). NET-EN: 200 mg for injections into the muscle.
- For each injection use a prefilled single-use syringe and needle from a new, sealed package (within expiration date and not damaged), if available.
- If a single-dose prefilled syringe is not available, use single-dose vials. Check expiration date. If using an open multidose vial, check that the vial is not leaking.
  - DMPA: A 2 ml syringe and a 21–23 gauge intramuscular needle.
  - NET-EN: A 2 or 5 ml syringe and a 19-gauge intramuscular needle. A narrower needle (21–23 gauge) also can be used.

2. Wash

- Wash hands with soap and water, if possible. Let your hands dry in the air.
- If injection site is dirty, wash it with soap and water.
- No need to wipe site with antiseptic.

If using a prefilled syringe, skip to step 5.

3. Prepare vial	• DMPA: Gently shake the vial. • NET-EN: Shaking the vial is not necessary. • No need to wipe top of vial with antiseptic. • If vial is cold, warm to skin temperature before giving the injection.
4. Fill syringe	• Pierce top of vial with sterile needle and fill syringe with proper dose.
5. Inject formula	• Insert sterile needle deep into the hip (ventro-gluteal muscle), the upper arm (deltoid muscle), or the buttocks (gluteal muscle, upper outer portion), whichever the woman prefers. Inject the contents of the syringe. • Do not massage injection site.

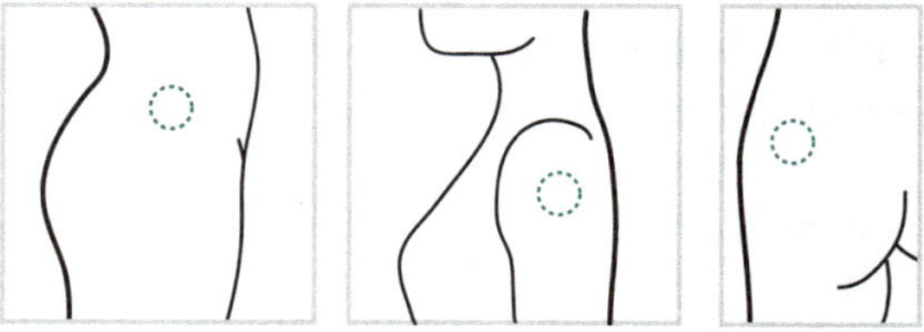

6. Dispose of disposable syringes and needles safely

- Do not recap, bend, or break needles before disposal.
- Place in a puncture-proof sharps container.
- Do not reuse disposable syringes and needles. They are meant to be destroyed after a single use. Because of their shape, they are very difficult to disinfect. Therefore, reuse might transmit diseases such as HIV and hepatitis.
- If reusable syringe and needle are used, they must be sterilized again after each use (see Infection Prevention in the Clinic, p. 376).

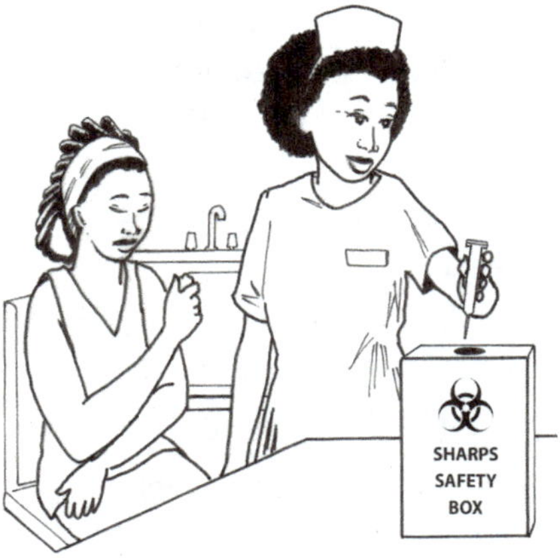

Giving the Injection with Subcutaneous DMPA in Uniject (Sayana Press)

1. Gather the supplies	Supplies include: • Uniject prefilled injection device at room temperature that has not passed its expiration date • Soap and clean water • Cotton swabs or cotton balls, if available • Safe puncture-proof container for sharps disposal
2. Wash	Wash hands with soap and water, if possible. • Let your hands dry in the air. • If injection site is dirty, wash it with soap and water. • No need to wipe site with antiseptic.
3. Ask where the client wants the injection	You can give the injection just under the skin: • in the back of the upper arm • in the abdomen (but not at the navel) • on the front of the thigh.
4. Open the pouch	• Open the foil pouch and remove the device.
5. Mix the solution	• Hold the device by the port (see picture 1). • Shake it hard for 30 seconds. • Check that the solution is mixed (granules distributed throughout the solution) and there is no damage or leaking.

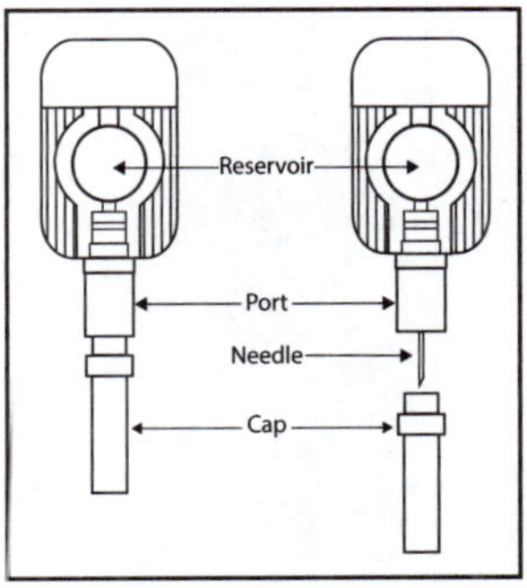

1. Parts of Uniject device

(Continued on next page)

6. Close the gap

- Hold the device by the port.
- Take care not to squeeze the reservoir during this step.
- Hold the device with the needle pointed upward to avoid spilling the drug.
- Push the cap into the port (see part A of picture 2, below).
- Continue to push firmly until the gap between the cap and port is closed (see part B of picture 2, below).
- Take off the cap (see part C of picture 2, below).

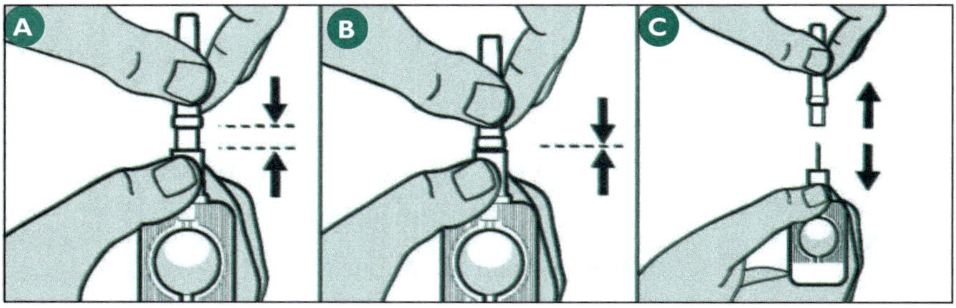

2. Close the gap and take off the cap

7. Give the injection

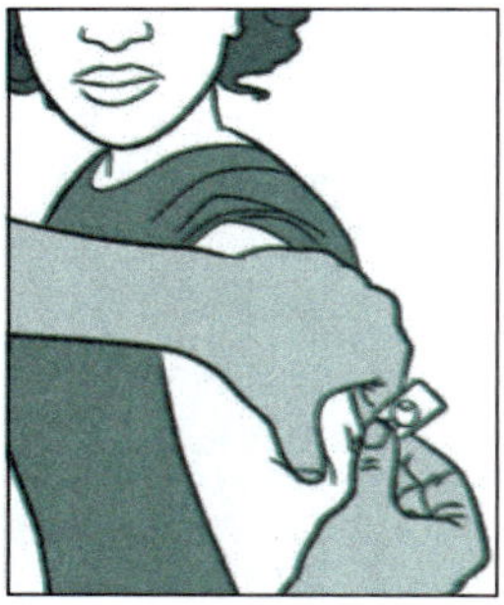

3. Pinch the skin and inject

- Gently pinch the skin at the injection site (see picture 3). This helps to make sure that the drug is injected into fatty tissue just under the skin and not into muscle.
- Hold the port. Gently push the needle straight into the skin with the needle pointing down (never upward) until the port touches the skin.
- Squeeze the reservoir slowly. Take 5 to 7 seconds.
- Pull out the needle and then release the skin.
- Do not clean or massage the site after injecting.

8. Discard the used device

- Do not replace the cap.
- Place the device in a safety box.

Supporting the User

Give specific instructions	• Tell her not to massage the injection site. • Tell the client the name of the injection. • Agree on a date for her next injection and give her a paper with the date written on it.

Self-injection Can Be an Option

Women can learn to inject themselves with the new subcutaneous formulation of DMPA. Some women like self-injection better than injections by health workers. Self-injection may save women time and money.

Research finds that 3 months after one-on-one training most women can competently give themselves their next injection. Women who inject themselves seem to be as likely to keep using injectable contraceptives as women who get their injections in clinics.

WHO recommends making self-injection an option where appropriate information and training are made available, referral links to a health care provider are strong, and women who self-inject are monitored and followed up. In addition, safe storage of injection devices at home and their safe disposal are important.

Teaching Clients to Self-Inject

Some clients will want to give themselves the injections. You can teach them how to do this. The following steps apply to self-injection with DMPA-SC in the Uniject injection system (Sayana Press).

1. Discuss plan for storage and disposal

Storage. Discuss where the client can store the devices for many months that is out of the reach of children and animals and in moderate temperatures (not in direct sunlight or in a refrigerator).

Disposal. Discuss how the client can dispose of the device in a container that has a lid and cannot be punctured and can be kept away from children. (Local programs should decide how to help women dispose of used needles.)

Note: The instructions on the next 2 pages can be copied and given to a client.

Steps in teaching clients to self-inject continue on p. 86.

How to give yourself an injection with Sayana Press

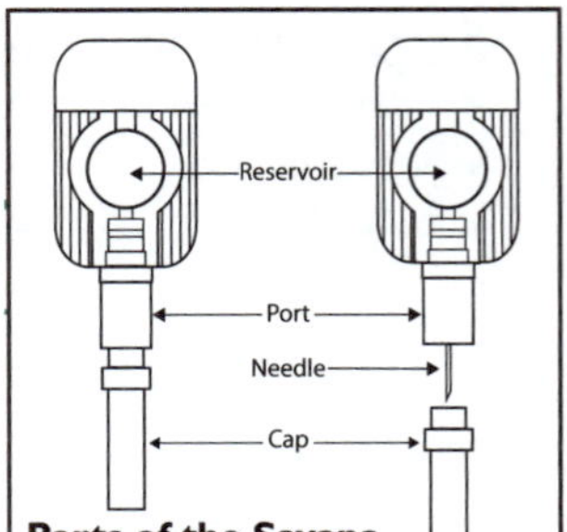

Parts of the Sayana Press injection device

Important steps	How to do it
1. Choose a correct injection site	Choose either: • the belly (but not the navel) OR • the front of the thigh.

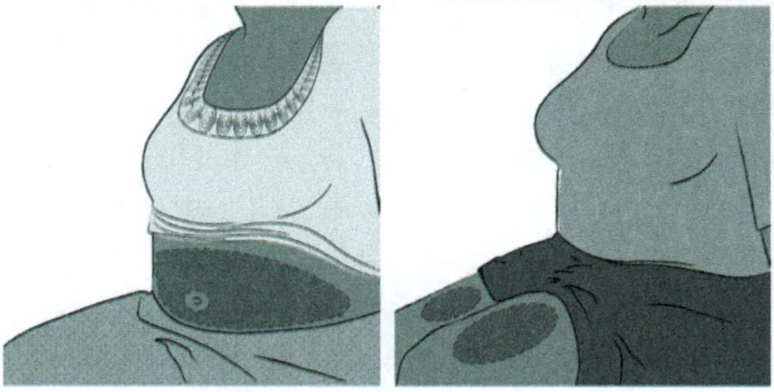

1. Where to give yourself the injection

Important steps	How to do it
2. Mix the solution	• After washing hands, open the pouch and take out the injection device. • Hold the device by the port (not the cap) and shake it hard for about 30 seconds. Make sure the solution is completely mixed.

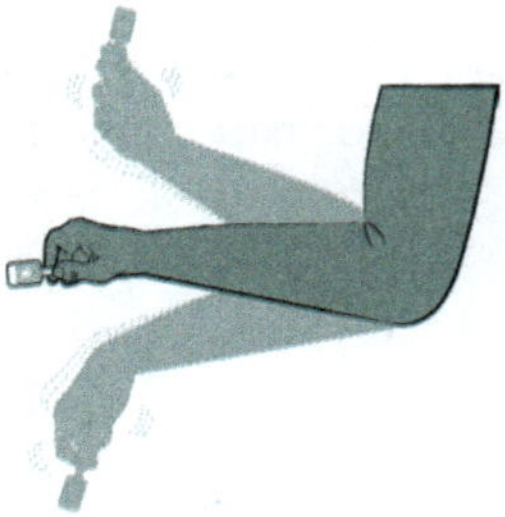

2. Mix the solution

Important steps	How to do it
3. Push the cap and the port together to close the gap	• Point the needle upward. • Hold the cap with one hand and the port with the other hand. • Press the cap down firmly until the gap is closed.

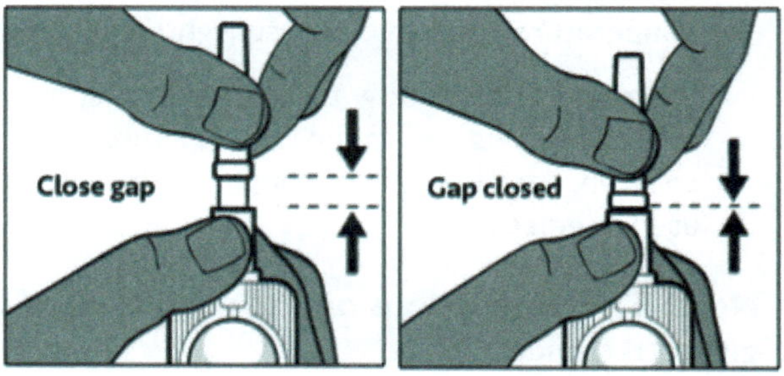

3. Close the gap

Important steps	How to do it
4. Pinch your skin into a "tent"	• Take the cap off the needle. Hold the device by the port. • With the other hand pinch about 4 cm (1½ inches) of skin.
5. Put the needle into the skin, and squeeze the reservoir slowly	• Press the needle straight into the skin with the needle pointing downward. • Press the needle in until the port touches the skin completely. • Squeeze the reservoir slowly, for 5 to 7 seconds.

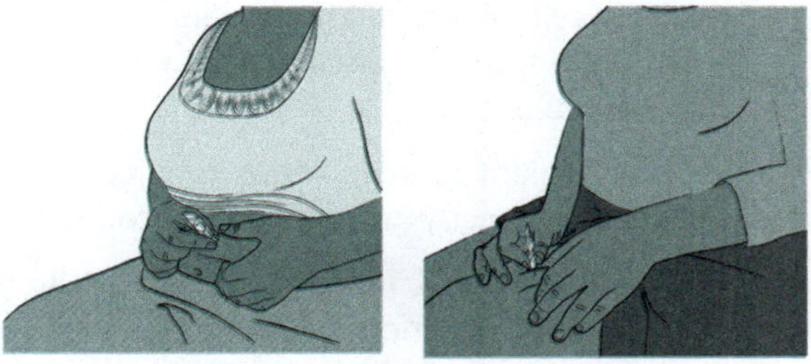

4 & 5. Pinch the skin and press in the needle

6. Dispose of the needle safely	• Pull the needle out and then let go of the skin. • Put the device in a container that can be closed and cannot be punctured.
7. Plan for your next injection	• Mark a calendar or other reminder for the same day of the month 3 months from today. • You can give yourself the next injection as early as 2 weeks before that date or as late as 4 weeks after. • If more than 4 weeks late, use another contraceptive method and see a health worker. • Make sure you have another device for the next injection and that it will not expire before then.

If you need help or more injection devices, contact:

____

at ____

2. **Explain and show how to self-inject.** Show the device and describe its parts. (See picture in instructions, p. 84.) Give the client a copy of the instructions and pictures on the previous 2 pages, a similar instruction sheet, or a booklet of more detailed instructions. Explain the important steps.

   Use an injection model to explain and show the client how to do each step while helping the client follow along on the instruction sheet. (If an injection model is not available, you can use a condom filled with salt or sugar. Or you can use fruit or bread.)

3. **Ask the client to try it.** After you have used the injection model to show self-injection, ask the client to practice injecting the model. Watch her and then discuss what went well and what did not. Answer her questions.

   Invite the client to keep trying to inject the model until she can do all the steps correctly and feels ready to inject herself.

4. **Ask the woman to inject herself while you are watching.** Then give her injection devices to take home so that she can inject herself in the future. Make sure that she understands when her future injection dates are, and how to calculate those dates by noting the same day of the month every 3 months.

   If she is unable to inject herself, give her the injection. When she returns for her next injection, ask if she wants to try self-injection again. If so, repeat the training.

5. **Tell the client where to get more injection devices.** Invite her to contact you if she has any questions or problems with self-injection or getting more injection devices.

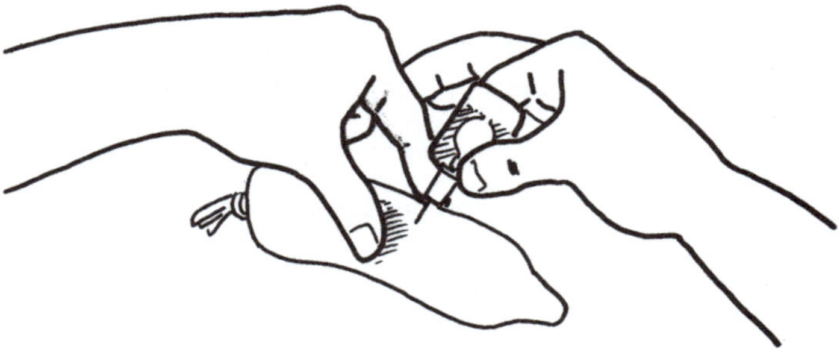

How Can a Partner Help?

The client's partner is welcome to participate in counseling and learn about the method and what support he can give to his partner. A male partner can:

- Support a woman's choice of a progestin-only injectable
- Show understanding and support if she has side effects
- Help her to remember to get her next injection on time
- Help to make sure she has ECPs on hand in case she is late for an injection by more than 4 weeks for DMPA or more than 2 weeks for NET-EN
- Use condoms consistently in addition to the progestin-only injectable if he has an STI/HIV or thinks he may be at risk of an STI/HIV

"Come Back Any Time": Reasons to Return Before the Next Injection

Assure every client that she is welcome to come back any time—for example, if she has problems, questions, or wants another method; she has a major change in health status; or she thinks she might be pregnant.

General health advice: Anyone who suddenly feels that something is seriously wrong with her health should immediately seek medical care from a nurse or doctor. Her contraceptive method is most likely not the cause of the condition, but she should tell the nurse or doctor what method she is using.

Planning the Next Injection

1. Agree on a date for her next injection in 3 months (13 weeks) for DMPA, or in 2 months (8 weeks) for NET-EN. Give her a paper with the date written on it (or dates, if she is self-injecting and taking home more than one injection device). Discuss how to remember the date, perhaps tying it to a holiday or other event or circling a date on a calendar.
2. Ask her to try to come on time. With DMPA she may come up to 4 weeks after the scheduled injection date and still get an injection. With NET-EN she may come up to 2 weeks after the scheduled injection date and still get an injection. With either DMPA or NET-EN, she can come up to 2 weeks before the scheduled injection date.
3. She should come back no matter how late she is for her next injection. If more than 4 weeks late for DMPA or 2 weeks late for NET-EN, she should abstain from sex or use condoms, spermicides, or withdrawal until she can get an injection. Also, if she has had sex in the past 5 days without using another contraceptive method, she can consider emergency contraceptive pills (see Emergency Contraceptive Pills, p. 49).

Helping Continuing Users

Repeat Injection Visits

1. Ask how the client is doing with the method and whether she is satisfied. Ask if she has any questions or anything to discuss.
2. Ask especially if she is concerned about bleeding changes. Give her any information or help that she needs (see Managing Any Problems, next page).
3. Give her the injection. **Injection of DMPA can be given up to 4 weeks late. Injection of NET-EN can be given up to 2 weeks late.**
4. Plan for her next injection. Agree on a date for her next injection (in 3 months or 13 weeks for DMPA, 2 months for NET-EN). Remind her that she should try to come on time, but she should come back no matter how late she is. (See Managing Late Injections, below.)
5. Every year or so, check her blood pressure if possible (see Medical Eligibility Criteria, Question 3, p. 72).
6. Ask a long-term client if she has had any new health problems. Address problems as appropriate. For new health problems that may require switching methods, see p. 91.
7. Ask a long-term client about major life changes that may affect her needs—particularly plans for having children and STI/HIV risk. Follow up as needed.

Managing Late Injections

- If the client is less than 4 weeks late for a repeat injection of DMPA, or less than 2 weeks late for a repeat injection of NET-EN, she can receive her next injection. No need for tests, evaluation, or a backup method.
- A client who is more than 4 weeks late for DMPA, or more than 2 weeks late for NET-EN, can receive her next injection if:
  - She has not had sex since 2 *weeks after* the scheduled date of her injection, or
  - She has used a backup method or has taken emergency contraceptive pills (ECPs) after any unprotected sex since 2 *weeks after* the scheduled date of her injection, or
  - She is fully or nearly fully breastfeeding and she gave birth less than 6 months ago.

  She will need a backup method for the first 7 days after the injection.
- If the client is more than 4 weeks late for DMPA, or more than 2 weeks late for NET-EN, and she does not meet these criteria, additional steps can be taken to be reasonably certain she is not pregnant (see Ruling Out

Pregnancy, p. 439). These steps are helpful because many women who have been using progestin-only injectables will have no monthly bleeding for at least a few months, even after discontinuation. Thus, asking her to come back during her next monthly bleeding means her next injection could be unnecessarily delayed. She may be left without contraceptive protection.

- Discuss why the client was late and solutions. Remind her that she should keep trying to come back every 3 months for DMPA, or every 2 months for NET-EN. If coming back on time is often a problem, discuss using a backup method when she is late for her next injection, taking ECPs, or choosing another method, such as an implant or IUD.

Managing Any Problems

Problems Reported as Side Effects

May or may not be due to the method.

- Problems with side effects affect women's satisfaction and use of injectables. They deserve the provider's attention. If the client reports side effects, listen to her concerns, give her advice and support, and, if appropriate, treat. Make sure she understands the advice and agrees.
- Offer to help the client choose another method—now, if she wishes, or if problems cannot be overcome.

No monthly bleeding

- Reassure her that most women using progestin-only injectables stop having monthly bleeding over time, and this is not harmful. There is no need to lose blood every month. It is similar to not having monthly bleeding during pregnancy. She is not infertile. Blood is not building up inside her. (Some women are happy to be free from monthly bleeding.)
- If not having monthly bleeding bothers her, she may want to switch to monthly injectables, if available.

Irregular bleeding (bleeding at unexpected times that bothers the client)

- Reassure her that many women using progestin-only injectables experience irregular bleeding. It is not harmful and usually becomes less or stops after the first few months of use.
- For modest short-term relief, she can take 500 mg mefenamic acid (NSAID) 2 times daily after meals for 5 days or 40 mg of valdecoxib daily for 5 days, beginning when irregular bleeding starts. (Bextra NSAID)
- If irregular bleeding continues or starts after several months of normal or no monthly bleeding, or you suspect that something may be wrong for other reasons, consider underlying conditions unrelated to method use (see Unexplained vaginal bleeding, p. 91).

Weight gain

- Review diet and counsel as needed.

Abdominal bloating and discomfort

- Consider locally available remedies.

Heavy or prolonged bleeding (twice as much as usual or longer than 8 days)

- Reassure her that some women using progestin-only injectables experience heavy or prolonged bleeding. It is not harmful and usually becomes less or stops after a few months.
- For modest short-term relief she can try (one at a time), beginning when heavy bleeding starts:
  - 500 mg of mefenamic acid twice daily after meals for 5 days
  - 40 mg of valdecoxib daily for 5 days
  - 50 µg of ethinyl estradiol daily for 21 days
- If bleeding becomes a health threat or if the woman wants, help her choose another method. In the meantime, she can use one of the treatments listed above to help reduce bleeding.
- To help prevent anemia, suggest she take iron tablets and tell her it is important to eat foods containing iron, such as meat and poultry (especially beef and chicken liver), fish, green leafy vegetables, and legumes (beans, bean curd, lentils, and peas).
- If heavy or prolonged bleeding continues or starts after several months of normal or no monthly bleeding, or you suspect that something may be wrong for other reasons, consider underlying conditions unrelated to method use (see Unexplained vaginal bleeding, next page).

Ordinary headaches (nonmigrainous)

- Suggest aspirin (325–650 mg), ibuprofen (200–400 mg), paracetamol (325–1000 mg), or other pain reliever.
- Any headaches that get worse or occur more often during use of injectables should be evaluated.

Mood changes or changes in sex drive

- Ask about changes in her life that could affect her mood or sex drive, including changes in her relationship with her partner. Give support as appropriate.
- Clients who have serious mood changes such as major depression should be referred for care.
- Consider locally available remedies.

Dizziness

- Consider locally available remedies.

New Problems That May Require Switching Methods

May or may not be due to the method.

Migraine headaches (see Identifying Migraine Headaches and Auras, p. 436)

- If she has migraine headaches without aura, she can continue to use the method if she wishes.
- If she has migraine aura, do not give the injection. Help her choose a method without hormones.

Unexplained vaginal bleeding (that suggests a medical condition not related to the method)

- Refer or evaluate by history and pelvic examination. Diagnose and treat as appropriate.
- If no cause of bleeding can be found, consider stopping progestin-only injectables to make diagnosis easier. Provide another method of her choice to use until the condition is evaluated and treated (not implants or a copper-bearing or LNG-IUD).
- If bleeding is caused by sexually transmitted infection or pelvic inflammatory disease, she can continue using progestin-only injectables during treatment.

Certain serious health conditions (suspected blocked or narrowed arteries, serious liver disease, severe high blood pressure, blood clots in deep veins of legs or lungs, stroke, breast cancer, or damage to arteries, vision, kidneys, or nervous system caused by diabetes). See Signs and Symptoms of Serious Health Conditions, p. 384.

- Do not give next injection.
- Give her a backup method to use until the condition is evaluated.
- Refer for diagnosis and care if not already under care.

Suspected pregnancy

- Assess for pregnancy.
- Stop injections if pregnancy is confirmed.
- There are no known risks to a fetus conceived while a woman is using injectables (see Question 12, p. 95) or to a woman who receives an injection while pregnant.

Questions and Answers About Progestin-Only Injectables

1. **Can women who could get sexually transmitted infections (STIs) use progestin-only injectables?**

   Yes. Women at risk for STIs can use progestin-only injectables. The few studies available have found that women using DMPA were more likely to acquire chlamydia than women not using hormonal contraception. The reason for this difference is not known. There are few studies available on use of NET-EN and STIs. Like anyone else at risk for STIs, a user of progestin-only injectables who may be at risk for STIs should be advised to use condoms correctly every time she has sex. Consistent and correct condom use will reduce her risk of becoming infected with an STI.

2. **Can women at high risk for HIV use progestin-only injectables?**

   Yes. Women at high risk of HIV infection can use any contraceptive method, including progestin-only injectables, except spermicide or diaphragm with spermicide (see Spermicides and Diaphragms, p. 271).

   In late 2016 a WHO assessment observed that some research finds that women who are at high risk of HIV infection and use a progestin-only injectable are slightly more likely to get HIV. It is not clear why studies find this. The injectable may or may not be responsible for increasing a woman's chances of becoming infected if exposed to HIV.

   An expert group convened by WHO concluded, "Women should not be denied the use of progestogen-only injectables because of concerns about the possible increased risk" of HIV infection. WHO classified progestin-only injectables, such as DMPA (including Sayana Press) and NET EN, as Medical Eligibility Criteria (MEC) category 2 for high risk of HIV. This classification means that women at high risk of HIV can generally use the method.

   WHO advises that, in countries and populations where HIV is common, providers should clearly inform women interested in progestin-only injectables about these research findings and their uncertainty, as well as how to protect themselves from HIV, so that each woman can make a fully informed choice (see Considering Progestin-Only Injectables Where HIV Risk Is High, p. 438, for counseling tips). In keeping with the MEC 2 classification, women should be told clearly that they can choose and use a progestin-only injectable if they wish. Women also should be told that other long-acting and effective methods are available if they would like to consider a different method.

3 . **If a woman does not have monthly bleeding while using progestin-only injectables, does this mean that she is pregnant?**

Probably not, especially if she is breastfeeding. Eventually, most women using progestin-only injectables will not have monthly bleeding. If a woman has been getting her injections on time, she is probably not pregnant and can keep using injectables. If she is still worried after being reassured, she can be offered a pregnancy test, if available, or referred for one. If not having monthly bleeding bothers her, switching to another method may help.

4. **Can a woman who is breastfeeding safely use progestin-only injectables?**

Yes. This is a good choice for a breastfeeding mother who wants a hormonal method. Progestin-only injectables are safe for both the mother and the baby starting as early as 6 weeks after childbirth. They do not affect milk production.

5. **How much weight do women gain when they use progestin-only injectables?**

Women gain an average of 1–2 kg per year when using DMPA. Some of the weight increase may be the usual weight gain as people age. Some women, particularly overweight adolescents, have gained much more than 1–2 kg per year. At the same time, some users of progestin-only injectables lose weight or have no significant change in weight. Asian women in particular do not tend to gain weight when using DMPA.

6. **Do DMPA and NET-EN cause abortion?**

No. Research on progestin-only injectables finds that they do not disrupt an existing pregnancy. They should not be used to try to cause an abortion. They will not do so.

7. **Do progestin-only injectables make a woman infertile?**

No. There may be a delay in regaining fertility after stopping progestin-only injectables, but in time the woman will be able to become pregnant as before, although fertility decreases as women get older. The bleeding pattern a woman had before she used progestin-only injectables generally returns several months after the last injection even if she had no monthly bleeding while using injectables.

8. How long does it take to become pregnant after stopping DMPA or NET-EN?

Women who stop using DMPA wait about 4 months longer on average to become pregnant than women who have used other methods. This means they become pregnant on average 10 months after their last injection. Women who stop using NET-EN wait about one month longer on average to become pregnant than women who have used other methods, or 6 months after their last injection. These are averages. A woman should not be worried if she has not become pregnant even as much as 12 months after stopping use. The length of time a woman has used injectables makes no difference to how quickly she becomes pregnant once she stops having injections.

After stopping progestin-only injectables, a woman may ovulate before her monthly bleeding returns—and thus can become pregnant. If she wants to continue avoiding pregnancy, she should start another method before monthly bleeding returns.

9. Does DMPA cause cancer?

Many studies show that DMPA does not cause cancer. DMPA use helps protect against cancer of the lining of the uterus (endometrial cancer). Findings of the few studies on DMPA use and breast cancer are similar to findings with combined oral contraceptives: Women using DMPA were slightly more likely to be diagnosed with breast cancer while using DMPA or within 10 years after they stopped. It is unclear whether these findings are explained by earlier detection of existing breast cancers among DMPA users or by a biologic effect of DMPA on breast cancer.

A few studies on DMPA use and cervical cancer suggest that there may be a slightly increased risk of cervical cancer among women using DMPA for 5 years or more. Cervical cancer cannot develop because of DMPA alone, however. It is caused by persistent infection with human papillomavirus (see Cervical Cancer, p. 340). Little information is available about NET-EN. It is assumed to be as safe as DMPA and other contraceptive methods containing only a progestin, such as progestin-only pills and implants.

10. Can a woman switch from one progestin-only injectable to another?

Switching injectables is safe, and it does not decrease effectiveness. If switching is necessary due to shortages of supplies, the first injection of the new injectable should be given when the next injection of the old formulation would have been given. Clients need to be told that they are switching, the name of the new injectable, and its injection schedule.

11. How does DMPA affect bone density?

During use, DMPA decreases bone mineral density slightly. This may increase the risk of developing osteoporosis and possibly having bone fractures later, after menopause. WHO has concluded that this decrease in bone mineral density does not place age or time limits on use of DMPA.

12. Do progestin-only injectables cause birth defects? Will the fetus be harmed if a woman accidentally uses progestin-only injectables while she is pregnant?

No. Good evidence shows that progestin-only injectables will not cause birth defects and will not otherwise harm the fetus if a woman becomes pregnant while using progestin-only injectables or accidentally starts injectables when she is already pregnant.

13. Do progestin-only injectables lower women's mood or sex drive?

Generally, no. Some women using injectables report these complaints. The great majority of injectables users do not report any such changes, however. It is difficult to tell whether such changes are due to progestin-only injectables or to other reasons. Providers can help a client with these problems (see Mood changes or changes in sex drive, p. 90). There is no evidence that progestin-only injectables affect women's sexual behavior.

14. What if a woman returns for her next injection late?

A woman can have her next DMPA injection even if she is up to 4 weeks late, without the need for further evidence that she is not pregnant. A woman can receive her next NET-EN injection if she is up to 2 weeks late. Some women return even later for their repeat injection, however. In such cases providers can use the instructions on p. 439, Ruling Out Pregnancy. Whether a woman is late for reinjection or not, her next injection of DMPA should be planned for 3 months later, or her next injection of NET-EN should be planned for 2 months later, as usual.

When a Woman Can Have Her Next Injection of DMPA or NET-EN

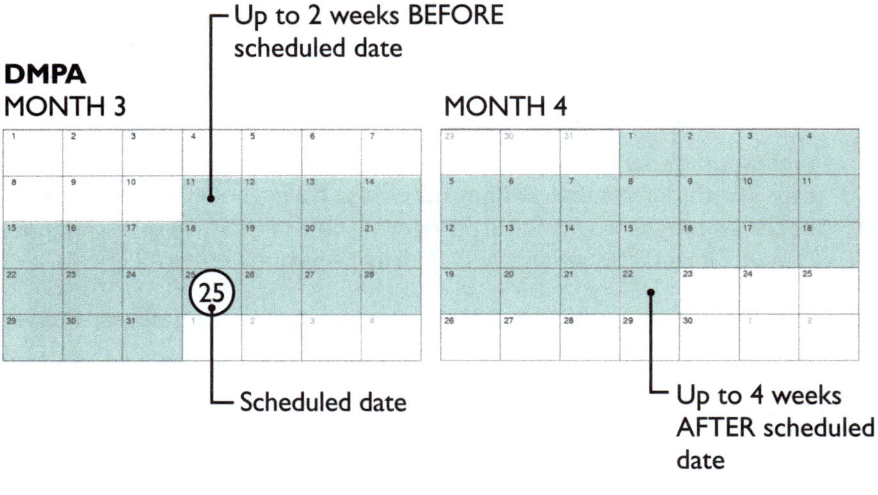

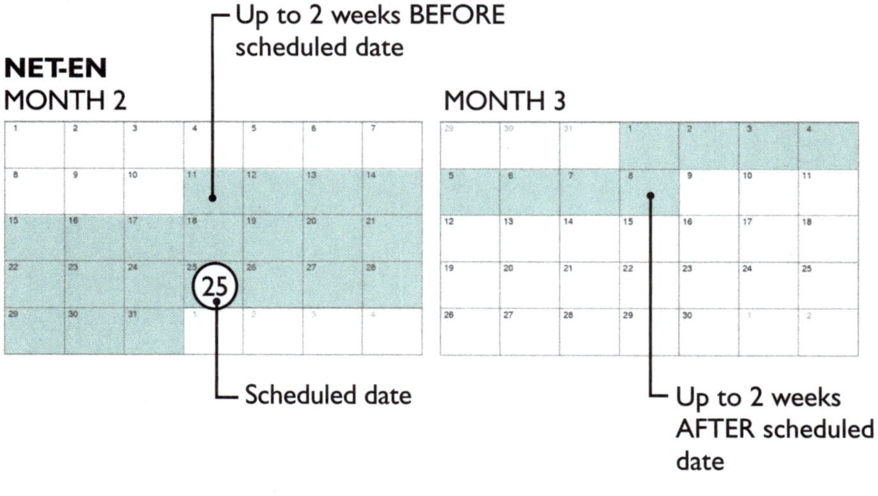

CHAPTER 5

Monthly Injectables

Key Points for Providers and Clients

- **Bleeding changes are common but not harmful.** Typically, lighter monthly bleeding, fewer days of bleeding, or irregular or infrequent bleeding.
- **Return on time.** Coming back every 4 weeks is important for greatest effectiveness.
- **Injection can be as much as 7 days early or late.** Even if later, she may still be able to have the injection.

What Are Monthly Injectables?

- Monthly injectables contain 2 hormones—a progestin and an estrogen—like the natural hormones progesterone and estrogen in a woman's body. (Combined oral contraceptives also contain these 2 types of hormones.)
- Also called combined injectable contraceptives, CICs, the injection.
- Information in this chapter applies to medroxyprogesterone acetate (MPA)/estradiol cypionate and to norethisterone enanthate (NET-EN)/estradiol valerate. The information may also apply to older formulations, about which less is known.
- MPA/estradiol cypionate is marketed under trade names such as Ciclofem, Ciclofemina, Cyclofem, Cyclo-Provera, Feminena, Lunella, Lunelle, and Novafem. NET-EN/estradiol valerate is marketed under trade names such as Mesigyna and Norigynon.
- Work primarily by preventing the release of eggs from the ovaries (ovulation).

How Effective?

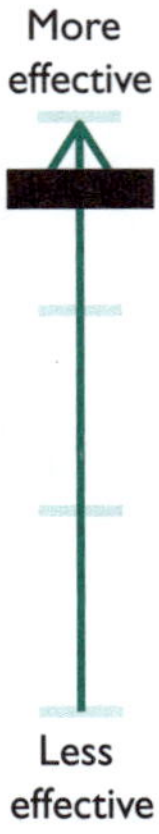

Effectiveness depends on returning on time: Risk of pregnancy is greatest when a woman is late for an injection or misses an injection.

- As commonly used, about 3 pregnancies per 100 women using monthly injectables over the first year. This means that 97 of every 100 women using injectables will not become pregnant.
- When women have injections on time, less than 1 pregnancy per 100 women using monthly injectables over the first year (5 per 10,000 women).

Return of fertility after injections are stopped: An average of about 5 months, one month longer than with most other methods (see Question 11, p. 100).

Protection against sexually transmitted infections (STIs): None

Why Some Women Say They Like Monthly Injectables

- Do not require daily action
- Are private: No one else can tell that a woman is using contraception
- Can be stopped at any time
- Are good for spacing births

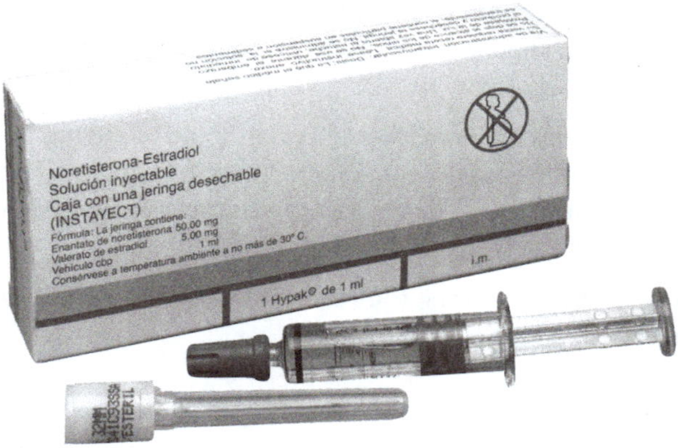

Side Effects, Health Benefits, and Health Risks

Side Effects (see also Managing Any Problems, p. 112)

Some users report the following:

- Changes in bleeding patterns,[†] including:
  - Lighter bleeding and fewer days of bleeding
  - Irregular bleeding
  - Infrequent bleeding
  - Prolonged bleeding
  - No monthly bleeding
- Weight gain
- Headaches
- Dizziness
- Breast tenderness

Bleeding changes are normal and not harmful. If a woman finds them bothersome, counseling and support can help.

Known Health Benefits and Health Risks

Long-term studies of monthly injectables are limited, but researchers expect that their health benefits and health risks are similar to those of combined oral contraceptives (see Combined Oral Contraceptives, Health Benefits and Health Risks, p. 3). There may be some differences in the effects on the liver, however (see Question 2, p. 116).

Correcting Misunderstandings (see also Questions and Answers, p. 116)

Monthly injectables:

- Can stop monthly bleeding, but this is not harmful. It is similar to not having monthly bleeding during pregnancy. Blood is not building up inside the woman.
- Do not make women infertile.
- Do not cause early menopause.
- Do not cause birth defects or multiple births.
- Do not cause itching.
- Do not change women's sexual behavior.

† *For definitions of bleeding patterns, see "vaginal bleeding," p. 407.*

Who Can and Cannot Use Monthly Injectables

Safe and Suitable for Nearly All Women

Nearly all women can use monthly injectables safely and effectively, including women who:

- Have or have not had children
- Are married or are not married
- Are of any age, including adolescents and women over 40 years old
- Have just had an abortion or miscarriage
- Smoke any number of cigarettes daily *and* are under 35 years old
- Smoke fewer than 15 cigarettes daily *and* are over 35 years old
- Have anemia now or had anemia in the past
- Have varicose veins
- Are living with HIV, whether or not on antiretroviral therapy

Avoid Unnecessary Procedures

Women can begin using monthly injectables:

- Without a pelvic examination
- Without any blood tests or other routine laboratory tests
- Without cervical cancer screening
- Without a breast examination
- Without a pregnancy test. A woman can begin using monthly injectables even when she is not having monthly bleeding at the time, if it is reasonably certain she is not pregnant (see Pregnancy Checklist, inside back cover).

Blood pressure measurement is desirable before starting a hormonal method. However, where the risks of pregnancy are high and few methods are available, a woman should not be denied a hormonal method simply because her blood pressure cannot be measured. If possible, she can have her blood pressure measured later at a time and place convenient for her.

Monthly Injectables for Women With HIV

- Women living with HIV or on antiretroviral therapy can safely use monthly injectables.
- Urge these women to use condoms along with monthly injectables. Used consistently and correctly, condoms help prevent transmission of HIV and other STIs.

Medical Eligibility Criteria for

Monthly Injectables

Ask the client the questions below about known medical conditions. Examinations and tests are not necessary. If she answers "no" to all of the questions, then she can start monthly injectables if she wants. If she answers "yes" to a question, follow the instructions. In some cases she can still start monthly injectables.

1. Are you breastfeeding a baby less than 6 months old?

❑ NO ❑ **YES**

- If fully or nearly fully breastfeeding: She can start 6 months after giving birth or when breast milk is no longer the baby's main food—whichever comes first (see Fully or nearly fully breastfeeding, p. 105).
- If partially breastfeeding: She can start monthly injectables as soon as 6 weeks after giving birth (see Partially breastfeeding, p. 106).

2. Have you had a baby in the last 3 weeks and you are not breastfeeding?

❑ NO ❑ **YES** She can start monthly injectables as soon as 3 weeks after childbirth. (If there is an additional risk that she might develop a blood clot in a deep vein [deep vein thrombosis, or VTE], then she should not start monthly injectables at 3 weeks after childbirth, but can start at 6 weeks instead. These additional risk factors include previous VTE, thrombophilia, caesarean delivery, blood transfusion at delivery, postpartum hemorrhage, pre-eclampsia, obesity [>_30 kg/m^2], smoking, and being bedridden for a prolonged time.)

3. Do you smoke 15 or more cigarettes a day?

❑ NO ❑ **YES** If she is 35 years of age or older and smokes more than 15 cigarettes a day, do not provide monthly injectables. Urge her to stop smoking and help her choose another method.

4. Do you have severe liver disease—active hepatitis, severe cirrhosis, or liver tumor?

❑ NO ❑ **YES** If she reports active hepatitis, severe cirrhosis, or liver tumor, do not provide monthly injectables. Help her choose a method without hormones. (If she has mild cirrhosis or gallbladder disease, she can use monthly injectables.)

(Continued on next page)

5. Do you have high blood pressure?

❑ NO ❑ **YES** If you cannot check blood pressure and she reports a history of high blood pressure, or if she is being treated for high blood pressure, do not provide monthly injectables. Refer her for a blood pressure check if possible or help her choose another method without estrogen.

Check her blood pressure if possible:

- If blood pressure is below 140/90 mm Hg, provide monthly injectables.
- If systolic blood pressure is 140 mm Hg or higher or diastolic blood pressure is 90 or higher, do not provide monthly injectables. Help her choose a method without estrogen, but not progestin-only injectables if systolic blood pressure is 160 or higher or diastolic pressure is 100 or higher.

(One blood pressure reading in the range of 140–159/ 90–99 mm Hg is not enough to diagnose high blood pressure. Provide a backup method* to use until she can return for another blood pressure check, or help her choose another method now if she prefers. If blood pressure at next check is below 140/90, she can use monthly injectables.)†

6. Have you had diabetes for more than 20 years or damage to your arteries, vision, kidneys, or nervous system caused by diabetes?

❑ NO ❑ **YES** Do not provide monthly injectables. Help her choose a method without estrogen but not progestin-only injectables.

7. Have you ever had a stroke, blood clot in your leg or lungs, heart attack, or other serious heart problems?

❑ NO ❑ **YES** If she reports heart attack, heart disease due to blocked or narrowed arteries, or stroke, do not provide monthly injectables. Help her choose a method without estrogen but not progestin-only injectables. If she reports a current blood clot in the deep veins of the leg (not a superficial clot) or in the lungs, help her choose a method without hormones.

* *Backup methods include abstinence, male and female condoms, spermicides, and withdrawal. Tell her that spermicides and withdrawal are the least effective contraceptive methods. If possible, give her condoms.*

† *For guidance on routine blood pressure testing, see Chapter 1, Question 18, p. 28.*

8. Do you have or have you ever had breast cancer?

❑ NO ❑ **YES** Do not provide monthly injectables. Help her choose a method without hormones.

9. Do you sometimes see a bright area of lost vision in the eye before a very bad headache (migraine aura)? Do you get throbbing, severe head pain, often on one side of the head, that can last from a few hours to several days and can cause nausea or vomiting (migraine headaches)? Such headaches are often made worse by light, noise, or moving about.

❑ NO ❑ **YES** If she has migraine aura at any age, do not provide monthly injectables. If she has migraine headaches *without* aura *and* is age 35 or older, do not provide monthly injectables. Help these women choose a method without estrogen. If she is under age 35 and has migraine headaches without aura, she can use monthly injectables (see Identifying Migraine Headaches and Auras, p. 436).

10. Are you planning major surgery that will keep you from walking for one week or more?

❑ NO ❑ **YES** If so, she can start monthly injectables 2 weeks after the surgery. Until she can start monthly injectables, she should use a backup method.

11. Do you have several conditions that could increase your chances of heart disease (coronary artery disease) or stroke, such as older age, smoking, high blood pressure, or diabetes?

❑ NO ❑ **YES** Do not provide monthly injectables. Help her choose a method without estrogen, but not progestin-only injectables.

12. Are you taking lamotrigine?

❑ NO ❑ **YES** Do not provide monthly injectables. Monthly injectables can make lamotrigine less effective. Help her choose a method without estrogen.

Also, women should not use monthly injectables if they report having thrombogenic mutations or lupus with positive (or unknown) antiphospholipid antibodies. For complete classifications, see Medical Eligibility Criteria for Contraceptive Use, p. 388.

Be sure to explain the health benefits and risks and the side effects of the method that the client will use. Also, point out any conditions that would make the method inadvisable, when relevant to the client.

Using Clinical Judgment in Special Cases

Usually, a woman with any of the conditions listed below should not use monthly injectables. In special circumstances, however, when other, more appropriate methods are not available or acceptable to her, a qualified provider who can carefully assess a specific woman's condition and situation may decide that she can use monthly injectables. The provider needs to consider the severity of her condition and, for most conditions, whether she will have access to follow-up.

- Not breastfeeding and less than 3 weeks since giving birth, without additional risk that she might develop a blood clot in a deep vein (VTE)
- Not breastfeeding and between 3 and 6 weeks postpartum with additional risk that she might develop VTE
- Primarily breastfeeding between 6 weeks and 6 months since giving birth
- Age 35 or older and smokes more than 15 cigarettes a day
- High blood pressure (systolic blood pressure between 140 and 159 mm Hg or diastolic blood pressure between 90 and 99 mm Hg)
- Controlled high blood pressure, where continuing evaluation is possible
- History of high blood pressure, where blood pressure cannot be taken (including pregnancy-related high blood pressure)
- Severe liver disease, infection, or tumor
- Age 35 or older and has migraine headaches without aura
- Younger than age 35 and has migraine headaches that have developed or have gotten worse while using monthly injectables
- Had breast cancer more than 5 years ago, and it has not returned
- Diabetes for more than 20 years or damage to arteries, vision, kidneys, or nervous system caused by diabetes
- Multiple risk factors for arterial cardiovascular disease, such as older age, smoking, diabetes, and high blood pressure
- Taking lamotrigine. Monthly injectables may reduce the effectiveness of lamotrigine.

Providing Monthly Injectables

When to Start

IMPORTANT: A woman can start injectables any time she wants if it is reasonably certain she is not pregnant. To be reasonably certain she is not pregnant, use the Pregnancy Checklist (see inside back cover).

Woman's situation	When to start
Having menstrual cycles or switching from a nonhormonal method	**Any time of the month** • If she is starting within 7 days after the start of her monthly bleeding, no need for a backup method. • If it is more than 7 days after the start of her monthly bleeding, she can start injectables any time if it is reasonably certain she is not pregnant. She will need a backup method* for the first 7 days after the injection. • If she is switching from an IUD, she can start injectables immediately (see Copper-Bearing IUD, Switching From an IUD to Another Method, p. 172).
Switching from a hormonal method	• Immediately, if she has been using the hormonal method consistently and correctly or if it is otherwise reasonably certain she is not pregnant. No need to wait for her next monthly bleeding. No need for a backup method. • If she is switching from another injectable, she can have the new injectable when the repeat injection would have been given. No need for a backup method.
Fully or nearly fully breastfeeding	
Less than 6 months after giving birth	• Delay her first injection until 6 months after giving birth or when breast milk is no longer the baby's main food—whichever comes first.

* *Backup methods include abstinence, male and female condoms, spermicides, and withdrawal. Tell her that spermicides and withdrawal are the least effective contraceptive methods. If possible, give her condoms.*

Woman's situation	When to start
Fully or nearly fully breastfeeding (continued)	
More than 6 months after giving birth	• If her monthly bleeding has not returned, she can start injectables any time if it is reasonably certain she is not pregnant. She will need a backup method for the first 7 days after the injection. • If her monthly bleeding has returned, she can start injectables as advised for women having menstrual cycles (see p. 105).
Partially breastfeeding	
Less than 6 weeks after giving birth	• Delay her first injection until at least 6 weeks after giving birth.
More than 6 weeks after giving birth	• If her monthly bleeding has not returned, she can start injectables any time if it is reasonably certain she is not pregnant.† She will need a backup method for the first 7 days after the injection. • If her monthly bleeding has returned, she can start injectables as advised for women having menstrual cycles (see p. 105).
Not breastfeeding	
Less than 4 weeks after giving birth	• She can start injectables at any time on days 21–28 after giving birth. No need for a backup method. (If additional risk for VTE, wait until 6 weeks. See p. 101, Question 2.)
More than 4 weeks after giving birth	• If her monthly bleeding has not returned, she can start injectables any time if it is reasonably certain she is not pregnant.† She will need a backup method for the first 7 days after the injection. • If her monthly bleeding has returned, she can start injectables as advised for women having menstrual cycles (see p. 105).

† *Where a visit 6 weeks after childbirth is routinely recommended and other opportunities to obtain contraception are limited, some providers and programs may give the first injection at the 6-week visit, without further evidence that the woman is not pregnant, if her monthly bleeding has not yet returned.*

Woman's situation	When to start
No monthly bleeding (not related to childbirth or breastfeeding)	• She can start injectables any time if it is reasonably certain she is not pregnant. She will need a backup method for the first 7 days after the injection.
After miscarriage or abortion	• Immediately. If she is starting within 7 days after first- or second-trimester miscarriage or abortion, no need for a backup method. • If it is more than 7 days after first- or second-trimester miscarriage or abortion, she can start injectables any time if it is reasonably certain she is not pregnant. She will need a backup method for the first 7 days after the injection.
After taking emergency contraceptive pills (ECPs)	**After taking progestin-only or combined ECPs:** • She can start or restart injectables on the same day as taking the ECPs. There is no need to wait for her next monthly bleeding to have the injection. • She will need to use a backup method for the first 7 days after the injection. • If she does not start immediately, but returns for injectables, she can start at any time if it is reasonably certain she is not pregnant. **After taking ulipristal acetate (UPA) ECPs:** • She can start or restart injectables on the 6th day after taking UPA-ECPs. *No need to wait for her next monthly bleeding.* Monthly injectables and UPA interact. If an injectable is started sooner, and thus both are present in the body, one or both may be less effective. • Make an appointment for her to return for the injection on the 6th day after taking UPA-ECPs, or as soon as possible after that. • She will need to use a backup method from the time she takes UPA-ECPs until 7 days after the injection. • If she does not start on the 6th day but returns later for injectables, she may start at any time if it is reasonably certain she is not pregnant.

Giving Advice on Side Effects

IMPORTANT: Thorough counseling about bleeding changes and other side effects must come before giving the injection. Counseling about bleeding changes may be the most important help a woman needs to keep using the method without concern.

Describe the most common side effects	• Lighter bleeding and fewer days of bleeding, irregular bleeding, and infrequent bleeding. • Weight gain, headaches, dizziness, breast tenderness, and possibly other side effects.
Explain about these side effects	• Side effects are not signs of illness. Lack of bleeding does not mean pregnancy. • Usually become less or stop within the first few months after starting injections. • Common, but some women do not have them. • The client can come back for help if side effects bother her or if she has other concerns.

Giving the Injection

1. Obtain one dose of injectable, needle, and syringe	• 25 mg MPA/estradiol cypionate or 50 mg NET-EN/estradiol valerate, intramuscular injection needle, and 2 ml or 5 ml syringe. (NET-EN/estradiol valerate is sometimes available in prefilled syringes.) • For each injection use a disposable auto-disable syringe and needle from a new sealed package (within expiration date and not damaged), if available.

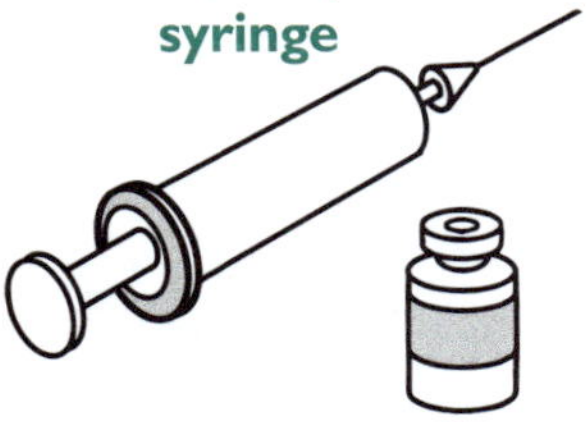

2. Wash	• Wash hands with soap and water, if possible. • If injection site is dirty, wash it with soap and water. • No need to wipe site with antiseptic.

If using a prefilled syringe, skip to step 5.

3. Prepare vial

- MPA/estradiol cypionate: Gently shake the vial.
- NET-EN/estradiol valerate: Shaking the vial is not necessary.
- No need to wipe top of vial with antiseptic.
- If vial is cold, warm to skin temperature before giving the injection.

4. Fill syringe

- Pierce top of vial with sterile needle and fill syringe with proper dose.

5. Inject formula

- Insert sterile needle deep into the hip (ventrogluteal muscle), the upper arm (deltoid muscle), the buttocks (gluteal muscle, upper outer portion), or outer (anterior) thigh, whichever the woman prefers. Inject the contents of the syringe.
- Do not massage injection site.

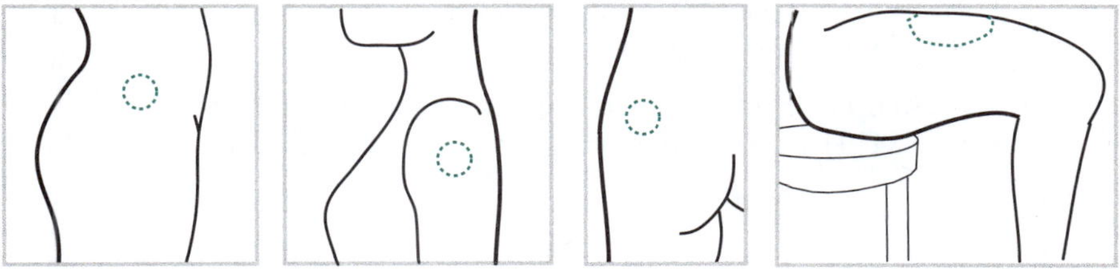

6. Dispose of disposable syringes and needles safely

- Do not recap, bend, or break needles before disposal.
- Place in a puncture-proof sharps container.

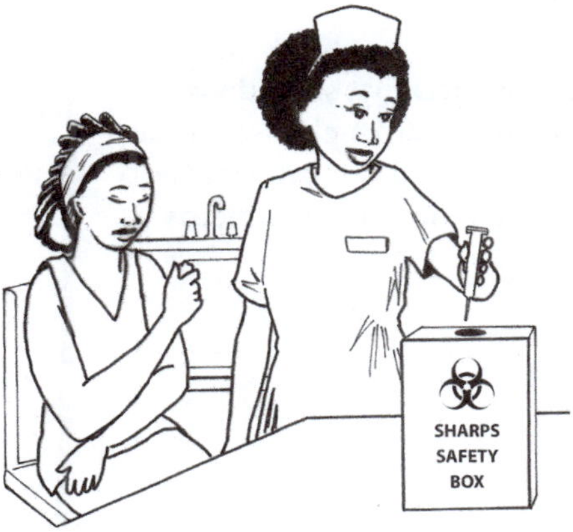

- Do not reuse disposable syringes and needles. They are meant to be destroyed after a single use. Because of their shape, they are very difficult to disinfect. Therefore, reuse might transmit diseases such as HIV and hepatitis.
- If reusable syringe and needle are used, they must be sterilized again after each use (see Infection Prevention in the Clinic, p. 376).

Supporting the User

Give specific instructions	• Tell her not to massage the injection site. • Tell the client the name of the injection and agree on a date for her next injection in about 4 weeks.

How Can a Partner Help?

The client's partner is welcome to participate in counseling and learn about the method and what support he can give to his partner. A male partner can:

- Support a woman's choice of a monthly injectable
- Show understanding and support if she has side effects
- Help her to remember to get her next injection on time
- Help to make sure she has ECPs on hand in case she is more than one week late for injection
- Use condoms consistently in addition to monthly injectables if he has an STI/HIV or thinks he may be at risk of an STI/HIV

"Come Back Any Time": Reasons to Return Before the Next Injection

Assure every client that she is welcome to come back any time—for example, if she has problems, questions, or wants another method; she has a major change in health status; or she thinks she might be pregnant.

General health advice: Anyone who suddenly feels that something is seriously wrong with her health should immediately seek medical care from a nurse or doctor. Her contraceptive method is most likely not the cause of the condition, but she should tell the nurse or doctor what method she is using.

Planning the Next Injection

1. Agree on a date for her next injection in 4 weeks.
2. Ask her to try to come on time. She may come up to 7 days before the scheduled date or 7 days late and still get an injection.
3. She should come back no matter how late she is for her next injection. If more than 7 days late, she should abstain from sex or use condoms, spermicides, or withdrawal until she can get an injection. She can also consider emergency contraceptive pills if she is more than 7 days late and she has had unprotected sex in the past 5 days (see Emergency Contraceptive Pills, p. 49).

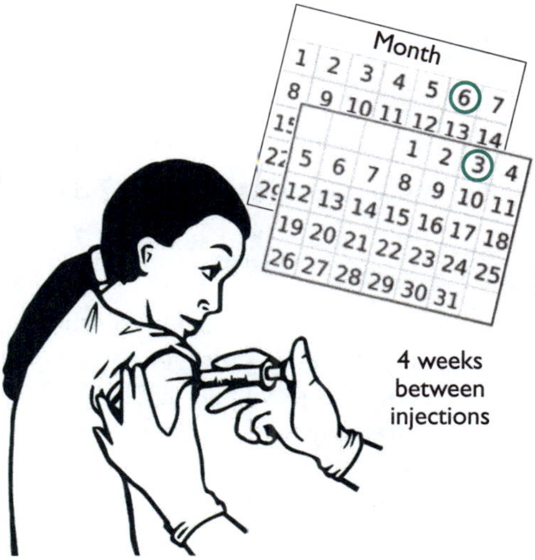

Helping Continuing Users

Repeat Injection Visits

1. Ask how the client is doing with the method and whether she is satisfied. Ask if she has any questions or anything to discuss.
2. Ask especially if she is concerned about bleeding changes. Give her any information or help that she needs (see Managing Any Problems, next page).
3. Give her the injection. Injection can be given up to 7 days early or late.
4. Plan for her next injection. Agree on a date for her next injection (in 4 weeks). Remind her that she should try to come on time, but she should come back no matter how late she is. She may still be able to have her injection.
5. Every year or so, check her blood pressure if possible (see Medical Eligibility Criteria, Question 5, p. 102).
6. Ask a long-term client if she has had any new health problems. Address problems as appropriate. For new health problems that may require switching methods, see p. 114.
7. Ask a long-term client about major life changes that may affect her needs—particularly plans for having children and STI/HIV risk. Follow up as needed.

Managing Late Injections

- If the client is less than 7 days late for a repeat injection, she can receive her next injection. No need for tests, evaluation, or a backup method.
- A client who is more than 7 days late can receive her next injection if:
  - She has not had sex since 7 *days after* the scheduled date of her injection, or
  - She has used a backup method or has taken emergency contraceptive pills (ECPs) after any unprotected sex since 7 *days after* the scheduled date of her injection.
  - She will need a backup method for the first 7 days after the injection.
- If the client is more than 7 days late and does not meet these criteria, additional steps can be taken to be reasonably certain she is not pregnant (see Ruling Out Pregnancy, p. 439).
- Discuss why the client was late and solutions. If coming back on time is often a problem, discuss using a backup method when she is late for her next injection, taking ECPs, or choosing another method.

When a Woman Can Have Her Next Injection of a Monthly Injectable

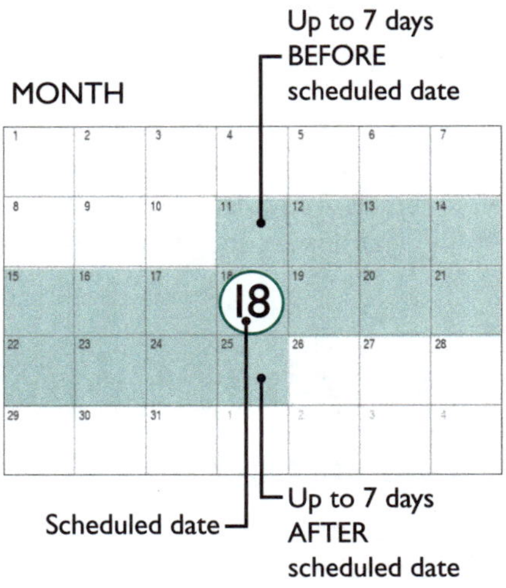

Managing Any Problems

Problems Reported as Side Effects

May or may not be due to the method.

- Problems with side effects affect women's satisfaction and use of injectables. They deserve the provider's attention. If the client reports side effects, listen to her concerns, give her advice and support, and, if appropriate, treat. Make sure she understands the advice and agrees.
- Offer to help the client choose another method—now, if she wishes, or if problems cannot be overcome.

Irregular bleeding (bleeding at unexpected times that bothers the client)

- Reassure her that many women using monthly injectables experience irregular bleeding. It is not harmful and usually becomes less or stops after the first few months of use.
- For modest short-term relief, she can try 800 mg ibuprofen 3 times daily after meals for 5 days, or other nonsteroidal anti-inflammatory drug (NSAID), beginning when irregular bleeding starts. NSAIDs provide some relief of irregular bleeding for implants, progestin-only injectables, and IUDs, and they may also help for monthly injectables.
- If irregular bleeding continues or starts after several months of normal or no monthly bleeding, or you suspect that something may be wrong for other reasons, consider underlying conditions unrelated to method use (see Unexplained vaginal bleeding, next page).

Heavy or prolonged bleeding (twice as much as usual or longer than 8 days)

- Reassure her that many women using monthly injectables experience heavy or prolonged bleeding. It is generally not harmful and usually becomes less or stops after a few months.
- For modest short-term relief, she can try 800 mg ibuprofen 3 times daily after meals for 5 days, or other NSAID, beginning when heavy bleeding starts. NSAIDs provide some relief of heavy bleeding for implants, progestin-only injectables, and IUDs, and they may also help for monthly injectables.
- To help prevent anemia, suggest she take iron tablets and tell her it is important to eat foods containing iron, such as meat and poultry (especially beef and chicken liver), fish, green leafy vegetables, and legumes (beans, bean curd, lentils, and peas).
- If heavy or prolonged bleeding continues or starts after several months of normal or no monthly bleeding, or you suspect that something may be wrong for other reasons, consider underlying conditions unrelated to method use (see Unexplained vaginal bleeding, next page).

No monthly bleeding

- Reassure her that some women using monthly injectables stop having monthly bleeding, and this not harmful. There is no need to lose blood every month. It is similar to not having monthly bleeding during pregnancy. She is not pregnant or infertile. Blood is not building up inside her. (Some women are happy to be free from monthly bleeding.)

Weight gain

- Review diet and counsel as needed.

Ordinary headaches (nonmigrainous)

- Suggest aspirin (325–650 mg), ibuprofen (200–400 mg), paracetamol (325–1000 mg), or other pain reliever.
- Any headaches that get worse or occur more often during use of injectables should be evaluated.

Breast tenderness

- Recommend that she wear a supportive bra (including during strenuous activity and sleep).
- Try hot or cold compresses.
- Suggest aspirin (325–650 mg), ibuprofen (200–400 mg), paracetamol (325–1000 mg), or other pain reliever.
- Consider locally available remedies.

Dizziness

- Consider locally available remedies.

New Problems That May Require Switching Methods

May or may not be due to the method.

Unexplained vaginal bleeding (that suggests a medical condition not related to the method)

- Refer or evaluate by history and pelvic examination. Diagnose and treat as appropriate.
- She can continue using monthly injectables while her condition is being evaluated.
- If bleeding is caused by sexually transmitted infection or pelvic inflammatory disease, she can continue using monthly injectables during treatment.

Migraine headaches (see Identifying Migraine Headaches and Auras, p. 436)

- Regardless of her age, a woman who develops migraine headaches, with or without aura, or whose migraine headaches become worse while using monthly injectables, should stop using injectables.
- Help her choose a method without estrogen.

Circumstances that will keep her from walking for one week or more

- If she is having major surgery, or her leg is in a cast, or for other reasons she will be unable to move about for several weeks, she should:
  - Tell her doctors that she is using monthly injectables.
  - Stop injections one month before scheduled surgery, if possible, and use a backup method during this period.
  - Restart monthly injectables 2 weeks after she can move about again.

Certain serious health conditions (suspected heart or liver disease, high blood pressure (systolic pressure of 140 mm Hg or higher or diastolic pressure of 90 mm Hg or higher), blood clots in deep veins of legs or lungs, stroke, breast cancer, or damage to arteries, vision, kidneys, or nervous system caused by diabetes). See Signs and Symptoms of Serious Health Conditions, p. 384.

- Do not give the next injection.
- Give her a backup method to use until the condition is evaluated.
- Refer for diagnosis and care if not already under care.

Suspected pregnancy

- Assess for pregnancy.
- Stop injections if pregnancy is confirmed.
- There are no known risks to a fetus conceived while a woman is using injectables (see Question 3, p. 116.)

Starting treatment with lamotrigine

- Combined hormonal methods, including monthly injectables, can make lamotrigine less effective. Unless she can use a different medication for seizures than lamotrigine, help her choose a method without estrogen.

Questions and Answers About Monthly Injectables

1. How are monthly injectables different from progestin-only injectables?

The major difference between monthly injectables and the progestin-only injectables DMPA or NET-EN is that the monthly injectables contain an estrogen as well as these progestins, making them a combined method. Also, monthly injectables contain less progestin. These differences result in more regular bleeding and fewer bleeding disturbances than with progestin-only injectables. Monthly injectables require a monthly injection, whereas NET-EN is injected every 2 months and DMPA, every 3 months. (See Comparing Injectables, p. 427.)

2. Do monthly injectables function like combined oral contraceptives?

Largely, yes. Monthly injectables (also called combined injectable contraceptives) are similar to combined oral contraceptives (COCs). There are few long-term studies done on monthly injectables, but researchers assume that most of the findings about COCs also apply to monthly injectables. Monthly injectables, however, do not pass through the liver first because they are not taken by mouth like COCs. Short-term studies have shown that monthly injectables have less effect than COCs on blood pressure, blood clotting, the breakdown of fatty substances (lipid metabolism), and liver function. Long-term studies of the health risks and benefits of monthly injectables are underway.

3. Do monthly injectables cause birth defects? Will the fetus be harmed if a woman accidentally uses monthly injectables while she is pregnant?

No. Good evidence from studies on other hormonal methods shows that hormonal contraception will not cause birth defects and will not otherwise harm the fetus if a woman becomes pregnant while using monthly injectables or accidentally starts injectables when she is already pregnant.

4. Do monthly injectables cause abortion?

No. Research on combined contraceptives finds that they do not disrupt an existing pregnancy. They should not be used to try to cause an abortion. They will not do so.

5. Should the dates for a woman's repeat injections be based on when monthly bleeding starts?

No. Some providers think that the next injection should be given only when the next monthly bleeding begins. Bleeding episodes should not guide the injection schedule, however. A woman should receive the injection every 4 weeks. The timing of injections should not be based on her monthly bleeding.

6. Can monthly injectables be used to bring on monthly bleeding?

No. A woman may experience some vaginal bleeding (a "withdrawal bleed") as a result of an injection, but there is no evidence that giving a woman who has irregular bleeding a single injection of a monthly injectable will cause her monthly bleeding to begin properly about one month later. Also, giving a pregnant woman an injection will not cause an abortion.

7. Can women who smoke use monthly injectables safely?

Women younger than age 35 who smoke any number of cigarettes and women 35 and older who smoke fewer than 15 cigarettes a day can safely use monthly injectables. (In contrast, women 35 and older who smoke any number of cigarettes should not use combined oral contraceptives.) Women age 35 and older who smoke more than 15 cigarettes a day should choose a method without estrogen such as progestin-only injectables, if available. All women who smoke should be urged to stop smoking.

8. Do monthly injectables lower women's mood or sex drive?

Generally, no. Some women using monthly injectables report these complaints. The great majority of injectables users do not report any such changes, however, and some report that both mood and sex drive improve. It is difficult to tell whether such changes are due to monthly injectables or to other reasons. There is no evidence that monthly injectables affect women's sexual behavior.

9. Can women with varicose veins use monthly injectables?

Yes. Monthly injectables are safe for women with varicose veins. Varicose veins are enlarged blood vessels close to the surface of the skin. They are not dangerous. They are not blood clots, nor are these veins the deep veins in the legs where a blood clot can be dangerous (deep vein thrombosis). A woman who has or has had deep vein thrombosis should not use monthly injectables.

10. Do monthly injectables make a woman infertile?

No. There may be a delay in regaining fertility after stopping monthly injectables, but in time the woman will be able to become pregnant as before, although fertility decreases as women get older. The bleeding pattern a woman had before she used monthly injectables generally returns a few months after the last injection.

11. How long does it take to become pregnant after stopping monthly injectables?

Women who stop using monthly injectables wait about one month longer on average to become pregnant than women who have used other methods. This means they become pregnant on average 5 months after their last injection. These are averages. A woman should not be worried if she has not become pregnant even as much as 12 months after stopping use. After stopping monthly injectables, a woman may ovulate before her monthly bleeding returns—and thus can become pregnant. If she wants to continue avoiding pregnancy, she should start another method before monthly bleeding returns.

Combined Patch

Key Points for Providers and Clients

- **A woman wears a small adhesive patch** on her body at all times, day and night. A new patch is put on each week for 3 weeks, and then no patch for the fourth week.
- **Replace each patch on time for greatest effectiveness.**
- **Bleeding changes are common but not harmful.** Typically, irregular bleeding for the first few months and then lighter and more regular bleeding.

What Is the Combined Patch?

- A small, thin, square of flexible plastic worn on the body.
- Continuously releases 2 hormones—a progestin and an estrogen, like the natural hormones progesterone and estrogen in a woman's body—directly through the skin into the bloodstream.
- The woman puts on a new patch every week for 3 weeks, then no patch for the fourth week. During this fourth week the woman will have monthly bleeding.
- Also called Ortho Evra and Evra.
- Works primarily by preventing the release of eggs from the ovaries (ovulation).

How Effective?

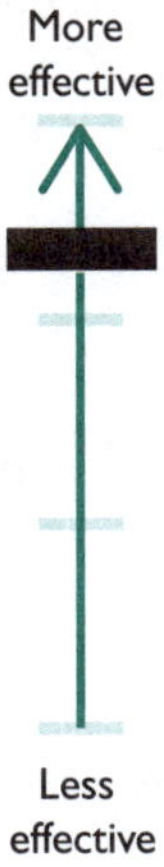

Effectiveness depends on the user: Risk of pregnancy is greatest when a woman is late to change the patch.

- As commonly used, about 7 pregnancies per 100 women using the combined patch over the first year. This means that 93 of every 100 women using the combined patch will not become pregnant.
- When no mistakes are made with use of the patch, less than 1 pregnancy per 100 women using a patch over the first year (3 per 1,000 women).

- Pregnancy rates may be slightly higher among women weighing 90 kg or more.

Return of fertility after patch use is stopped: No delay

Protection against sexually transmitted infections: None

Side Effects, Health Benefits, and Health Risks

Side Effects

Some users report the following:

- Skin irritation or rash where the patch is applied
- Changes in bleeding patterns[†]:
  - Lighter bleeding and fewer days of bleeding
  - Irregular bleeding
  - Prolonged bleeding
  - No monthly bleeding
- Headaches
- Nausea
- Vomiting
- Breast tenderness and pain
- Abdominal pain
- Flu symptoms/upper respiratory infection
- Irritation, redness, or inflammation of the vagina (vaginitis)

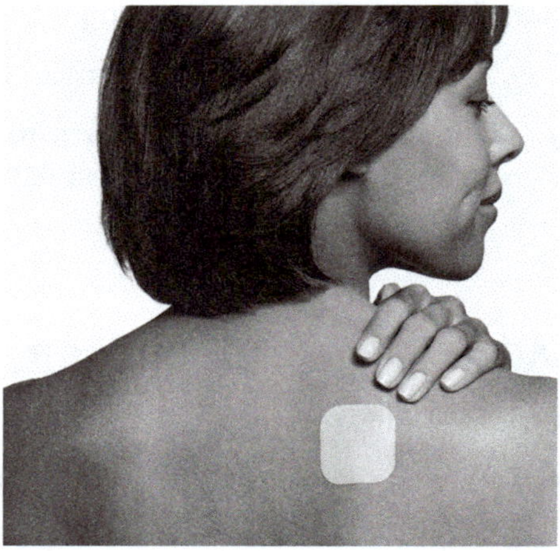

Known Health Benefits and Health Risks

Long-term studies of the patch are limited, but researchers expect that its health benefits and risks are like those of combined oral contraceptives (see Combined Oral Contraceptives, Side Effects, Health Benefits, and Health Risks, p. 3).

> Medical eligibility criteria guidelines for when to start and helping continuing users for the combined patch are the same as for combined oral contraceptives and the combined vaginal ring. See Chapter 1, Combined Oral Contraceptives, pp. 6, 11, and 19.

† *For definitions of bleeding patterns, see "vaginal bleeding," p. 407.*

Providing the Combined Patch

Explaining How to Use

Explain how to remove the patch from the pouch and remove backing	• Explain to the user that she should tear the foil pouch along the edge. • She should then pull out the patch and peel away the backing without touching the sticky surface.
Show her where and how to apply the patch	• Explain that she can apply it on the upper outer arm, back, stomach, abdomen, or buttocks, wherever it is clean and dry, but not on the breasts. • She must press the sticky, medicated part against her skin for 10 seconds. She should run her finger along the edge to make sure it sticks. • The patch will stay on even during work, exercise, swimming, and bathing.
She must change the patch every week for 3 weeks in a row	• She should apply each new patch on the same day of each week—the "patch-change day." For example, if she puts on her first patch on a Sunday, all of her patches should be applied on a Sunday. • Explain that to avoid irritation, she should not apply the new patch to the same place on the skin where the previous patch was.
She should not wear a patch on the fourth week	• She will probably have monthly bleeding this week.
After the patch-free week, she should apply a new patch	• She should never go without wearing a patch for more than 7 days. Doing so risks pregnancy.

Supporting the User

Instructions for Late Replacement or Removal, or if the Patch Comes Off

Forgot to apply a new patch after the 7-day patch-free interval?	• Apply a new patch as soon as possible. • Keep the same patch-change day. • If late by only 1 or 2 days (48 hours or less), there is no need for a backup method.

(Continued on next page)

Forgot to apply a new patch after the 7-day patch-free interval? (continued)	• If more than 2 days late (more than 48 hours) (that is, no patch was worn for 10 days or more in a row), use a backup method* for the first 7 days of patch use. • Also, if more than 2 days late and unprotected sex occurred in the past 5 days, consider taking emergency contraceptive pills (see Emergency Contraceptive Pills, p. 49).
Late changing the patch at the end of week 1 or 2?	• If late by only 1 or 2 days (48 hours or less), apply a new patch as soon as possible. Keep the same patch-change day. No need for a backup method. • If more than 2 days late (more than 48 hours), apply a new patch as soon as possible. This patch will begin a new 4-week patch cycle, and this day of the week will become the new patch-change day. Also use a backup method for the next 7 days. • Also, if more than 2 days late and unprotected sex occurred in the past 5 days, consider taking emergency contraceptive pills (see Emergency Contraceptive Pills, p. 49).
Late taking off the patch at the end of week 3?	• Remove the patch. • Start the next cycle on the usual patch-change day. • No need for a backup method.
The patch came off and was off for less than 2 days (48 hours or less)**?**	• Apply a new patch as soon as possible. (The same patch can be re-used if it was off less than 24 hours.) • No need for a backup method. • Keep the same patch change day.
The patch came off and was off for more than 2 days (more than 48 hours)?	• Apply a new patch as soon as possible. • Use a backup method* for the next 7 days. • Keep the same patch-change day. • If during week 3, skip the patch-free week and start a new patch immediately after week 3. If a new patch cannot be started immediately, use a backup method* and keep using it through the first 7 days of patch use. • If during week one and unprotected sex occurred in the past 5 days, consider taking emergency contraceptive pills (see Emergency Contraceptive Pills, p. 49).

* *Backup methods include abstinence, male and female condoms, spermicides, and withdrawal. Tell her that spermicides and withdrawal are the least effective contraceptive methods. If possible, give her condoms.*

Combined Vaginal Ring

Key Points for Providers and Clients

- **A woman places a flexible ring in her vagina.** She leaves it there at all times, every day and night for 3 weeks. Then, she removes the ring. Seven days later she inserts a new ring.
- **Start each new ring on time for greatest effectiveness.**
- **Bleeding changes are common but not harmful.** Typically, irregular bleeding for the first few months and then lighter and more regular bleeding.

What Is the Combined Vaginal Ring?

- A flexible ring that a woman places in her vagina.
- Continuously releases 2 hormones—a progestin and an estrogen, like the natural hormones progesterone and estrogen in a woman's body—from inside the ring. Hormones are absorbed through the wall of the vagina directly into the bloodstream.
- She leaves the ring in place for 3 weeks, then removes it for the fourth week. During this fourth week the woman will have monthly bleeding.
- Also called NuvaRing.
- Works primarily by preventing the release of eggs from the ovaries (ovulation).

How Effective?

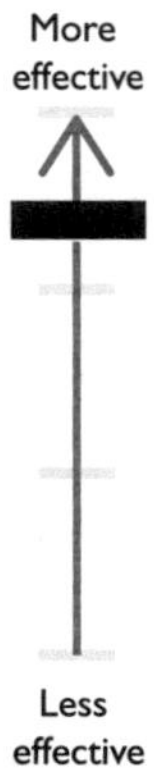

Effectiveness depends on the user: Risk of pregnancy is greatest when a woman is late to start a new ring.

- As commonly used, about 7 pregnancies per 100 women using the combined vaginal ring over the first year. This means that 93 of every 100 women using the combined vaginal ring will not become pregnant.
- When no mistakes are made with use of the combined vaginal ring, less than 1 pregnancy per 100 women using the combined vaginal ring over the first year (3 per 1,000 women).

Return of fertility after ring use is stopped: No delay

Protection against sexually transmitted infections: None

Side Effects, Health Benefits, and Health Risks

Side Effects

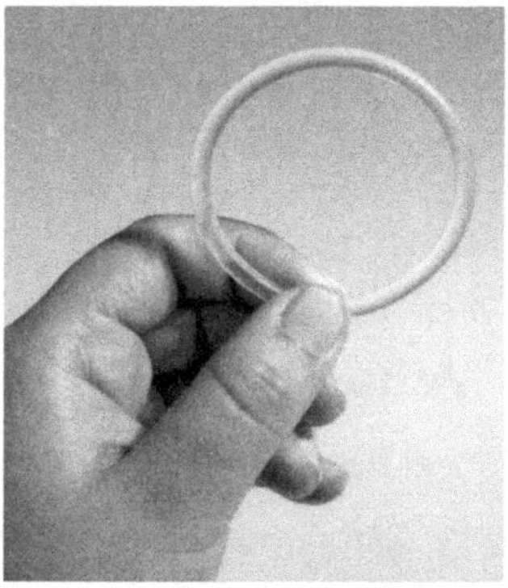

Some users report the following:

- Changes in bleeding patterns,[†] including:
  - Lighter bleeding and fewer days of bleeding
  - Irregular bleeding
  - Infrequent bleeding
  - Prolonged bleeding
  - No monthly bleeding
- Headaches
- Irritation, redness, or inflammation of the vagina (vaginitis)
- White vaginal discharge

Known Health Benefits and Health Risks

Long-term studies of the vaginal ring are limited, but researchers expect that its health benefits and risks are like those of combined oral contraceptives (see Combined Oral Contraceptives, Side Effects, Health Benefits, and Health Risks, p. 3). Evidence to date has not shown adverse effects.

> Medical eligibility criteria, guidelines for when to start, and helping continuing users for the combined ring are the same as for combined oral contraceptives and the combined patch. See Chapter 1, Combined Oral Contraceptives, pp. 6, 11, and 19.

† *For definitions of bleeding patterns, see "vaginal bleeding," p. 407.*

Providing the Combined Vaginal Ring

Explaining How to Use

Explain how to insert the ring

- The user can choose the position most comfortable for her—for example, standing with one leg up, squatting, or lying down.
- She should press opposite sides of the ring together and gently push the folded ring entirely inside the vagina.
- The exact position is not important, but inserting it deeply helps it to stay in place, and she is less likely to feel it. The muscles of the vagina naturally keep the ring in place.

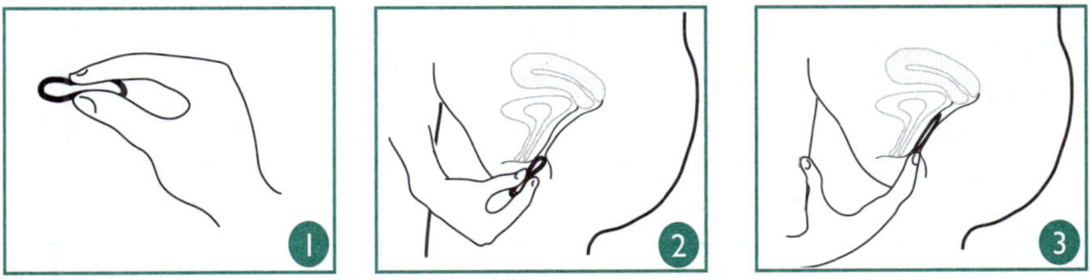

Explain that the ring must be left in place for 3 weeks

- She should leave the ring in place at all times, every day and night for 3 weeks.
- She can take the ring out at the end of the third week and dispose of it in a waste receptacle.

She should take out the ring for the fourth week

- To remove the ring, she can hook her index finger inside it, or squeeze the ring between her index and middle fingers, and pull it out.
- She will probably have monthly bleeding this week.
- If she forgets and leaves the ring in for as long as a fourth week, no special action is needed.

Ring should never be left out for more than 48 hours until the fourth week

- The ring can be removed for sex, cleaning, or other reasons, although removing it is not necessary and is not recommended because some women forget to put it back within 48 hours.
- If the ring slips out, she should rinse it in clean water and immediately reinsert it.

Supporting the User

Instructions for Late Replacement or Removal

Left ring out for 48 hours or less during weeks 1 through 3?	• Put the ring back in as soon as possible. • No need for a backup method.
Left ring out for more than 48 hours during weeks 1 or 2?	• Put the ring back in as soon as possible. • Use a backup method* for the next 7 days. • If the ring was left out for more than 48 hours in the first week and unprotected sex occurred in the previous 5 days, consider taking emergency contraceptive pills (see Emergency Contraceptive Pills, p. 49).
Left ring out for more than 48 hours during week 3?	• Put the ring back in as soon as possible. • Use a backup method* for the next 7 days. • Start a new ring at the end of the third week and skip the ring-free week. If unable to start the new ring at the end of the third week, use a backup method and keep using it through the first 7 days after starting a new ring.
Forgot to insert a new ring at beginning of the cycle?	• Insert a new ring as soon as possible. If late by only 1 or 2 days (48 hours or less)—that is, the ring is left out no longer than 9 days in a row—no need for a backup method. • Keep the same ring removal day. • If the new ring is inserted more than 2 days (more than 48 hours) late—that is, the ring is left out 10 days or more in a row—use a backup method for the first 7 days of ring use. • Also, if unprotected sex occurred in the past 5 days, consider taking emergency contraceptive pills (see Emergency Contraceptive Pills, p. 49).
Kept ring in longer than 3 weeks?	• If the same ring is used for up to 28 days (4 weeks), no backup method is needed. She can take a ring-free week or start a new ring immediately. • If the same ring is used for 28 to 35 days (more than 4 weeks but less than 5 weeks), insert a new ring and skip the ring-free week. No backup method is needed.

* *Backup methods include abstinence, male and female condoms, spermicides, and withdrawal. Tell her that spermicides and withdrawal are the least effective contraceptive methods. If possible, give her condoms.*

Progesterone-Releasing Vaginal Ring

Key Points for Providers and Clients

- **Suitable for postpartum women who are actively breastfeeding, at least 4 times per day.**
- **A woman places a flexible ring in her vagina.** She leaves it in place at all times, every day and night for 90 days. Four rings can be used, one after another, for approximately one year after giving birth.
- **Start each new ring immediately after removal of the previous ring for greatest effectiveness.**
- **Easy for a woman to insert and remove from her vagina.** If her reproductive plans change, she can take out the ring at any time without a provider's help.

What Is the Progesterone-Releasing Vaginal Ring?

- A smooth, soft, flexible silicone ring placed in the vagina to prolong lactational amenorrhea (postponing the return of monthly bleeding) and help breastfeeding women space pregnancies.
- Continuously releases natural progesterone hormone—like that in a woman's body—from inside the ring. The hormone passes through the wall of the vagina directly into the bloodstream. This ring does not contain estrogen.

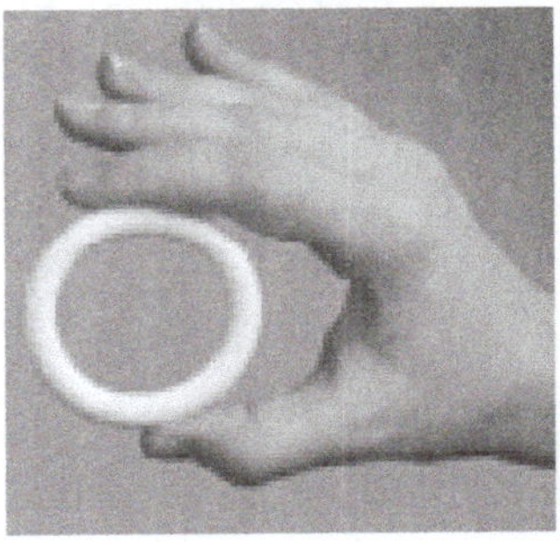

- Use of the ring starts 4 to 9 weeks after giving birth. Each ring is kept in place for 90 days. The woman can then replace it with a new ring immediately. Up to 4 rings can be used, one after another, with no breaks.

- Works by preventing release of an egg from the ovaries (ovulation). Progesterone extends the postpartum amenorrhea of the breastfeeding woman. That is, it delays the return of monthly bleeding.
- Safe and effective option for a woman:
  - Who has a baby at least 4 weeks old
  - Who is breastfeeding her baby at least 4 times per day and plans to continue breastfeeding
  - Whose monthly bleeding has not returned

How Effective?

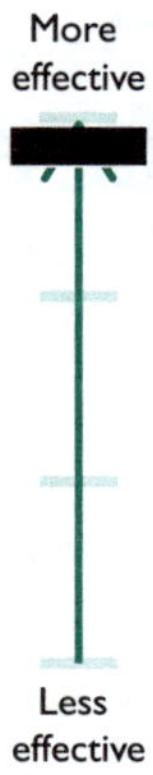

One or 2 pregnancies per 100 women using the progesterone-releasing vaginal ring for a year.

- *Return of fertility after use is stopped:* No delay
- *Protection against sexually transmitted infections:* None

Side Effects, Health Benefits, and Health Risks

Side Effects

Some users report the following:

- Spotting or irregular bleeding
- Low abdominal pain
- Breast pain
- Vaginal discharge

Known Health Benefits and Health Risks

- No change in breast milk production or composition; the method supports continued breastfeeding and healthy infant nutrition.
- Safe and effective, based on several 1-year studies. Its health risks may be like those of progestin-only pills (see Progestin-Only Pills, Side Effects, Health Benefits, and Health Risks, p. 31).
- Women who are actively breastfeeding and are at least 4 weeks postpartum can safely use the progesterone-releasing vaginal ring (MEC Category 1).

Providing the Progesterone-Releasing Vaginal Ring

Explain How to Use

Explain how to insert the ring

- The user can choose the position most comfortable for her—for example, standing with one leg up, squatting, or lying down.
- She should press opposite sides of the ring together and, with her index finger, gently push the ring entirely inside the vagina as far as she can (see picture 1). It can help to push down with the muscles of the vagina while inserting the ring.

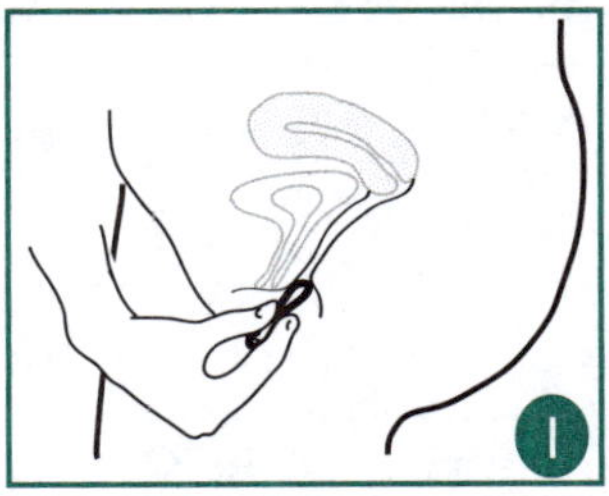

- The exact position of the ring in the vagina is not important, but inserting it deeply helps it to stay in place (see picture 2), and the user is less likely to feel it. The muscles of the vagina naturally keep the ring in place.

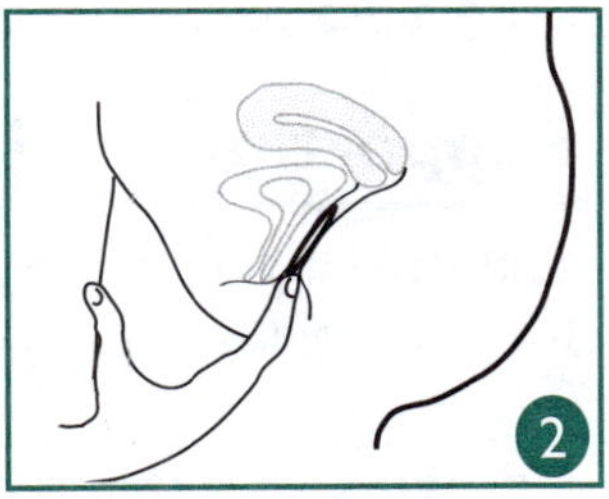

- She should not feel the ring after she places it into her vagina. If she feels the ring in her vagina, she has a sensation of it slipping, or it feels uncomfortable, she may not have pushed it back into her vagina far enough. Instruct her to use a clean finger to gently push the ring as far as she can into her vagina. There is no danger of the ring being pushed too far up in the vagina, breaking during insertion, or getting lost.

(Continued on next page)

Explain that the ring must be left in for 90 days	• She should keep the ring in place at all times to maintain effectiveness. • To continue avoiding pregnancy, the user can take the ring out at the end of the 90 days and replace it immediately with a new ring. She can use 4 rings, for up to one year of use in the postpartum period. • The ring can be disposed of in a waste receptacle. Disposing of the ring in a flush toilet is not recommended.
The ring should never be left out for more than 2 hours	• The ring should be left in place always. Some women may remove the ring for sex or for cleaning, but this is not necessary and not recommended because some women forget to put it back within 2 hours. • If the ring slips out completely, she should rinse it in clean water and immediately put it back in place.
Explain that her partner may be able to feel the ring	• This generally does not interfere with sex or decrease sexual pleasure.

Supporting the User: What to Do if You…

Left the ring out for more than 2 hours	• Put the ring back in the vagina as soon as possible. Contact your health care provider to discuss any concerns.
Left the ring out for more than 24 hours	• Put the ring back in as soon as possible. Use a condom if you have sex in the next 48 hours. Contact your health care provider to discuss any concerns.
Feel the ring slipping	• Use a clean finger to push the ring up as far into the vagina as possible.
After one year of use or if no longer breastfeeding at least 4 times per day	• For longer birth spacing, she can plan ahead to switch to another family planning method. At least 2 years between giving birth and the next pregnancy is healthy for both mother and child.

CHAPTER 9

Implants

Key Points for Providers and Clients

- **Implants are small flexible rods** that are placed just under the skin of the upper arm.
- **Provide long-term pregnancy protection.** Very effective for 3 to 5 years, depending on the type of implant. Immediately reversible.
- **Require specifically trained provider to insert and remove.** A woman cannot start or stop implants on her own.
- **Little required of the client once implants are in place.** Avoids user errors and problems with resupply.
- **Bleeding changes are common but not harmful.** Typically, prolonged irregular bleeding over the first year, and then lighter, more regular bleeding, infrequent bleeding, or no bleeding.

What Are Implants?

- Small plastic rods, each about the size of a matchstick, that release a progestin like the natural hormone progesterone in a woman's body.
- A specifically trained provider performs a minor surgical procedure to place one or 2 rods under the skin on the inside of a woman's upper arm.
- Do not contain estrogen, and so can be used throughout breastfeeding and by women who cannot use methods with estrogen.
- Types of implants:
  - Jadelle: 2 rods containing levonorgestrel, highly effective for 5 years
  - Implanon NXT (Nexplanon): 1 rod containing etonogestrel, labeled for up to 3 years of use (a recent study shows it may be highly effective for 5 years). Replaces Implanon; Implanon NXT can be seen on X-ray and has an improved insertion device.
  - Levoplant (Sino-Implant (II)), 2 rods containing levonorgestrel. Labeled for up to 4 years of use.

- Norplant, which consisted of 6 capsules and was effective for 5–7 years, was discontinued in 2008 and is no longer available for insertion. A small number of women, however, may still need Norplant capsules removed.

- Work primarily by:
  - Preventing the release of eggs from the ovaries (ovulation)
  - Thickening cervical mucus (this blocks sperm from reaching an egg)

How Effective?

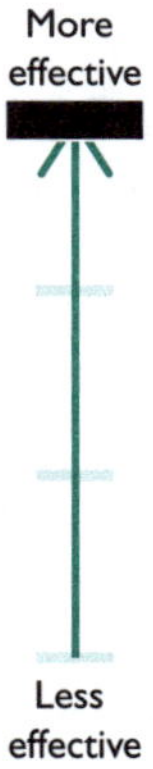

One of the most effective and long-lasting methods:

- Far less than 1 pregnancy per 100 women using implants over the first year (1 per 1,000 women). This means that 999 of every 1,000 women using implants will not become pregnant. Less than 1 pregnancy per 100 women over the duration of use.
- A small risk of pregnancy remains beyond the first year of use and continues as long as the woman is using implants.
- For heavier women, the effectiveness of Jadelle and Levoplant may decrease near the end of the duration of use stated on the label. These users may want to replace their implants sooner (see Question 9, p. 153).

Return of fertility after implants are removed: No delay

Protection against sexually transmitted infections (STIs): None

Why Some Women Say They Like Implants

- Do not require the user to do anything once they are inserted
- Prevent pregnancy very effectively
- Are both long-lasting and reversible
- Do not interfere with sex

Side Effects, Health Benefits, Health Risks, and Complications

Side Effects (see also Managing Any Problems, p. 146)

Some users report the following:

- Changes in bleeding patterns,[†] including:

  First several months to a year:
  - Lighter bleeding and fewer days of bleeding
  - Prolonged bleeding
  - Irregular bleeding
  - Infrequent bleeding
  - No monthly bleeding

  After about one year:
  - Lighter bleeding and fewer days of bleeding
  - Irregular bleeding
  - Infrequent bleeding
  - No monthly bleeding

- Users of Implanon and Implanon NXT are more likely to have infrequent bleeding, prolonged bleeding, or no monthly bleeding than irregular bleeding.
- Headaches
- Abdominal pain
- Acne (can improve or worsen)
- Weight change
- Breast tenderness
- Dizziness
- Mood changes
- Nausea

> Bleeding changes are normal and not harmful. If a woman finds them bothersome, counseling and support can help.

Other possible physical changes:

- Enlarged ovarian follicles

[†] *For definitions of bleeding patterns, see "vaginal bleeding," page 407.*

Known Health Benefits

Help protect against:

- Risks of pregnancy, including ectopic pregnancy
- Symptomatic pelvic inflammatory disease

May help protect against:

- Iron-deficiency anemia

Reduces:

- Risk of ectopic pregnancy

Known Health Risks

None

Complications

Uncommon:

- Infection at insertion site (most infections occur within the first 2 months after insertion)
- Difficult removal (rare if properly inserted and the provider is skilled at removal)

Rare:

- Expulsion of implant (expulsions most often occur within the first 4 months after insertion)

Extremely rare:

- There are a few reports of implants found in another place in the body due to improper insertion, for example, in a blood vessel.

Correcting Misunderstandings (see also Questions and Answers, p.152)

Implants:

- Do not work once they are removed. Their hormones do not remain in a woman's body.
- Do not cause any harm if they stop monthly bleeding. This is similar to not having monthly bleeding during pregnancy. Blood is not building up inside the woman.
- Do not make women infertile.
- Do not increase the risk of ectopic pregnancy (see Question 7, p.153).

Who Can and Cannot Use Implants

Safe and Suitable for Nearly All Women

Nearly all women can use implants safely and effectively, including women who:

- Have or have not had children
- Are married or are not married
- Are of any age, including adolescents and women over 40 years old (see Question 13, p. 154)
- Have just had an abortion, miscarriage, or ectopic pregnancy
- Smoke cigarettes, regardless of woman's age or number of cigarettes smoked
- Are breastfeeding
- Have anemia now or in the past
- Have varicose veins
- Are living with HIV, whether or not on antiretroviral therapy (see Implants for Women With HIV, p. 137)

Avoid Unnecessary Procedures

(see Importance of Procedures, p. 368)

Women can begin using implants:

- Without a pelvic examination
- Without any blood tests or other routine laboratory tests
- Without cervical cancer screening
- Without a breast examination
- Without a pregnancy test. A woman can have implants inserted at any time, even when she is not having monthly bleeding, if it is reasonably certain she is not pregnant (see Pregnancy Checklist, inside back cover).

Blood pressure measurement is desirable before starting a hormonal method. However, where the risks of pregnancy are high and few methods are available, a woman should not be denied a hormonal method simply because her blood pressure cannot be measured. If possible, she can have her blood pressure measured later at a time and place convenient for her.

Medical Eligibility Criteria for

Implants

Ask the client the questions below about known medical conditions. Examinations and tests are not necessary. If she answers "no" to all of the questions, then she can have implants inserted if she wants. If she answers "yes" to a question, follow the instructions. In some cases she can still start using implants.

1. Do you have severe cirrhosis of the liver or a severe liver tumor?

❑ NO ❑ **YES** If she reports severe cirrhosis or severe liver tumor, such as liver cancer, do not provide implants. Help her choose a method without hormones.

2. Do you have a serious problem now with a blood clot in your leg or lungs?

❑ NO ❑ **YES** If she reports a current blood clot in legs (affecting deep veins, not superficial veins) or in a lung and she is not on anticoagulant therapy, do not provide implants. Help her choose a method without hormones.

3. Are you having vaginal bleeding that is unusual for you?

❑ NO ❑ **YES** If she has unexplained vaginal bleeding that suggests pregnancy or an underlying medical condition, implants could make diagnosis and monitoring of any treatment more difficult. Help her choose a method to use until the condition is evaluated (not progestin-only injectables or a copper-bearing or LNG-IUD). After evaluation, reconsider the use of implants.

4. Do you have or have you ever had breast cancer?

❑ NO ❑ **YES** Do not provide implants. Help her choose a method without hormones.

Also, women should not use implants if they report having lupus with positive (or unknown) antiphospholipid antibodies and are not on immunosuppressive therapy. For complete classifications, see Medical Eligibility Criteria for Contraceptive Use, p. 388.

Be sure to explain the health benefits and risks and the side effects of the method that the client will use. Also, point out any conditions that would make the method inadvisable, when relevant to the client.

Using Clinical Judgment in Special Cases

Usually, a woman with any of the conditions listed below should not use implants. In special circumstances, however, when other, more appropriate methods are not available or acceptable to her, a qualified provider who can carefully assess a specific woman's condition and situation may decide that she can use implants. The provider needs to consider the severity of her condition and, for most conditions, whether she will have access to follow-up.

- Acute blood clot in deep veins of legs or lungs
- Unexplained vaginal bleeding before evaluation for possible serious underlying condition
- Had breast cancer more than 5 years ago, and it has not returned
- Severe cirrhosis of the liver or liver tumor
- Systemic lupus erythematosus with positive (or unknown) antiphospholipid antibodies, and not on immunosuppressive therapy

Implants for Women With HIV

- Women who are living with HIV or are on antiretroviral (ARV) therapy can safely use implants.
- Efavirenz may reduce the effectiveness of implants. Urge women taking this ARV to use condoms along with implants to provide better protection from pregnancy. (See Question 14, p. 154.)

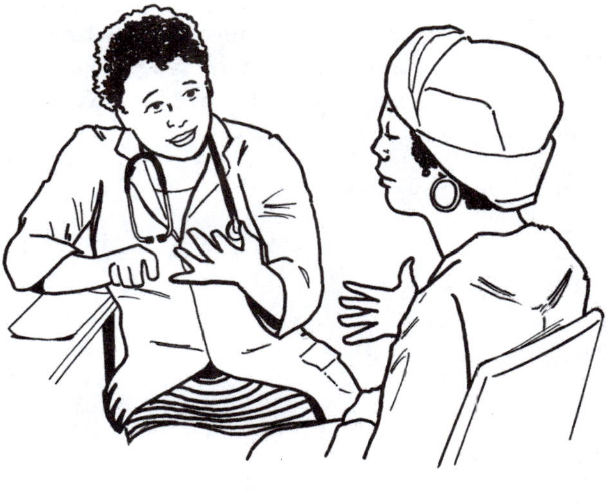

Providing Implants

When to Start

IMPORTANT: A woman can start using implants any time she wants if it is reasonably certain she is not pregnant. To be reasonably certain she is not pregnant, use the Pregnancy Checklist (see inside back cover). No tests or examinations are necessary before starting implants, although blood pressure measurement is desirable.

Woman's situation	When to start
Having menstrual cycles or switching from a nonhormonal method	**Any time of the month** • If she is starting within 7 days after the start of her monthly bleeding, no need for a backup method. • If it is more than 7 days after the start of her monthly bleeding, she can have implants inserted any time if it is reasonably certain she is not pregnant. She will need a backup method* for the first 7 days after insertion. • If she is switching from an IUD, also see Copper-Bearing IUD, Switching From an IUD to Another Method, p. 172.
Switching from another hormonal method	• Immediately, if she has been using the hormonal method consistently and correctly or if it is otherwise reasonably certain she is not pregnant. No need to wait for her next monthly bleeding. No need for a backup method. • If she is switching from a progestin-only or monthly injectable, she can have implants inserted when the repeat injection would have been given. No need for a backup method.

* *Backup methods include abstinence, male and female condoms, spermicides, and withdrawal. Tell her that spermicides and withdrawal are the least effective contraceptive methods. If possible, give her condoms.*

Woman's situation	When to start
Fully or nearly fully breastfeeding	
Less than 6 months after giving birth	• If her monthly bleeding has not returned, she can have implants inserted any time between giving birth and 6 months. No need for a backup method. • If her monthly bleeding has returned, she can have implants inserted as advised for women having menstrual cycles (see previous page).
More than 6 months after giving birth	• If her monthly bleeding has not returned, she can have implants inserted any time if it is reasonably certain she is not pregnant. She will need a backup method for the first 7 days after insertion. • If her monthly bleeding has returned, she can have implants inserted as advised for women having menstrual cycles (see previous page).
Partially breastfeeding	
If her monthly bleeding has not returned	• She can have implants inserted any time if it is reasonably certain she is not pregnant.† She will need a backup method for the first 7 days after insertion.
If her monthly bleeding has returned	• If her monthly bleeding has returned, she can have implants inserted as advised for women having menstrual cycles (see previous page).
Not breastfeeding	
Less than 4 weeks after giving birth	• She can have implants inserted at any time. No need for a backup method.

† *Where a visit 6 weeks after childbirth is routinely recommended and other opportunities to obtain contraception are limited, some providers and programs may insert implants at the 6-week visit, without further evidence that the woman is not pregnant, if her monthly bleeding has not yet returned.*

Woman's situation	When to start
Not breastfeeding (continued)	
More than 4 weeks after giving birth	• If her monthly bleeding has not returned, she can have implants inserted any time if it is reasonably certain she is not pregnant.† She will need a backup method for the first 7 days after insertion. • If her monthly bleeding has returned, she can have implants inserted as advised for women having menstrual cycles (see p. 138).
No monthly bleeding (not related to childbirth or breastfeeding)	• She can have implants inserted any time if it is reasonably certain she is not pregnant. She will need a backup method for the first 7 days after insertion.
After miscarriage or abortion	• Immediately. If implants are inserted within 7 days after first- or second-trimester miscarriage or abortion, no need for a backup method. • If it is more than 7 days after first- or second-trimester miscarriage or abortion, she can have implants inserted any time if it is reasonably certain she is not pregnant. She will need a backup method for the first 7 days after insertion.
After taking emergency contraceptive pills (ECPs)	**After taking progestin-only or combined ECPs:** • Implants can be inserted on the same day as she takes the ECPs. – She will need to use a backup method for the first 7 days. • If she does not start immediately, but returns for an implant, she can start at any time if it is reasonably certain she is not pregnant. **After taking ulipristal acetate ECPs:** • Implants can be inserted on the 6th day after taking UPA-ECPs. No need to wait for her next monthly bleeding. Implants and UPA interact. If an implant is inserted sooner, and thus both are present in the body, one or both may be less effective.

† *Where a visit 6 weeks after childbirth is routinely recommended and other opportunities to obtain contraception are limited, some providers and programs may insert implants at the 6-week visit, without further evidence that the woman is not pregnant, if her monthly bleeding has not yet returned.*

Woman's situation	When to start
After taking emergency contraceptive pills (ECPs) (continued)	• Make an appointment for her to return on the 6th day to have the implant inserted, or as soon as possible after that. • She will need to use a backup method from the time she takes UPA-ECPs until 7 days after the implant is inserted. • If she does not start on the 6th day but returns later for implants, she can start at any time if it is reasonably certain she is not pregnant.

Giving Advice on Side Effects

IMPORTANT: Thorough counseling about bleeding changes and other side effects must come before inserting implants. Counseling about bleeding changes may be the most important help a woman needs to keep using the method without concern.

Describe the most common side effects	• Changes in her bleeding pattern: – Irregular bleeding that lasts more than 8 days at a time over the first year. – Later, regular, infrequent, or no bleeding at all. • Headaches, abdominal pain, breast tenderness, and possibly other side effects.
Explain about these side effects	• Side effects are not signs of illness. Lack of bleeding does not mean pregnancy. • Most side effects usually become less or stop within the first year. • Common, but some women do not have them. • Client can come back for help if side effects bother her or if she has other concerns.

Inserting Implants

Explaining the Insertion Procedure

A woman who has chosen implants needs to know what will happen during insertion. The following description can help explain the procedure to her. Learning to insert and remove implants requires training and practice under direct supervision. Therefore, this description is a summary and not detailed instructions.

Inserting implants usually takes only a few minutes but can sometimes take longer, depending on the skill of the provider. Related complications are rare. How often complications occur also depends on the skill of the provider.

1. The provider uses proper infection-prevention procedures.
2. The provider marks the skin where the implant will be inserted on the inner side of the woman's upper arm (usually the arm she uses less often).
3. The woman receives an injection of local anesthetic under the skin of her arm to prevent pain while the implant is being inserted. This injection may sting, but she should not feel any pain when the implant is inserted. She stays fully awake throughout the procedure.
4. The provider uses a specially designed applicator to make an incision and insert the implant under the skin.
5. After the implant is inserted, the provider closes the incision with surgical tape and an adhesive bandage. Stitches are not needed. The incision is covered with a dry piece of gauze (a pressure dressing), and the arm is wrapped snugly with gauze.

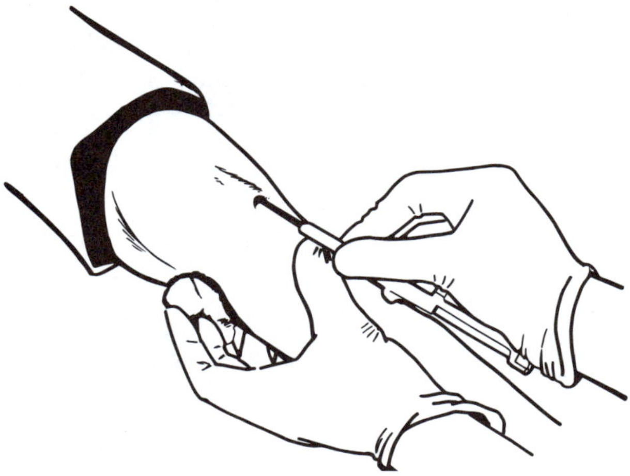

Supporting the User

Giving Specific Instructions

Keep arm dry	• The user should keep the insertion area dry for 4 days. She can take off the gauze after 2 days and the adhesive bandage and surgical tape when the incision heals, usually after 3 to 5 days.
Expect soreness, bruising	• After the anesthetic wears off, her arm may be sore for a few days. She also may have swelling and bruising at the insertion site. This is common and will go away without treatment.
Length of pregnancy protection	• Explain that it is important to have implants removed before they start to lose effectiveness. She can have a new set of implants inserted if she wants. • Discuss how to remember the date to return for implant removal and possible replacement. • Give each woman the following information in writing on a reminder card, like the one shown below, if possible, and explain: – The type of implant she has and in which arm – Date of insertion – Month and year when implants will need to be removed or replaced – Where to go if she has problems or questions about her implants

Implant Reminder Card

Client's name: ______________________________

Type of implant: ______________________ Arm: L ____ R ____

Date inserted: ______________________________

Remove or replace by: Month: ______ Year: ______

If you have any problems or questions, go to:

(name and location of facility)

How Can a Partner Help?

The client's partner is welcome to participate in counseling and learn about the method and what support he can give to his partner. A male partner can:

- Support a woman's choice of implants
- Show understanding and support if she has side effects
- Use condoms consistently in addition to the implant if he has an STI/HIV or thinks he may be at risk of an STI/HIV
- Help to remember when the implant is due for removal

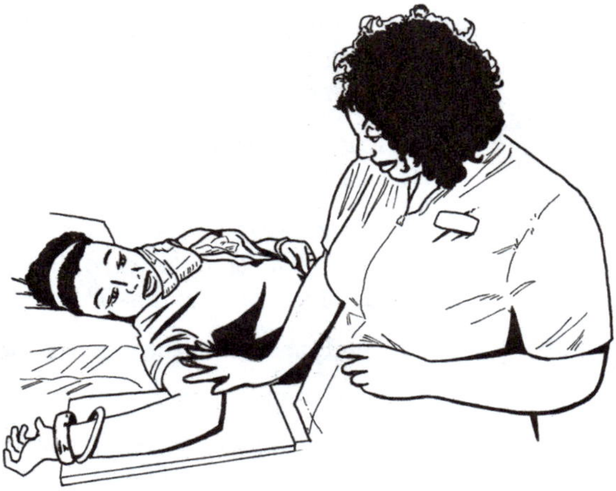

"Come Back Any Time": Reasons to Return

Assure every client that she is welcome to come back any time—for example, if she has problems, questions, or wants another method; she has a major change in health status; or she thinks she might be pregnant. Also if:

- She has pain, heat, pus, or redness at the insertion site that becomes worse or does not go away, or she sees a rod coming out.
- She wants the implants taken out, for whatever reason.
- It is time for the implants to be removed and, if she wishes, for new implants to be put in.

General health advice: Anyone who suddenly feels that something is seriously wrong with her health should immediately seek medical care from a nurse or doctor. Her contraceptive method is most likely not the cause of the condition, but she should tell the nurse or doctor what method she is using.

Removing Implants

IMPORTANT: Providers must not refuse or delay when a woman asks to have her implants removed, whatever her reason, whether it is personal or medical. All staff must understand and agree that she must not be pressured or forced to continue using implants. If the implants may be difficult to remove, a provider with the necessary skills should be available. Removals should be provided free of charge if possible.

Explaining the Removal Procedure

A woman needs to know what will happen during removal. The following description can help explain the procedure to her. The same removal procedure is used for all types of implants.

1. The provider uses proper infection-prevention procedures.

2. The provider marks the location of the implant.

3. The woman receives an injection of local anesthetic under the skin of her arm at the incision site to prevent pain during implant removal. This injection may sting. She stays fully awake throughout the procedure.

4. The health care provider makes a small incision in the skin near the site of insertion.

5. With the fingers, the provider pushes the implant toward the incision and then uses forceps to pull out the implant. A woman may feel tugging, slight pain, or soreness during the procedure and for a few days after.

6. The provider closes the incision with an adhesive bandage. Stitches are not needed. An elastic bandage may be placed over the adhesive bandage to apply gentle pressure for 2 or 3 days and keep down swelling.

The provider should ask whether the woman wants to continue preventing pregnancy and discuss her options. If she wants new implants, they are placed above or below the site of the previous implants or in the other arm.

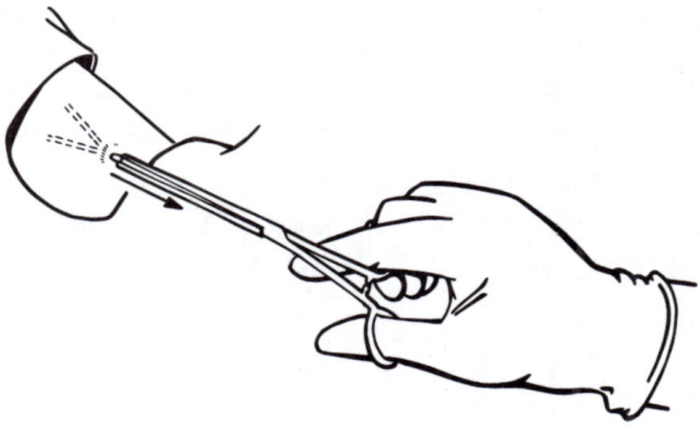

Helping Continuing Users

IMPORTANT: No routine return visit is required until it is time to remove the implants. The client should be clearly invited to return any time she wishes, however. At any future visit:

1. Ask how the client is doing with the method and whether she is satisfied. Ask if she has any questions or anything to discuss.
2. Ask especially if she is concerned about bleeding changes. Give her any information or help that she needs (see Managing Any Problems, below).
3. Ask a long-term client if she has had any new health problems since her last visit. Address problems as appropriate. For new health problems that may require switching methods, see p. 151.
4. Ask a long-term client about major life changes that may affect her needs—particularly plans for having children and STI/HIV risk. Follow up as needed.
5. If she wants to keep using implants and no new medical condition prevents it, remind her how much longer her implants will protect her from pregnancy.

Managing Any Problems

Problems Reported as Side Effects or Complications

May or may not be due to the method.

- Problems with side effects and complications affect women's satisfaction and use of implants. They deserve the provider's attention. If the client reports any side effects or complications, listen to her concerns, give her advice and support, and, if appropriate, treat. Make sure she understands the advice and agrees.
- Offer to help the client choose another method—now, if she wishes, or if problems cannot be overcome.

Irregular bleeding (bleeding at unexpected times that bothers the client)

- Reassure her that many women using implants experience irregular bleeding. It is not harmful and usually becomes less or stops after the first year of use.
- For modest short-term relief, she can take 800 mg ibuprofen or 500 mg mefenamic acid 3 times daily after meals for 5 days, beginning when irregular bleeding starts.

- If these drugs do not help her, she can try one of the following, beginning when irregular bleeding starts:
  - Combined oral contraceptives that contain the progestin levonorgestrel. Ask her to take one pill daily for 21 days.
  - 50 µg ethinyl estradiol daily for 21 days.
- If irregular bleeding continues or starts after several months of normal or no monthly bleeding, or you suspect that something may be wrong for other reasons, consider underlying conditions unrelated to method use (see Unexplained vaginal bleeding, p. 151).

No monthly bleeding

- If she has no monthly bleeding soon after implant insertion, rule out pregnancy. She might have been pregnant at the time of insertion. If she is pregnant, remove the implant.
- Reassure her that some women stop having monthly bleeding when using implants, and this is not harmful. It is similar to not having monthly bleeding during pregnancy because of the effect of the hormones. She is not pregnant or infertile. Blood is not building up inside her. (Some women are happy to be free from monthly bleeding.) Also, not bleeding can have health benefits, for example, reducing the risk of anemia.

Heavy or prolonged bleeding (twice as much as usual or longer than 8 days)

- Reassure her that some women using implants experience heavy or prolonged bleeding. It is generally not harmful and usually becomes less or stops after a few months.
- For modest short-term relief, she can try any of the treatments for irregular bleeding, above, beginning when heavy bleeding starts. Combined oral contraceptives with 50 µg of ethinyl estradiol may work better than lower-dose combined pills.
- To help prevent anemia, suggest she take iron tablets and tell her it is important to eat foods containing iron, such as meat and poultry (especially beef and chicken liver), fish, green leafy vegetables, and legumes (beans, bean curd, lentils, and peas).
- If heavy or prolonged bleeding continues or starts after several months of normal or no monthly bleeding, or you suspect that something may be wrong for other reasons, consider underlying conditions unrelated to method use (see Unexplained vaginal bleeding, p. 151).

Ordinary headaches (nonmigrainous)

- Suggest aspirin (325–650 mg), ibuprofen (200–400 mg), paracetamol (325–1000 mg), or other pain reliever.
- Any headaches that get worse or occur more often during use of implants should be evaluated.

Mild abdominal pain

- Suggest paracetamol (325–1000 mg), aspirin (325–650 mg), ibuprofen (200–400 mg), or other pain reliever.
- Consider locally available remedies.

Acne

- Consider locally available remedies.
- If client wants to stop using implants because of acne, she can consider switching to COCs. Many women's acne improves with COC use.

Weight change

- Review diet and counsel as needed.

Breast tenderness

- Recommend that she wear a supportive bra (including during strenuous activity and sleep).
- Try hot or cold compresses.
- Suggest aspirin (325–650 mg), ibuprofen (200–400 mg), paracetamol (325–1000 mg), or other pain reliever.
- Consider locally available remedies.

Mood changes or changes in sex drive

- Ask about changes in her life that could affect her mood or sex drive, including changes in her relationship with her partner. Give her support as appropriate.
- Clients who have serious mood changes such as major depression should be referred for care.
- Consider locally available remedies.

Nausea or dizziness

- Consider locally available remedies.

Pain after insertion or removal

- For pain after insertion, check that the bandage or gauze on her arm is not too tight.
- Put a new bandage on the arm and advise her to avoid pressing on the site for a few days.
- Give her aspirin (325–650 mg), ibuprofen (200–400 mg), paracetamol (325–1000 mg), or other pain reliever.

Infection at the insertion site (redness, heat, pain, pus)

- Do not remove the implants.
- Clean the infected area with soap and water or antiseptic.
- Give oral antibiotics for 7 to 10 days.
- Ask the client to return after taking all antibiotics if the infection does not clear. If infection has not cleared, remove the implants or refer for removal.
- Expulsion or partial expulsion often follows infection. Ask the client to return if she notices an implant coming out.

Abscess (pocket of pus under the skin due to infection)

- Do not remove the implants.
- Clean the area with antiseptic.
- Cut open (incise) and drain the abscess.
- Treat the wound.
- Give oral antibiotics for 7 to 10 days.
- Ask the client to return after taking all antibiotics if she has heat, redness, pain, or drainage of the wound. If infection is present when she returns, remove the implants or refer for removal.

Expulsion (when one or more implants begin to come out of the arm)

- Rare. Usually occurs within a few months of insertion or with infection.
- If no infection is present, after explanation and counseling replace the expelled rod or capsule through a new incision near the other rods or capsules, or refer for replacement.

Severe pain in lower abdomen

- Abdominal pain may be due to various problems, such as enlarged ovarian follicles or cysts.
  - A woman can continue to use implants during evaluation.
  - There is no need to treat enlarged ovarian follicles or cysts unless they grow abnormally large, twist, or burst. Reassure the client that they usually disappear on their own. To be sure the problem is resolving, see the client again in 6 weeks, if possible.
- With severe abdominal pain, be particularly alert for additional signs or symptoms of ectopic pregnancy. Ectopic pregnancy is rare and not caused by implants, but it can be life-threatening (see Question 7, p. 129). In the early stages of ectopic pregnancy, symptoms may be absent or mild, but eventually they will become severe. A combination of these signs or symptoms should increase suspicion of ectopic pregnancy:
  - Unusual abdominal pain or tenderness
  - Abnormal vaginal bleeding or no monthly bleeding—especially if this is a change from her usual bleeding pattern
  - Light-headedness or dizziness
  - Fainting
- If ectopic pregnancy or other serious health condition is suspected, refer at once for immediate diagnosis and care. (See Female Sterilization, Managing Ectopic Pregnancy, p. 227, for more on ectopic pregnancies.)

New Problems That May Require Switching Methods

May or may not be due to method.

Unexplained vaginal bleeding (that suggests a medical condition not related to the method)

- Refer or evaluate by history and pelvic examination. Diagnose and treat as appropriate.
- If no cause of bleeding can be found, consider stopping implants to make diagnosis easier. Provide another method of her choice to use until the condition is evaluated and treated (not progestin-only injectable or a copper-bearing or hormonal IUD).
- If bleeding is caused by sexually transmitted infection or pelvic inflammatory disease, she can continue using implants during treatment.

Migraine headaches (see Identifying Migraine Headaches and Auras, p. 436)

- If she has migraine headaches without aura, she can continue to use implants if she wishes.
- If she has migraine aura, remove the implants. Help her choose a method without hormones.

Certain serious health conditions (suspected blood clots in deep veins of legs or lungs, serious liver disease, or breast cancer). See Signs and Symptoms of Serious Health Conditions, p. 384.

- Remove the implants or refer for removal.
- Give her a backup method to use until her condition is evaluated.
- Refer for diagnosis and care if not already under care.

Heart disease due to blocked or narrowed arteries (ischemic heart disease) **or stroke**

- A woman who has one of these conditions can safely start implants. If, however, the condition develops while she is using implants:
  - Remove the implants or refer for removal.
  - Help her choose a method without hormones.
  - Refer for diagnosis and care if not already under care.

Suspected pregnancy

- Assess for pregnancy, including ectopic pregnancy (see Severe pain in lower abdomen, previous page).
- Remove the implants or refer for removal if she will carry the pregnancy to term.
- There are no known risks to a fetus conceived while a woman has implants in place (see Question 5, next page).

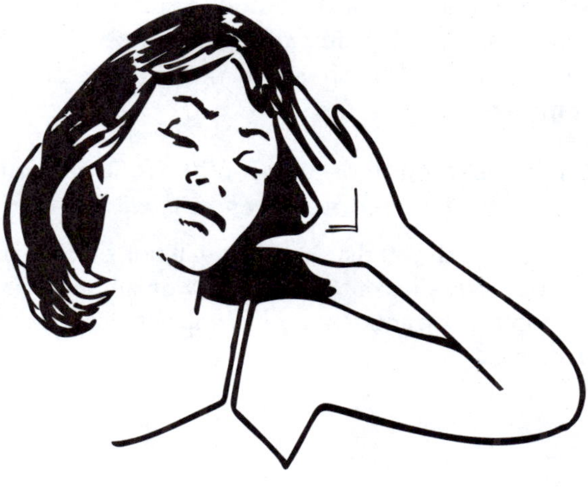

Questions and Answers About Implants

1. Do users of implants require follow-up visits?

No. Routine periodic visits are not necessary for implant users. Annual visits may be helpful for other preventive care, but they are not necessary or required. Of course, women are welcome to return at any time with questions or to have implants removed.

2. Can implants be left in a woman's arm?

Leaving the implants in place beyond their effective lifespan is generally not recommended if the woman continues to be at risk of pregnancy. The implants themselves are not dangerous, but as the hormone levels in the implants drop, they become less and less effective. After they lose effectiveness, they may still release a small dose of hormone for several more years, which serves no purpose.

If a woman wants to continue using implants, she may have a new implant inserted in the other arm even if the first implant is not removed at that time, for example, if removal services are not immediately available.

3. Do implants cause cancer?

No. Studies have not found increased risk of any cancer with use of implants.

4. How long does it take to become pregnant after the implants are removed?

Women who stop using implants can become pregnant as quickly as women who stop nonhormonal methods. Implants do not delay the return of a woman's fertility after they are removed. The bleeding pattern a woman had before she used implants generally returns after they are removed.

5. Do implants cause birth defects? Will the fetus be harmed if a woman accidentally becomes pregnant with implants in place?

No. Good evidence shows that implants will not cause birth defects and will not otherwise harm the fetus if a woman becomes pregnant while using implants or accidentally has implants inserted when she is already pregnant.

6. Can implants come out of a woman's arm?

Rarely, a rod may start to come out, most often in the first 4 weeks after insertion. This usually happens because they were not inserted well or because of an infection where they were inserted. In these cases, the woman will see the implants coming out. Some women may have a sudden change in bleeding pattern. If a woman notices a rod coming out, she should start using a backup method and return to the clinic at once.

7. Do implants increase the risk of ectopic pregnancy?

No. On the contrary, implants greatly reduce the risk of ectopic pregnancy. Ectopic pregnancies are extremely rare among implant users. The rate of ectopic pregnancy among women with implants is 6 per 100,000 women per year. The rate of ectopic pregnancy among women in the United States using no contraceptive method is 650 per 100,000 women per year.

On the very rare occasions that implants fail and pregnancy occurs, 10 to 17 of every 100 of these pregnancies are ectopic. Thus, the great majority of pregnancies after implants fail are not ectopic. Still, ectopic pregnancy can be life-threatening, and so a provider should be aware that ectopic pregnancy is possible if implants fail.

8. When can a breastfeeding woman start implants?

In 2015 WHO considered this question and updated its guidance to allow a woman to use progestin-only implants after childbirth regardless of how recently she gave birth. She does not need to wait until 6 weeks postpartum. This change in guidance also applies to progestin-only pills and the LNG-IUD. For details on when breastfeeding women can start implants, see p. 139.

9. Should heavy women avoid implants?

No. Some but not all studies have found that Jadelle implants became slightly less effective for heavier women after 4 or more years of use. As a precaution, women weighing over 80 kg may want to have their implants replaced after 4 years for greatest effectiveness. Studies of Implanon have not found that effectiveness decreases for heavier women within the lifespan approved for this type of implant.

10. What should be done if an implant user has an ovarian cyst?

The great majority of cysts are not true cysts but actually fluid-filled structures in the ovary (follicles) that continue to grow beyond the usual size in a normal menstrual cycle. They may cause some mild abdominal pain, but they require treatment only if they grow abnormally large, twist, or burst. These follicles usually go away without treatment (see Severe pain in lower abdomen, p. 150).

11. Can a woman work soon after having implants inserted?

Yes, a woman can do her usual work immediately after leaving the clinic as long as she does not bump the insertion site or get it wet.

12. Must a woman have a pelvic examination before she can have implants inserted?

No. Instead, asking the right questions can help the provider be reasonably certain she is not pregnant (see Pregnancy Checklist, inside back cover). No condition that can be detected by a pelvic examination rules out use of implants.

13. Can young women, including adolescents, use implants?

Yes. If a young woman wants to use implants, she can. In fact, implants and IUDs can be good methods for young women who want to be sure to avoid pregnancy for a number of years. They are highly effective and long-lasting methods. According to the Medical Eligibility Criteria, age is not relevant to implant use. Implant use will not affect a young woman's future fertility, whether or not she has already had children.

All young women seeking contraception, whether married or not and whether or not they have had children, can safely choose from the full range of available contraceptive methods. This includes implants, copper-bearing IUDs, and LNG-IUDs. If women want to have children in the future, however, they should not choose female sterilization, which is a permanent method.

14. Should women who are taking efavirenz be offered implants?

Yes. Women taking the antiretroviral (ARV) drug efavirenz as HIV treatment should be offered implants along with the full range of contraceptive methods. However, it is important to tell women who are taking efavirenz that efavirenz is likely to make the implants less effective. For women taking efavirenz, implants may be about as effective as combined oral contraceptives or male condoms as typically used. Women taking efavirenz who choose implants should be encouraged to use condoms in addition to implants to enhance protection from pregnancy. Or they also can consider effective contraceptive methods that do not interact with efavirenz or other ARVs. These methods include progestin-only injectables, the copper-bearing IUD, and the LNG-IUD or, if they want no more children, female sterilization or vasectomy.

A user of implants who is starting on efavirenz or already taking it can be told about this reduced effectiveness. A provider then can help her decide whether to keep using implants or to switch to another, more effective method. If she prefers another method, the provider can remove the implants and help her start another method.

CHAPTER 10

Copper-Bearing Intrauterine Device

This chapter describes primarily the TCu-380A intrauterine device. (For the levonorgestrel intrauterine device, see p. 181.)

Key Points for Providers and Clients

- **Long-term pregnancy protection.** Shown to be very effective for up to 12 years, immediately reversible.
- **Inserted into the uterus by a specifically trained provider.**
- **Little required of the client once the IUD is in place.**
- **Bleeding changes are common.** Typically, longer and heavier bleeding and more cramps or pain during monthly bleeding, especially in the first 3 to 6 months.

What Is the Copper-Bearing Intrauterine Device?

- The copper-bearing intrauterine device (IUD) is a small, flexible plastic frame with copper sleeves or wire around it. A specifically trained health care provider inserts it into a woman's uterus through her vagina and cervix.
- Almost all types of IUDs have one or two strings, or threads, tied to them. The strings hang through the cervix into the vagina.
- Works by causing a chemical change that damages sperm and egg before they can meet.

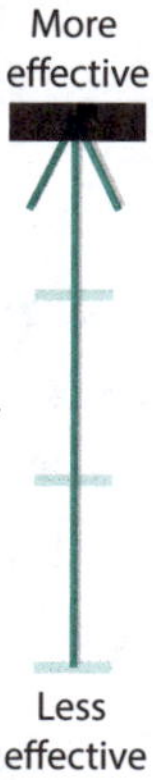

How Effective?

One of the most effective and long-lasting methods:

- Less than 1 pregnancy per 100 women using an IUD over the first year (6 per 1,000 women who use the IUD perfectly, and 8 per 1,000 women as commonly used). This means that 992 to 994 of every 1,000 women using IUDs will not become pregnant.
- A small risk of pregnancy remains beyond the first year of use and continues as long as the woman is using the IUD.
  - Over 10 years of IUD use: About 2 pregnancies per 100 women

- Studies have found that the TCu-380A is effective for 12 years. The TCu-380A is labeled for up to 10 years of use, however. (Providers should follow national guidelines as to when the IUD should be removed.)

Return of fertility after IUD is removed: No delay

Protection against sexually transmitted infections (STIs): None

Side Effects, Health Benefits, Health Risks, and Complications

Side Effects (see also Managing Any Problems, p. 173)

Some users report the following:

- Changes in bleeding patterns† (especially in the first 3 to 6 months), including:
  - Prolonged and heavy monthly bleeding
  - Irregular bleeding
  - More cramps and pain during monthly bleeding

> Bleeding changes are normal and not harmful. If a woman finds them bothersome, counseling and support can help.

Known Health Benefits

Helps protect against:

- Risks of pregnancy

May help protect against:

- Cancer of the lining of the uterus (endometrial cancer)
- Cervical cancer

Reduces:

- Risk of ectopic pregnancy

Known Health Risks

Uncommon:

- May contribute to anemia if a woman already has low iron blood stores before insertion and the IUD causes heavier monthly bleeding

Rare:

- Pelvic inflammatory disease (PID) may occur if the woman has chlamydia or gonorrhea at the time of IUD insertion

Complications

Rare:

- Puncturing (perforation) of the wall of the uterus by the IUD or an instrument used for insertion. Usually heals without treatment.
- Miscarriage, preterm birth, or infection in the rare case that the woman becomes pregnant with the IUD in place.

† *For definitions of bleeding patterns, see "vaginal bleeding," p. 407.*

Correcting Misunderstandings (see also Questions and Answers, p.178)

Intrauterine devices:

- Can be used by women of any age, including adolescents.
- Can be used by women who have had children and those who have not.
- Rarely lead to PID.
- Do not increase the risk of contracting STIs, including HIV.
- Do not increase the risk of miscarriage when a woman becomes pregnant after the IUD is removed.
- Do not make women infertile.
- Do not cause birth defects.
- Do not cause cancer.
- Do not move to the heart or brain.
- Do not cause discomfort or pain for the woman or the man during sex.
- Substantially reduce the risk of ectopic pregnancy.

Why Some Women Say They Like the IUD

- Prevents pregnancy very effectively
- Is long-lasting
- Is private—usually no one else can tell a woman is using contraception (sometimes a partner may feel the strings during sex)
- Has no further costs for supplies after the IUD is inserted
- Does not require the user to do anything once the IUD is inserted

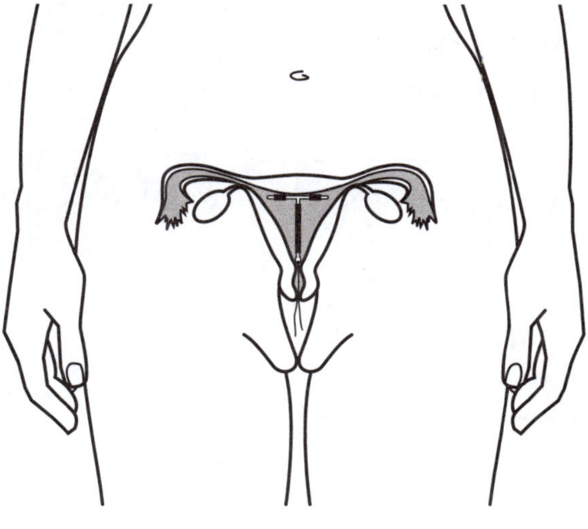

Who Can and Cannot Use the Copper-Bearing IUD

Safe and Suitable for Nearly All Women

Most women can use IUDs safely and effectively, including women who:

- Have or have not had children
- Are married or are not married
- Are of any age, including adolescents and women over 40 years old
- Have just had an abortion or miscarriage (if no evidence of infection)
- Are breastfeeding
- Do hard physical work
- Have had ectopic pregnancy
- Have had pelvic inflammatory disease (PID)
- Have vaginal infections
- Have anemia
- Have HIV clinical disease that is mild or with no symptoms whether or not they are on antiretroviral therapy (see IUDs for Women With HIV, p. 162)

Avoid Unnecessary Procedures

(see Importance of Procedures, p. 368)

Women can begin using IUDs:

- Without cervical cancer screening
- Without a breast examination
- Without a blood pressure check

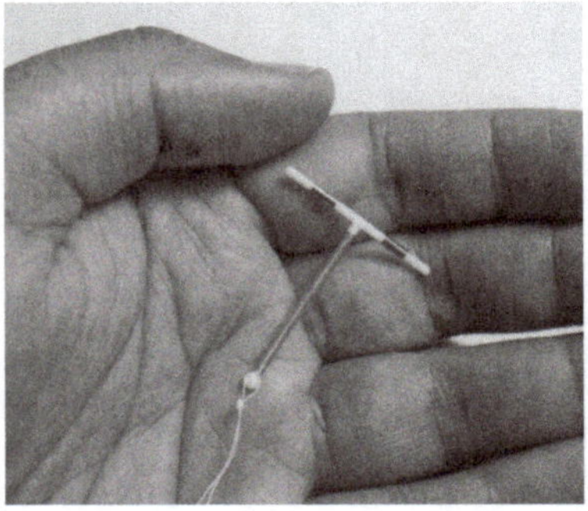

A pelvic examination and an STI risk assessment are essential. When available, a hemoglobin test and laboratory tests for STIs including HIV can contribute to safe and effective use.

Medical Eligibility Criteria for

Copper-Bearing IUDs

Ask the client the questions below about known medical conditions. If she answers "no" to all of the questions, then she can have an IUD inserted if she wants. If she answers "yes" to a question, follow the instructions. In some cases she can still have an IUD inserted.

1. Did you give birth more than 48 hours ago but less than 4 weeks ago?

❏ NO ❏ **YES** Delay inserting an IUD until 4 or more weeks after childbirth (see Soon after childbirth, p. 164).

2. Do you have an infection following childbirth or abortion?

❏ NO ❏ **YES** If she currently has infection of the reproductive organs during the first 6 weeks after childbirth (puerperal sepsis) or she just had an abortion-related infection in the uterus (septic abortion), do not insert the IUD. Treat or refer if she is not already receiving care. Help her choose another method or offer a backup method.* After treatment, re-evaluate for IUD use.

3. Are you having vaginal bleeding that is unusual for you?

❏ NO ❏ **YES** If she has unexplained vaginal bleeding that suggests pregnancy or an underlying medical condition, use of an IUD could make diagnosis and monitoring of any treatment more difficult. Help her choose a method to use while being evaluated and treated (but not a hormonal IUD, progestin-only injectable, or implant). After treatment, re-evaluate for IUD use.

4. Do you have any female conditions or problems (gynecologic or obstetric conditions or problems), such as genital cancer or pelvic tuberculosis? If so, what problems?

❏ NO ❏ **YES** Known current cervical, endometrial, or ovarian cancer; gestational trophoblast disease; pelvic tuberculosis: Do not insert an IUD. Treat or refer for care if she is not already receiving care. Help her choose another method. In case of pelvic tuberculosis, re-evaluate for IUD use after treatment.

(Continued on next page)

* *Backup methods include abstinence, male and female condoms, spermicides, and withdrawal. Tell her that spermicides and withdrawal are the least effective contraceptive methods. If possible, give her condoms.*

Medical Eligibility Criteria for Copper-Bearing IUDs (continued)

5. Do you have HIV or AIDS? Do you have any health conditions associated with HIV infection?

❑ NO ❑ **YES** If a woman has HIV infection with severe or advanced clinical disease, do not insert an IUD. In contrast, a woman living with HIV who has mild clinical disease or no clinical disease can have an IUD inserted, whether or not she is on antretroviral therapy. See IUDs for Women With HIV, p. 162.

6. Assess whether she is at very high individual risk for STIs.

Women who have a very high individual likelihood of STI infection should not have an IUD inserted unless gonorrhea and chlamydia are ruled out by lab tests (see Assessing Women for Risk of Sexually Transmitted Infections, p. 162).

7. Rule out pregnancy.

Ask the client the questions in the Pregnancy Checklist (see inside back cover). If she answers "yes" to any of these questions, you can be reasonably certain that she is not pregnant, and she can have an IUD inserted. If the Pregnancy Checklist cannot rule out pregnancy, use another tool before inserting an IUD (see Ruling Out Pregnancy, p. 439).

Also, women should not use the IUD if they report having systemic lupus erythematosus with severe thrombocytopenia. For complete classifications, see Medical Eligibility Criteria for Contraceptive Use, p. 388.

Be sure to explain the health benefits and risks and the side effects of the method that the client will use. Also, point out any conditions that would make the method inadvisable, when relevant to the client.

Using Clinical Judgment in Special Cases

Usually, a woman with any of the conditions listed below should not have an IUD inserted. In special circumstances, however, when other, more appropriate methods are not available or acceptable to her, a qualified provider who can carefully assess a specific woman's condition and situation may decide that she can use an IUD. The provider needs to consider the severity of her condition and, for most conditions, whether she will have access to follow-up.

- Between 48 hours and 4 weeks since giving birth
- Noncancerous (benign) gestational trophoblast disease
- Current ovarian cancer
- Is at very high individual risk for STIs at the time of insertion
- Has severe or advanced HIV clinical disease
- Has systemic lupus erythematosus with severe thrombocytopenia

Screening Questions for Pelvic Examination Before IUD Insertion

A pelvic examination and STI risk assessment should be done before IUD insertion. (For STI risk assessment, see next page.) When performing the pelvic examination, asking yourself the questions below helps you check for signs of conditions that would rule out IUD insertion. If the answer to all of the questions is "no," then the client can have an IUD inserted. If the answer to any question is "yes," do not insert an IUD.

For questions 1 through 5, if the answer is "yes," refer for diagnosis and treatment as appropriate. Help her choose another method and counsel her about condom use if she faces any risk of sexually transmitted infections (STIs). Give her condoms, if possible. If an STI or pelvic inflammatory disease (PID) is confirmed and she still wants an IUD, it may be inserted as soon as she finishes treatment, if she is not at risk for reinfection before insertion.

1. Is there any type of ulcer on the vulva, vagina, or cervix?

❑ NO ❑ **YES** Possible STI.

2. Does the client feel pain in her lower abdomen when you move the cervix?

❑ NO ❑ **YES** Possible PID.

3. Is there tenderness in the uterus, ovaries, or fallopian tubes (adnexal tenderness)?

❑ NO ❑ **YES** Possible PID.

4. Is there a purulent cervical discharge?

❑ NO ❑ **YES** Possible STI or PID.

5. Does the cervix bleed easily when touched?

❑ NO ❑ **YES** Possible STI or cervical cancer.

6. Is there an anatomical abnormality of the uterine cavity that will prevent correct IUD placement?

❑ NO ❑ **YES** If an anatomical abnormality distorts the uterine cavity, proper IUD placement may not be possible. Help her choose another method.

7. Were you unable to determine the size and/or position of the uterus?

❑ NO ❑ **YES** Determining the size and position of the uterus before IUD insertion is essential to ensure high placement of the IUD and to minimize risk of perforation. If size and position cannot be determined, do not insert an IUD. Help her choose another method.

Intrauterine Devices for Women With HIV

- Women living with HIV can safely have an IUD inserted if they have mild or no clinical disease, whether or not they are on antiretroviral therapy.
- Women who have HIV infection with advanced or severe clinical disease should *not* have an IUD inserted.
- If a woman becomes infected with HIV while she has an IUD in place, it does not need to be removed.
- An IUD user living with HIV who develops advanced or severe clinical disease can keep the IUD but should be closely monitored for pelvic inflammatory disease.
- Urge women who have HIV or are at risk for HIV to use condoms along with the IUD. Used consistently and correctly, condoms help prevent transmission of HIV and other STIs.
- Women who are at risk of HIV but not infected with HIV can have an IUD inserted. The IUD does not increase the risk of becoming infected with HIV.

Assessing Women for Risk of Sexually Transmitted Infections

A woman who has gonorrhea or chlamydia now should not have an IUD inserted. Having these sexually transmitted infections (STIs) at the time of insertion may increase the risk of pelvic inflammatory disease. These STIs may be difficult to diagnose clinically, however, and reliable laboratory tests are time-consuming, expensive, and sometimes unavailable. Without clinical signs or symptoms and without laboratory testing, the only indication that a woman might already have an STI is whether her behavior or her situation places her at *very high individual likelihood* of infection. If this risk for the *individual* client is very high, she generally should not have an IUD inserted.[‡] (Local STI prevalence rates are not a basis for judging individual risk.)

There is no universal set of questions that will determine if a woman is at very high individual risk for STIs. Instead of asking questions, providers can discuss with the client the personal behaviors and the situations in their community that are most likely to expose women to STIs.

‡ In contrast, if a *current* IUD user's situation changes and she finds herself at very high individual risk for gonorrhea or chlamydia, she can keep using her IUD.

Steps to take:

1. Tell the client that a woman who faces a very high individual risk of STIs usually should not have an IUD inserted.

2. Ask the woman to consider her own risk and to think about whether she might have an STI. A woman is often the best judge of her own risk.[§] She does not have to tell the provider about her behavior or her partner's behavior. Providers can explain possibly risky situations that may place a woman at very high individual risk. The client can think about whether such situations occurred recently (in the past 3 months or so). If so, she may have an STI now, whether or not she has noticed symptoms, and may want to choose a method other than the IUD.

Possibly risky situations include:

- A sexual partner has STI symptoms such as pus coming from his penis, pain or burning during urination, or an open sore in the genital area
- She or a sexual partner was diagnosed with an STI recently
- She has had more than one sexual partner recently
- She has a sexual partner who has had other partners recently

All of these situations pose less risk if a woman or her partner uses condoms consistently and correctly.

Also, a provider can mention other high-risk situations that exist locally.

3. Ask if she thinks she is a good candidate for an IUD or would like to consider other contraceptive methods, including other long-acting methods. If, after considering her individual risk, she thinks she is a good candidate, and she is eligible, provide her with an IUD. If she wants to consider other methods or if you have strong reason to believe that the client is at very high individual risk of infection, help her choose another method.

Note: If she still wants the IUD while at very high individual risk of STIs, and reliable laboratory testing for gonorrhea and chlamydia is available, a woman who tests negative can have an IUD inserted. A woman who tests positive can have an IUD inserted as soon as she finishes treatment, if she is not at risk of reinfection by the time of insertion.

In special circumstances, if other, more appropriate methods are not available or not acceptable, a health care provider who can carefully assess a specific woman's condition and situation may decide that a woman at very high individual risk can have the IUD inserted even if STI testing is not available. (Depending on the circumstances, the provider may consider presumptively treating her with a full curative dose of antibiotics effective against both gonorrhea and chlamydia and inserting the IUD after she finishes treatment.) Whether or not she receives presumptive treatment, the provider should be sure that the client can return for the follow-up visit, will be carefully checked for infection, and will be treated immediately if needed. She should be asked to return at once if she develops a fever and either lower abdominal pain or abnormal vaginal discharge or both.

[§] Any woman who thinks she might have an STI should seek care immediately.

Providing the Intrauterine Device

When to Start

IMPORTANT: In many cases a woman can start the IUD any time if it is reasonably certain she is not pregnant. To be reasonably certain she is not pregnant, use the Pregnancy Checklist (see inside back cover).

Woman's situation	When to start
Having menstrual cycles	**Any time of the month** • If she is starting within 12 days after the start of her monthly bleeding, no need for a backup method. • If it is more than 12 days after the start of her monthly bleeding, she can have the IUD inserted any time if it is reasonably certain she is not pregnant. No need for a backup method.
Switching from another method	• Immediately, if she has been using the method consistently and correctly or if it is otherwise reasonably certain she is not pregnant. No need to wait for her next monthly bleeding. No need for a backup method. • If she is switching from an injectable, she can have the IUD inserted when the next injection would have been given. No need for a backup method.
Soon after childbirth (regardless of breastfeeding status)	• Any time within 48 hours after giving birth, including by caesarean delivery. (Provider needs specific training in postpartum insertion by hand or using a ring forceps.) • If it is more than 48 hours after giving birth, delay until 4 weeks or more after giving birth.
Fully or nearly fully breastfeeding	
Less than 6 months after giving birth	• If the IUD is not inserted within the first 48 hours and her monthly bleeding has not returned, she can have the IUD inserted any time between 4 weeks and 6 months after giving birth. No need for a backup method. • If her monthly bleeding has returned, she can have the IUD inserted as advised for women having menstrual cycles (see above).

Woman's situation	When to start
Fully or nearly fully breastfeeding (continued)	
More than 6 months after giving birth	• If her monthly bleeding has not returned, she can have the IUD inserted any time it is reasonably certain she is not pregnant. No need for a backup method. • If her monthly bleeding has returned, she can have the IUD inserted as advised for women having menstrual cycles (see previous page).
Partially breastfeeding or not breastfeeding	
More than 4 weeks after giving birth	• If her monthly bleeding has not returned, she can have the IUD inserted *if it can be determined that she is not pregnant* (see Ruling Out Pregnancy, p. 439). No need for a backup method. • If her monthly bleeding has returned, she can have the IUD inserted as advised for women having menstrual cycles (see previous page).
No monthly bleeding (not related to childbirth or breastfeeding)	• Any time *if it can be determined that she is not pregnant* (see Ruling Out Pregnancy, p. 439). No need for a backup method.
After miscarriage or abortion	• Immediately, if the IUD is inserted within 12 days after first- or second-trimester abortion or miscarriage and if no infection is present. No need for a backup method. • If it is more than 12 days after first- or second-trimester miscarriage or abortion and no infection is present, she can have the IUD inserted any time if it is reasonably certain she is not pregnant. No need for a backup method. • If infection is present, treat or refer, and help the client choose another method. If she still wants the IUD, it can be inserted after the infection has completely cleared. • IUD insertion after second-trimester abortion or miscarriage requires specific training. If not specifically trained, delay insertion until at least 4 weeks after miscarriage or abortion.

Woman's situation	When to start
For emergency contraception	• Within 5 days after unprotected sex. • When the time of ovulation can be estimated, she can have an IUD inserted up to 5 days after ovulation. Sometimes this may be more than 5 days after unprotected sex.
After taking emergency contraceptive pills (ECPs)	• The IUD can be inserted on the same day that she takes the ECPs (progestin-only, combined, or ulipristal acetate ECPs). No need for a backup method. • If she does not have it inserted immediately, but returns for an IUD, she can have it inserted any time *if it can be determined that she is not pregnant* (see Ruling Out Pregnancy, p. 439).

Preventing Infection at IUD Insertion

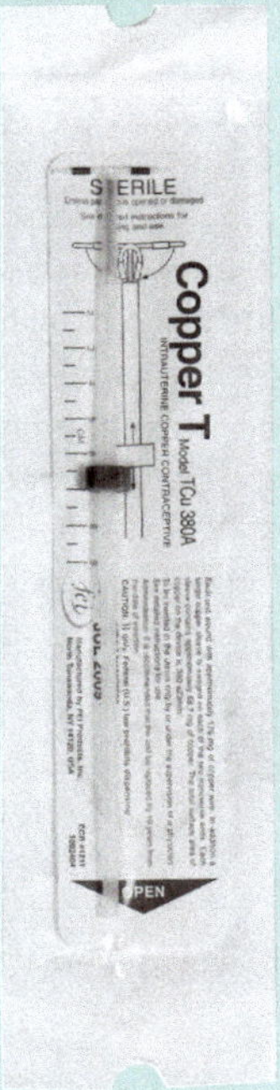

Proper insertion technique can help prevent many problems, such as infection, expulsion, and perforation.

- Follow proper infection-prevention procedures.
- Use high-level disinfected or sterile instruments. High-level disinfect by boiling, steaming, or soaking them in disinfectant chemicals.
- Use a new, presterilized IUD that is packaged with its inserter.
- The "no-touch" insertion technique is safest. This includes not letting the loaded IUD or uterine sound touch any unsterile surfaces (for example, hands, speculum, vagina, table top). The no-touch technique involves:
  - Loading the IUD into the inserter while the IUD is still in the sterile package, to avoid touching the IUD directly
  - Cleaning the cervix thoroughly with antiseptic before IUD insertion
  - Being careful not to touch the vaginal wall or speculum blades with the uterine sound or loaded IUD inserter
  - Passing both the uterine sound and the loaded IUD inserter only once each through the cervical canal
- Giving antibiotics routinely is generally not recommended for women at low risk of STIs.

Giving Advice on Side Effects

IMPORTANT: Thorough counseling about bleeding changes must come before IUD insertion. Counseling about bleeding changes may be the most important help a woman needs to keep using the method without concern.

Describe the most common side effects	• Changes in her bleeding pattern: – Prolonged and heavy monthly bleeding – Irregular bleeding – More cramps and pain during monthly bleeding
Explain about these side effects	• Bleeding changes are not signs of illness. • Usually become less after the first several months after insertion. • Client can come back for help if problems bother her or if she has other concerns.

Inserting the IUD

Talk with the client before the procedure	• Explain the insertion procedure (see next page). • Show her the speculum, tenaculum, and the IUD and inserter in the package. • Tell her that she will experience some discomfort or cramping during the procedure, and that this is to be expected. • Ask her to tell you any time that she feels discomfort or pain. • Ibuprofen (200–400 mg), paracetamol (325–1000 mg), or other pain reliever may be given 30 minutes before insertion to help reduce cramping and pain. Do not give aspirin, which slows blood clotting.
Talk with the client during the procedure	• Tell her what is happening, step by step, and reassure her. • Alert her before a step that may cause pain or might startle her. • Ask from time to time if she is feeling pain.
Talk with the client after the procedure	• Ask her how she is doing. • Tell her that the procedure was successful and that the IUD is in place. • Tell her that she can rest for a while and then slowly sit up before getting up and dressing. • Remind her that the two of you will be discussing next steps and follow-up.

Explaining the Insertion Procedure

A woman who has chosen the IUD needs to know what will happen during insertion. The following description can help explain the procedure to her. Learning IUD insertion requires training and practice under direct supervision. Therefore, this description is a summary and not detailed instructions.

1. The provider uses proper infection-prevention procedures.
2. The provider conducts a pelvic examination to determine the position of the uterus and assess eligibility (see Screening Questions for Pelvic Examination Before IUD Insertion, p. 161). The provider first does the bimanual examination and then inserts a speculum into the vagina to inspect the cervix.
3. The provider cleans the cervix and vagina with appropriate antiseptic.
4. The provider slowly inserts the tenaculum through the speculum and closes the tenaculum just enough to gently hold the cervix and uterus steady.
5. The provider slowly and gently passes the uterine sound through the cervix to measure the depth and position of the uterus.
6. The provider loads the IUD into the inserter while both are still in the unopened sterile package.
7. The provider slowly and gently inserts the IUD into the uterus and removes the inserter.
8. The provider cuts the strings on the IUD, leaving about 3 centimeters hanging out of the cervix.
9. After the insertion, the woman rests. She remains on the examination table until she feels ready to get dressed.

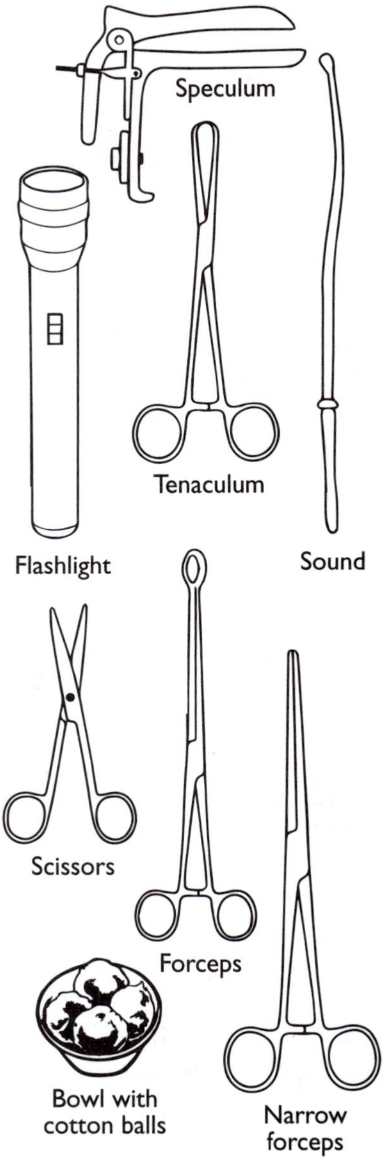

Supporting the User

Giving Specific Instructions

Expect cramping and pain

- She can expect some cramping and pain for a few days after insertion.
- Suggest ibuprofen (200–400 mg), paracetamol (325–1000 mg), or other pain reliever as needed.
- Also, she can expect some bleeding or spotting immediately after insertion. **Irregular spotting can continue during the first month after insertion.**

Length of pregnancy protection

- Discuss how to remember the date to return for removal or replacement.
- Give each woman the following information in writing on a reminder card, like the one shown below, if possible, and explain:
  - The type of IUD she has
  - Date of IUD insertion
  - Month and year when IUD will need to be removed or replaced
  - Where to go if she has problems or questions about her IUD

Follow-up visit

- A follow-up visit after her first monthly bleeding or 3 to 6 weeks after IUD insertion is recommended. No woman should be denied an IUD, however, because follow-up would be difficult or not possible.

IUD Reminder Card

Client's name: ______________________

Type of IUD: ______________________

Date inserted: ______________________

Remove or replace by: Month ______ Year ______

If you have any problems or questions, go to:

(name and location of facility)

How Can a Partner Help?

The client's partner is welcome to participate in counseling and learn about the method and what support he can give to his partner. A male partner can:

- Support a woman's choice of the IUD
- Show understanding and support if she has side effects
- Use condoms consistently in addition to the IUD if he has an STI/HIV or thinks he may be at risk of an STI/HIV
- Help to remember when the IUD is due for removal

"Come Back Any Time": Reasons to Return

Assure every client that she is welcome to come back any time—for example, if she has problems, questions, or wants another method; or she has a major change in health status. Also if:

- The IUD was expelled or she thinks it may have been expelled from her uterus.
- She has symptoms of pelvic inflammatory disease (increasing or severe pain in the lower abdomen, pain during sex, unusual vaginal discharge, fever, chills, nausea, and/or vomiting), especially in the first 20 days after insertion.
- She thinks she might be pregnant.
- She wants the IUD removed, for whatever reason.

General health advice: Anyone who suddenly feels that something is seriously wrong with her health should immediately seek medical care from a nurse or doctor. Her contraceptive method is most likely not the cause of the condition, but she should tell the nurse or doctor what method she is using.

Helping Continuing Users

Post-Insertion Follow-Up Visit (3 to 6 Weeks)

1. Ask how the client is doing with the method and whether she is satisfied. Ask if she has any questions or anything to discuss.
2. Ask especially if she is concerned about bleeding changes. Give her any information or help that she needs (see Managing Any Problems, p. 173).
3. Ask her if she has:
    - Increasing or severe abdominal pain or pain during sex or urination
    - Unusual vaginal discharge
    - Fever or chills

- Signs or symptoms of pregnancy
- Felt the hard plastic of an IUD that has partially come out
- A routine pelvic examination at the follow-up visit is not required. It may be appropriate in some settings or for some clients, however. Conduct a pelvic examination particularly if the client's answers lead you to suspect infection or that the IUD has partially or completely come out.

Any Visit

1. Ask how the client is doing with the method and about bleeding changes (see Post-Insertion Follow-Up Visit, Items 1 and 2, previous page).
2. Ask a long-term client if she has had any new health problems. Address problems as appropriate. For new health problems that may require switching methods, see p. 177.
3. Ask a long-term client about major life changes that may affect her needs—particularly plans for having children and STI/HIV risk. Follow up as needed.
4. Remind her how much longer the IUD will protect her from pregnancy and when she will need to have the IUD removed or replaced.

Removing the Intrauterine Device

IMPORTANT: Providers must not refuse or delay when a woman asks to have her IUD removed, whatever her reason, whether it is personal or medical. All staff must understand and agree that she must not be pressured or forced to continue using the IUD.

If a woman is finding side effects difficult to tolerate, first discuss the problems she is having (see Managing Any Problems, p. 173). Ask if she would rather try to manage the problem or to have the IUD removed immediately.

Removing an IUD is usually simple. It can be done any time of the month. Removal may be easier during monthly bleeding, when the cervix is naturally softened. In cases of uterine perforation or if removal is not easy (for example, when IUD strings are missing), refer the woman to an experienced clinician who can use an appropriate removal technique.

Explaining the Removal Procedure

Before removing the IUD, explain what will happen during removal:

1. The provider inserts a speculum to see the cervix and IUD strings and carefully cleans the cervix and vagina with an antiseptic solution such as iodine.
2. The provider asks the woman to take slow, deep breaths and to relax. The woman should say if she feels pain during the procedure.
3. Using narrow forceps, the provider pulls the IUD strings slowly and gently until the IUD comes completely out of the cervix.

Switching From an IUD to Another Method

These guidelines ensure that the client is protected from pregnancy without interruption when switching from a copper-bearing IUD or a hormonal IUD to another method. See also When to Start for each method.

Switching to	When to start
A hormonal method: combined oral contraceptives (COCs), **progestin-only pills** (POPs), **progestin-only injectables, monthly injectables, combined patch, combined vaginal ring, or implants**	• If starting during the first 7 days of monthly bleeding (first 5 days for COCs and POPs), start the hormonal method now and remove the IUD. No need for a backup method. • If starting after the first 7 days of monthly bleeding (after the first 5 days for COCs and POPs) and she has had sex since her last monthly bleeding, start the hormonal method now. It is recommended that the IUD be left in place until her next monthly bleeding. • If starting after the first 7 days of monthly bleeding (after the first 5 days for COCs and POPs) and she has *not* had sex since her last monthly bleeding, the IUD can stay in place and be removed during her next monthly bleeding, or the IUD can be removed and she can use a backup method* for the next 7 days (2 days for POPs).
Male or female condoms, spermicides, diaphragms, cervical caps, or withdrawal	• The next time she has sex after the IUD is removed.
Fertility awareness methods	• In the same cycle that the IUD is removed.
Female sterilization	• If during the first 7 days of monthly bleeding, remove the IUD and perform the female sterilization procedure. No need for a backup method. • If after the first 7 days of monthly bleeding, perform the sterilization procedure. Ideally, the IUD should stay in place until her follow-up visit or her next monthly bleeding. If a follow-up visit is not possible, remove the IUD at the time of sterilization. No need for a backup method.

* *Backup methods include abstinence, male and female condoms, spermicides, and withdrawal. Tell her that spermicides and withdrawal are the least effective contraceptive methods. If possible, give her condoms.*

Switching to	When to start
Vasectomy	• Any time • The woman can keep the IUD until a test of her partner's semen shows that the vasectomy is working, or for 3 months, when the vasectomy will be fully effective.

Managing Any Problems

Problems Reported As Side Effects or Complications

May or may not be due to the method.

- Problems with side effects or complications affect women's satisfaction and use of IUDs. They deserve the provider's attention. If the client reports any side effects or complications, listen to her concerns, give her advice and support, and, if appropriate, treat. Make sure she understands the advice and agrees.
- Offer to help her choose another method—now, if she wishes, or if problems cannot be overcome.

Heavy or prolonged bleeding (twice as much as usual or longer than 8 days)

- Reassure her that many women using IUDs experience heavy or prolonged bleeding. It is generally not harmful and usually becomes less or stops after the first several months of use.
- For modest short-term relief she can try (one at a time):
  - Tranexamic acid (1500 mg) 3 times daily for 3 days, then 1000 mg once daily for 2 days, beginning when heavy bleeding starts.
  - Nonsteroidal anti-inflammatory drugs (NSAIDs) such as ibuprofen (400 mg) or indomethacin (25 mg) 2 times daily after meals for 5 days, beginning when heavy bleeding starts. Other NSAIDs—except aspirin—also may provide some relief of heavy or prolonged bleeding. Aspirin could increase bleeding.
- Provide iron tablets if possible and tell her it is important for her to eat foods containing iron (see Possible anemia, next page).
- If heavy or prolonged bleeding continues or starts after several months of normal bleeding or long after the IUD was inserted, or if you suspect that something may be wrong for other reasons, consider underlying conditions unrelated to method use (see Unexplained vaginal bleeding, p. 177).

Irregular bleeding (bleeding at unexpected times that bothers the client)

- Reassure her that many women using IUDs experience irregular bleeding. It is not harmful and usually becomes less or stops after the first several months of use.

- For modest short-term relief she can try NSAIDs such as ibuprofen (400 mg) or indomethacin (25 mg) 2 times daily after meals for 5 days, beginning when irregular bleeding starts.
- If irregular bleeding continues or starts after several months of normal bleeding, or you suspect that something may be wrong for other reasons, consider underlying conditions unrelated to method use (see Unexplained vaginal bleeding, p. 177).

Cramping and pain

- She can expect some cramping and pain for the first day or two after IUD insertion.
- Explain that some cramping also is common in the first 3 to 6 months of IUD use, particularly during monthly bleeding. Generally, this is not harmful and usually decreases over time.
  - Suggest aspirin (325–650 mg), ibuprofen (200–400 mg), paracetamol (325–1000 mg), or other pain reliever. If she also has heavy or prolonged bleeding, aspirin should not be used because it may increase bleeding.
- If severe cramping continues beyond the first 2 days after insertion, evaluate for partial expulsion or perforation.

Possible anemia

- The copper-bearing IUD may contribute to anemia if a woman already has low iron blood stores before insertion and the IUD causes heavier monthly bleeding.
- Pay special attention to IUD users with any of the following signs and symptoms:
  - Inside of eyelids or underneath fingernails looks pale, pale skin, fatigue or weakness, dizziness, irritability, headache, ringing in the ears, sore tongue, and brittle nails.
  - If blood testing is available, hemoglobin less than 9 g/dl or hematocrit less than 30.
- Provide iron tablets if possible.
- Tell her it is important to eat foods containing iron, such as meat and poultry (especially beef and chicken liver), fish, green leafy vegetables, and legumes (beans, bean curd, lentils, and peas).

Partner can feel IUD strings during sex

- Explain that this happens sometimes when strings are cut too short.
- If her partner finds the strings bothersome, describe and discuss this option:
  - Strings can be cut even shorter so they are not coming out of the cervical canal. Her partner will not feel the strings, but it will make the removal procedure somewhat more difficult (may require a specially trained provider).

Severe pain in lower abdomen (suspected pelvic inflammatory disease [PID])

- Some common signs and symptoms of PID often also occur with other abdominal conditions, such as ectopic pregnancy. If ectopic pregnancy is ruled out, assess for PID.
- If possible, do abdominal and pelvic examinations (see Signs and Symptoms of Serious Health Conditions, p. 384, for signs from the pelvic examination that would indicate PID).
- If a pelvic examination is not possible, and she has a combination of the following signs and symptoms in addition to lower abdominal pain, suspect PID:
  - Unusual vaginal discharge
  - Fever or chills
  - Pain during sex or urination
  - Bleeding after sex or between monthly bleeding
  - Nausea and vomiting
  - A tender pelvic mass
  - Pain when the abdomen is gently pressed (direct abdominal tenderness) or when gently pressed and then suddenly released (rebound abdominal tenderness)
- Treat PID or immediately refer for treatment:
  - Because of the serious consequences of PID, health care providers should treat all suspected cases, based on the signs and symptoms above. Treatment should be started as soon as possible. Treatment is more effective at preventing long-term complications when appropriate antibiotics are given immediately.
  - Treat for gonorrhea, chlamydia, and anaerobic bacterial infections. Counsel the client about prevention and treatment of STIs and about condom use. If possible, give her condoms.
  - There is no need to remove the IUD if she wants to continue using it. If she wants it removed, take it out after starting antibiotic treatment. (If the IUD is removed, consider emergency contraceptive pills and discuss choosing another method. See Switching from an IUD to Another Method, p. 172.)
  - If the infection does not improve, consider removing the IUD while continuing antibiotics. If the IUD is not removed, antibiotics should still be continued. In both cases the woman's health should be closely monitored.

Severe pain in lower abdomen (suspected ectopic pregnancy)

- Many conditions can cause severe abdominal pain. Be particularly alert for additional signs or symptoms of ectopic pregnancy, which is rare but can be life-threatening. While the IUD reduces risk of ectopic pregnancy, it does not eliminate it (see Question 10, p. 180).

- In the early stages of ectopic pregnancy, symptoms may be absent or mild, but eventually they will become severe. A combination of these signs or symptoms should increase suspicion of ectopic pregnancy:
  - Unusual abdominal pain or tenderness
  - Abnormal vaginal bleeding or no monthly bleeding—especially if this is a change from her usual bleeding pattern
  - Light-headedness or dizziness
  - Fainting
- If ectopic pregnancy or other serious health condition is suspected, refer at once for immediate diagnosis and care. (See Female Sterilization, Managing Ectopic Pregnancy, p. 227, for more on ectopic pregnancies.)
- If the client does not have these additional symptoms or signs, assess for pelvic inflammatory disease (see Severe pain in lower abdomen, p. 175).

Suspected uterine puncturing (perforation)

- If puncturing is suspected at the time of insertion or sounding of the uterus, stop the procedure immediately (and remove the IUD if inserted). Observe the client in the clinic carefully:
  - For the first hour, keep the woman at bed rest and check her vital signs (blood pressure, pulse, respiration, and temperature) every 5 to 10 minutes.
  - If the woman remains stable after one hour, check for signs of intra-abdominal bleeding, such as low hematocrit or hemoglobin or rebound on abdominal examination, if possible, and her vital signs. Observe for several more hours. If she has no signs or symptoms, she can be sent home, but she should avoid sex for 2 weeks. Help her choose another method.
  - If she has a rapid pulse and falling blood pressure, or new pain or increasing pain around the uterus, refer her to a higher level of care.
  - If uterine perforation is suspected within 6 weeks or more after insertion based on clinical symptoms, refer the client for evaluation to a clinician experienced at removing such IUDs (see Question 6, p. 179).

IUD partially comes out (partial expulsion)

- If the IUD partially comes out, remove the IUD. Discuss with the client whether she wants another IUD or a different method. If she wants another IUD, she can have one inserted right away if it is reasonably certain she is not pregnant. If the client does not want to continue using an IUD, help her choose another method.

IUD completely comes out (complete expulsion)

- If the client reports that the IUD came out, discuss with her whether she wants another IUD or a different method. If she wants another IUD, she can have one inserted at any time it is reasonably certain she is not pregnant.

- If complete expulsion is suspected (for example, strings cannot be found on pelvic exam) and the client does not know whether the IUD came out, refer for ultrasound (or x-ray, if pregnancy can be ruled out) to assess whether the IUD might have moved to the abdominal cavity. Give her a backup method to use in the meantime.

Missing strings (suggesting possible pregnancy, uterine perforation, or expulsion)

- Ask the client:
  - Whether and when she saw the IUD come out
  - When she had her last monthly bleeding
  - If she has any symptoms of pregnancy
  - If she has used a backup method since she noticed that the IUD came out
- Always start with minor and safe procedures and be gentle. Check for the strings in the folds of the cervical canal with forceps. About half of missing IUD strings can be found in the cervical canal.
- If strings cannot be located in the cervical canal, either they have gone up into the uterus or the IUD has been expelled unnoticed. Refer for ultrasound (or x-ray, if pregnancy can be ruled out). Give her a backup method to use in the meantime, in case the IUD came out.

New Problems That May Require Switching Methods

May or may not be due to the method.

Unexplained vaginal bleeding (that suggests a medical condition not related to the method)

- Refer or evaluate by history or pelvic examination. Diagnose and treat as appropriate.
- She can continue using the IUD while her condition is being evaluated.
- If bleeding is caused by sexually transmitted infection or pelvic inflammatory disease, she can continue using the IUD during treatment.

Suspected Pregnancy

- Assess for pregnancy, including ectopic pregnancy.
- Explain that an IUD in the uterus during pregnancy increases the risk of preterm delivery or miscarriage, including infected (septic) miscarriage during the first or second trimester, which can be life-threatening.
- If the woman does not want to continue the pregnancy, counsel her according to program guidelines.

(Continued on next page)

- If she continues the pregnancy:
  - Advise her that it is best to remove the IUD.
  - Explain the risks of pregnancy with an IUD in place. Early removal of the IUD reduces these risks, although the removal procedure itself involves a small risk of miscarriage.
  - If she agrees to removal, gently remove the IUD or refer for removal.
  - Explain that she should return at once if she develops any signs of miscarriage or septic miscarriage (vaginal bleeding, cramping, pain, abnormal vaginal discharge, or fever).
  - If she chooses to keep the IUD, a nurse or doctor should follow her pregnancy closely. She should see a nurse or doctor at once if she develops any signs of septic miscarriage.
- If the IUD strings are not visible and cannot be found in the cervical canal, the IUD cannot be safely retrieved. Refer for ultrasound, if possible, to determine whether the IUD is still in the uterus. If it is, or if ultrasound is not available, her pregnancy should be followed closely. She should seek care at once if she develops any signs of septic miscarriage.

Questions and Answers About the Copper-Bearing IUD

1. Does the IUD cause pelvic inflammatory disease (PID)?

By itself, the IUD does not cause PID. Gonorrhea and chlamydia are the primary direct causes of PID. IUD *insertion* when a woman has gonorrhea or chlamydia may lead to PID, however. This does not happen often. When it does, it is most likely to occur in the first 20 days after IUD insertion. It has been estimated that, in a group of clients where STIs are common and screening questions identify half the STI cases, there might be 1 case of PID in every 666 IUD insertions (or less than 2 per 1,000) (see Assessing Women for Risk of Sexually Transmitted Infections, p. 162).

2. Can young women and older women use IUDs?

Yes. There is no minimum or maximum age limit. An IUD should be removed after menopause has occurred—within 12 months after her last monthly bleeding (see Women Near Menopause, p. 325).

3. **If a current IUD user has a sexually transmitted infection (STI) or has become at very high individual risk of infection with an STI, should her IUD be removed?**

No. If a woman develops a new STI after her IUD has been inserted, she is not especially at risk of developing PID because of the IUD. She can continue to use the IUD while she is being treated for the STI. Removing the IUD has no benefit and may leave her at risk of unwanted pregnancy. Counsel her on condom use and other strategies to avoid STIs in the future.

4. **Does the IUD make a woman infertile?**

No. A woman can become pregnant once the IUD is removed just as quickly as a woman who has never used an IUD, although fertility decreases as women get older. Good studies find no increased risk of infertility among women who have used IUDs, including young women and women with no children. Whether or not a woman has an IUD, however, if she develops PID and it is not treated, there is some chance that she will become infertile.

5. **Can a woman who has never had a baby use an IUD?**

Yes. A woman who has not had children generally can use an IUD, but she should understand that the IUD is more likely to come out because her uterus may be smaller than the uterus of a woman who has given birth.

6. **Can the IUD travel from the woman's uterus to other parts of her body, such as her heart or her brain?**

The IUD never travels to the heart, brain, or any other part of the body outside the abdomen. The IUD normally stays within the uterus like a seed within a shell. Rarely, the IUD may come through the wall of the uterus into the abdominal cavity. This is most often due to a mistake during insertion. If it is discovered within 6 weeks or so after insertion or if it is causing symptoms at any time, the IUD will need to be removed by laparoscopic or laparotomic surgery. Usually, however, the out-of-place IUD causes no problems and should be left where it is. The woman will need another contraceptive method.

7. **Should a woman have a "rest period" after using her IUD for several years or after the IUD reaches its recommended time for removal?**

No. This is not necessary, and it could be harmful. Removing the old IUD and immediately inserting a new IUD poses less risk of infection than 2 separate procedures. Also, a woman could become pregnant during a "rest period" before her new IUD is inserted.

8. Should antibiotics be routinely given before IUD insertion?

No, usually not. Most recent research done where STIs are not common suggests that PID risk is low with or without antibiotics. When appropriate questions to screen for STI risk are used and IUD insertion is done with proper infection-prevention procedures (including the no-touch insertion technique), there is little risk of infection. Antibiotics may be considered, however, in areas where STIs are common and STI screening is limited.

9. Must an IUD be inserted only during a woman's monthly bleeding?

No. For a woman having menstrual cycles, an IUD can be inserted at any time during her menstrual cycle if it is reasonably certain that she is not pregnant. Inserting the IUD during her monthly bleeding may be a good time because she is not likely to be pregnant, and insertion may be easier. It is not as easy to see signs of infection during monthly bleeding, however.

10. Do IUDs increase the risk of ectopic pregnancy?

No. On the contrary, IUDs greatly reduce the risk of ectopic pregnancy. Ectopic pregnancies are rare among IUD users. The rate of ectopic pregnancy among women with IUDs is 12 per 10,000 women per year. The rate of ectopic pregnancy among women in the United States using no contraceptive method is 65 per 10,000 women per year.

On the rare occasions that the IUD fails and pregnancy occurs, 6 to 8 of every 100 of these pregnancies are ectopic. Thus, the great majority of pregnancies after IUD failure are not ectopic. Still, ectopic pregnancy can be life-threatening, and so a provider should be aware that ectopic pregnancy is possible if the IUD fails.

CHAPTER 11

Levonorgestrel Intrauterine Device

Key Points for Providers and Clients

- **Long-term pregnancy protection.** Very effective for 5 years, immediately reversible.
- **Inserted into the uterus by a specifically trained provider.**
- **Little required of the client once the LNG-IUD is in place.**
- **Bleeding changes are common but not harmful.** Typically, lighter and fewer days of bleeding, or infrequent or irregular bleeding.

What Is the Levonorgestrel Intrauterine Device?

- The levonorgestrel intrauterine device (LNG-IUD) is a T-shaped plastic device that steadily releases a small amount of levonorgestrel each day. (Levonorgestrel is a progestin hormone also used in some contraceptive implants and oral contraceptive pills.)
- A specifically trained health care provider inserts it into a woman's uterus through her vagina and cervix.
- Also called the levonorgestrel-releasing intrauterine system, LNG-IUS, or hormonal IUD.
- Marketed under such brand names as Mirena, Liletta, Kyleena, Skyla, and Jaydess. The Kyleena, Skyla, and Jaydess IUDs and their inserters are slightly smaller than the Mirena and Liletta.
- Works by preventing sperm from fertilizing an egg.

How Effective?

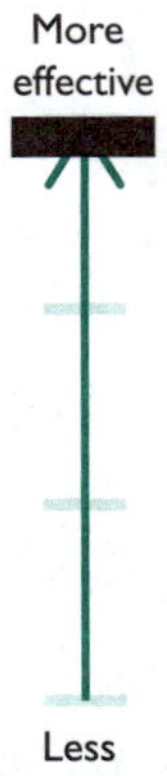

One of the most effective and long-lasting methods:

- Less than 1 pregnancy per 100 women using an LNG-IUD over the first year (2 per 1,000 women). This means that 998 of every 1,000 women using LNG-IUDs will not become pregnant.
- A small risk of pregnancy remains beyond the first year of use and continues as long as the woman is using the LNG-IUD.
  - Over 5 years of use of the Mirena LNG-IUD: Less than 1 pregnancy per 100 women (5 to 8 per 1,000 women).
- Mirena and Kyleena are approved for up to 5 years of use. Research suggests that Mirena may remain highly effective for up to 7 years. Liletta, Skyla, and Jaydess are approved for up to 3 years of use.

Return of fertility after LNG-IUD is removed: No delay

Protection against sexually transmitted infections (STIs): None

Side Effects, Health Benefits, Health Risks, and Complications

Side Effects (see also Managing Any Problems, p. 202)

Some users report the following:

- Most commonly, changes in bleeding patterns,[†] including:
  - Lighter bleeding and fewer days of bleeding
  - Infrequent bleeding
  - Irregular bleeding
  - No monthly bleeding
  - Prolonged bleeding
- Acne
- Headaches
- Breast tenderness or pain
- Nausea
- Weight gain
- Dizziness
- Mood changes

> Bleeding changes are normal and not harmful. If a woman finds them bothersome, counseling and support can help.

Other possible physical changes:

- Ovarian cysts

[†] *For definitions of bleeding patterns, see "vaginal bleeding," p. 407.*

Known Health Benefits

Helps protect against:

- Risks of pregnancy
- Iron-deficiency anemia

May help protect against:

- Endometrial cancer
- Cervical cancer

Reduces:

- Menstrual cramps
- Heavy monthly bleeding
- Symptoms of endometriosis (pelvic pain, irregular bleeding)
- Risk of ectopic pregnancy

Known Health Risks

Rare:

- In the short term PID may occur if the woman has gonorrhea or chlamydia at the time of insertion.

Complications

Rare:

- Puncturing (perforation) of the wall of the uterus by the LNG-IUD or an instrument used for insertion. Usually heals without treatment.

Very rare:

- Miscarriage, preterm birth, or infection in the very rare case that the woman becomes pregnant with the LNG-IUD in place.

Correcting Misunderstandings

LNG-IUDs:

- Can be used by women of any age, including adolescents.
- Can be used by women who have had children and those who have not.
- Do not increase the risk of contracting STIs, including HIV.
- Do not increase the risk of miscarriage when a woman becomes pregnant after the IUD is removed.
- Do not make women infertile.
- Do not cause birth defects.
- Do not cause cancer.
- Do not move to the heart or brain.
- Do not cause discomfort or pain for the woman or the man during sex.

Why Some Women Say They Like the LNG-IUD

- Prevents pregnancy very effectively
- Makes bleeding lighter and can prevent monthly bleeding for many months (amenorrhea)
- Is long-lasting
- Is private—usually no one else can tell a woman is using contraception (sometimes a partner may feel the strings during sex)
- Has no further costs for supplies after the IUD is inserted
- Does not require the user to do anything once the IUD is inserted

Who Can and Cannot Use Levonorgestrel IUDs

Nearly All Women Can Use LNG-IUDs

LNG-IUDs are safe and effective for nearly all women, including women who:

- Have or have not had children
- Are married or are not married
- Are of any age, including adolescents and women over 40 years old
- Have just had an abortion or miscarriage (if no evidence of infection)
- Are breastfeeding
- Do hard physical work
- Have had ectopic pregnancy
- Have had pelvic inflammatory disease (PID)
- Have vaginal infections
- Have anemia
- Have HIV clinical disease that is mild or with no symptoms, whether or not they are on antiretroviral therapy (see LNG-IUD for Women With HIV, p. 189)

Avoid Unnecessary Procedures

(see Importance of Procedures, p. 368)

Women can begin using IUDs:

- Without cervical cancer screening
- Without a breast examination
- Without a blood pressure check

A pelvic examination and an STI risk assessment are essential. When available, a hemoglobin test and laboratory tests for STIs including HIV can contribute to safe and effective use.

Medical Eligibility Criteria for

Levonorgestrel IUDs

Ask the client the questions below about known medical conditions. If she answers "no" to all of the questions (and no contraindications are found on pelvic exam; see p. 188), then she can have an LNG-IUD inserted. If she answers "yes" to a question, follow the instructions. In some cases she can still have an LNG-IUD inserted.

1. Did you give birth more than 48 hours ago but less than 4 weeks ago?

❑ NO ❑ **YES** Delay inserting an LNG-IUD until 4 or more weeks after childbirth (see Soon after childbirth, p. 193).

2. Do you have an infection following childbirth or abortion?

❑ NO ❑ **YES** If she currently has infection of the reproductive organs during the first 6 weeks after childbirth (puerperal sepsis) or she just had an abortion-related infection in the uterus (septic abortion), do not insert the LNG-IUD. Treat or refer if she is not already receiving care. Help her choose another method or offer a backup method.* After treatment, re-evaluate for LNG-IUD use.

3. Do you now have a blood clot in the deep veins of your leg or lungs?

❑ NO ❑ **YES** If she was recently diagnosed with a blood clot in legs (affecting deep veins, not superficial veins) or in a lung, and she is not on anticoagulant therapy, help her choose a method without hormones.

4. Do you have severe cirrhosis or severe liver tumor?

❑ NO ❑ **YES** If she reports severe cirrhosis or severe liver tumor such as liver cancer, do not provide the LNG-IUD. Help her choose a method without hormones.

5. Do you have or have you ever had breast cancer?

❑ NO ❑ **YES** Do not insert the LNG-IUD. Help her choose a method without hormones.

(Continued on next page)

* *Backup methods include abstinence, male and female condoms, spermicides, and withdrawal. Tell her that spermicides and withdrawal are the least effective contraceptive methods. If possible, give her condoms.*

6. Are you having vaginal bleeding that is unusual for you?

❑ NO ❑ **YES** If she has unexplained vaginal bleeding that suggests pregnancy or an underlying medical condition, use of an LNG-IUD could make diagnosis and monitoring of any treatment more difficult. Help her choose a method to use while being evaluated (but not a copper-bearing IUD, progestin-only injectable, or implant) and, if indicated, treated. After diagnosis/treatment, re-evaluate for IUD use.

7. Do you have any female conditions or problems (gynecologic or obstetric conditions or problems), such as genital cancer, pelvic tuberculosis, or gestational trophoblastic disease?

❑ NO ❑ **YES** If she has current cervical, endometrial, or ovarian cancer; pelvic tuberculosis; or gestational trophoblastic disease, do not insert an LNG-IUD. Treat or refer for care if she is not already receiving care. Help her choose another method. In case of pelvic tuberculosis, re-evaluate for LNG-IUD use after treatment.

8. Do you have HIV or AIDS? Do you have any health conditions associated with HIV infection?

❑ NO ❑ **YES** If a woman has HIV infection with severe or advanced clinical disease, do not insert an LNG-IUD. In contrast, a woman living with HIV who has mild clinical disease or no clinical disease can have an IUD inserted, whether or not she is on antretroviral therapy. (See LNG-IUD for Women With HIV, p. 189.)

9. Assess whether she is at very high individual risk for STIs.

Women who have a very high individual likelihood of STIs should not have an LNG-IUD inserted unless gonorrhea and chlamydia are ruled out by lab tests (see Assessing Women for Risk of Sexually Transmitted Infections, p. 190).

10. Rule out pregnancy.

Ask the client the questions in the Pregnancy Checklist (see inside back cover). If she answers "yes" to any of these questions, you can be reasonably certain that she is not pregnant and she can have an LNG-IUD inserted.

If the Pregnancy Checklist cannot rule out pregnancy, use another tool before inserting an LNG-IUD (see Ruling Out Pregnancy, p. 439).

Also, women should not use LNG-IUDs if they report having systemic lupus erythematosus with positive (or unknown) anti-phospholipid antibodies, but are not receiving immunosuppressive treatment. For complete classifications, see Medical Eligibility Criteria for Contraceptive Use, p. 388.

Be sure to explain the health benefits and risks and the side effects of the method that the client will use. Also, point out any conditions that would make the method inadvisable, when relevant to the client.

Using Clinical Judgment in Special Cases

Usually, a woman with any of the conditions listed below should not use an LNG-IUD. In special circumstances, however, when other, more appropriate methods are not available or acceptable to her, a qualified provider who can carefully assess a specific woman's condition and situation may decide that she can use an LNG-IUD. The provider needs to consider the severity of her condition and, for most conditions, whether she will have access to follow-up.

- Between 48 hours and 4 weeks since giving birth
- Acute blood clot in deep veins of legs or lungs
- Had breast cancer more than 5 years ago, and it has not returned
- Severe cirrhosis or severe liver tumor
- Noncancerous (benign) gestational trophoblast disease
- Has current ovarian cancer
- Is at very high individual risk for STIs at the time of insertion
- Has severe or advanced HIV clinical disease
- Has systemic lupus erythematosus with positive (or unknown) antiphospholipid antibodies and is not receiving immunosuppressive treatment

Screening Questions for Pelvic Examination Before IUD Insertion

A pelvic examination and STI risk assessment should be done before IUD insertion. (For STI risk assessment see page 190.) When performing the pelvic examination (both bimanual and speculum), asking yourself the questions below helps you check for signs of conditions that would rule out IUD insertion. If the answer to all of the questions is "no," then the client can have an IUD inserted. If the answer to any question is "yes," do not insert an IUD.

For questions 1 through 5, if the answer is "yes," refer for diagnosis and treatment as appropriate. Help her choose another contraceptive method and counsel her about condom use if she faces any risk of STIs. Give her condoms, if possible. If an STI or pelvic inflammatory disease (PID) is confirmed and she still wants an IUD, it may be inserted as soon as she finishes treatment, if she is not at risk for reinfection before insertion.

1. Is there any type of ulcer on the vulva, vagina, or cervix?

❑ NO ❑ **YES** Possible STI.

2. Does the client feel pain in her lower abdomen when you move the cervix?

❑ NO ❑ **YES** Possible PID.

3. Is there tenderness in the uterus, ovaries, or fallopian tubes (adnexal tenderness)?

❑ NO ❑ **YES** Possible PID.

4. Is there a purulent cervical discharge?

❑ NO ❑ **YES** Possible STI or PID.

5. Does the cervix bleed easily when touched?

❑ NO ❑ **YES** Possible STI or cervical cancer.

6. Is there an anatomical abnormality of the uterine cavity that will prevent correct IUD placement?

❑ NO ❑ **YES** If an anatomical abnormality distorts the uterine cavity, proper IUD placement may not be possible. If available, an ultrasound examination can help determine if proper IUD placement is possible. If not, help her choose another method.

7. Were you unable to determine the size and/or position of the uterus?

❑ NO ❑ **YES** Determining the size and position of the uterus before IUD insertion is essential to ensure high placement of the IUD and to minimize risk of perforation. If size and position cannot be determined, do not insert an IUD. Help her choose another method.

LNG-IUD for Women With HIV

- Women living with HIV can safely have an LNG-IUD inserted if they have mild or no clinical disease, whether or not they are on antiretroviral therapy.
- Women who have HIV infection with advanced or severe clinical disease should *not* have an IUD inserted.
- If a woman becomes infected with HIV while she has an IUD in place, it does not need to be removed.
- An IUD user living with HIV who develops advanced or severe clinical disease can keep the IUD but should be closely monitored for pelvic inflammatory disease.
- Urge women who have HIV or are at risk for HIV to use condoms along with the IUD. Used consistently and correctly, condoms help prevent transmission of HIV and other STIs.
- Women who are at risk of HIV but not infected with HIV can have an IUD inserted. The IUD does not increase the risk of becoming infected with HIV.

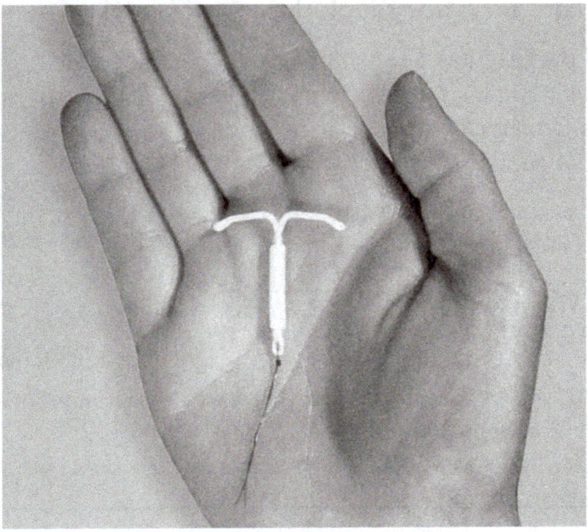

Assessing Women for Risk of Sexually Transmitted Infections

A woman who has gonorrhea or chlamydia now should not have an IUD inserted. Having these sexually transmitted infections (STIs) at the time of insertion may increase the risk of pelvic inflammatory disease. These STIs may be difficult to diagnose clinically, however, and reliable laboratory tests are time-consuming, expensive, and sometimes unavailable. Without clinical signs or symptoms and without laboratory testing, the only indication that a woman might already have an STI is whether her behavior or her situation places her at *very high individual risk* of infection. If this risk for the *individual* client is very high, she generally should not have an IUD inserted.‡ (Local STI prevalence rates are not a basis for judging individual risk.)

There is no universal set of questions that will determine if a woman is at very high individual risk for STIs. Instead of asking questions, providers can discuss with the client the personal behaviors and the situations in their community that are most likely to expose women to STIs.

Steps to take:

1. Tell the client that a woman who faces a very high individual risk of STIs usually should not have an IUD inserted.
2. Ask the woman to consider her own risk and to think about whether she might have an STI. A woman is often the best judge of her own risk.§ She does not have to tell the provider about her behavior or her partner's behavior. Providers can explain possibly risky situations that may place a woman at very high individual risk. The client can think about whether such situations occurred recently (in the past 3 months or so). If so, she may have an STI now, whether or not she has noticed symptoms, and may want to choose a method other than the IUD.

Possibly risky situations include:

- A sexual partner has STI symptoms such as pus coming from his penis, pain or burning during urination, or an open sore in the genital area
- She or a sexual partner was diagnosed with an STI recently
- She has had more than one sexual partner recently

All of these situations pose less risk if a woman or her partner uses condoms consistently and correctly.

‡ In contrast, if a current IUD user's situation changes and she finds herself at very high individual risk for gonorrhea or chlamydia, she can keep using her IUD.

§ Any woman who thinks she might have an STI should seek care immediately.

- She has a sexual partner who has had other partners recently

Also, a provider can mention other high-risk situations that exist locally.

3. Ask if she thinks she is a good candidate for an IUD or would like to consider other contraceptive methods, including other long-acting methods. If, after considering her individual risk, she thinks she is a good candidate, and she is eligible, provide her with an IUD. If she wants to consider other methods or if you have strong reason to believe that the client is at very high individual risk of infection, help her choose another method.

Note: If she still wants the IUD while at very high individual risk of STIs, and reliable laboratory testing for gonorrhea and chlamydia is available, a woman who tests negative can have an IUD inserted. A woman who tests positive can have an IUD inserted as soon as she finishes treatment, if she is not at risk of reinfection by the time of insertion.

In special circumstances, if other, more appropriate methods are not available or not acceptable, a health care provider who can carefully assess a specific woman's condition and situation may decide that a woman at very high individual risk can have the IUD inserted even if STI testing is not available. (Depending on the circumstances, the provider may consider presumptively treating her with a full curative dose of antibiotics effective against both gonorrhea and chlamydia and inserting the IUD after she finishes treatment.) Whether or not she receives presumptive treatment, the provider should be sure that the client can return for the follow-up visit, will be carefully checked for infection, and will be treated immediately if needed. She should be asked to return at once if she develops a fever and either lower abdominal pain or abnormal vaginal discharge or both.

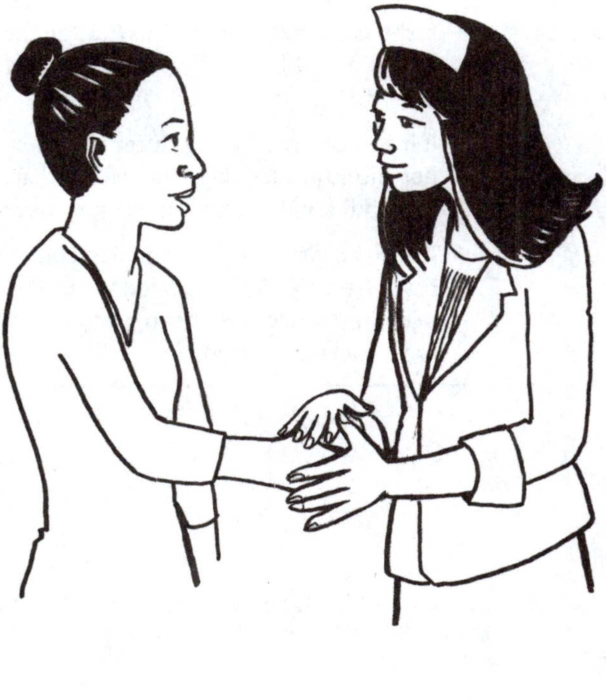

Providing the Levonorgestrel Intrauterine Device

When to Start

IMPORTANT: In many cases a woman can start the LNG-IUD any time if it is reasonably certain she is not pregnant. To be reasonably certain she is not pregnant, use the Pregnancy Checklist (see inside back cover).

Woman's situation	When to start
Having menstrual cycles or switching from a nonhormonal method	**Any time of the month** • If she is starting within 7 days after the start of her monthly bleeding, no need for a backup method. • If it is more than 7 days after the start of her monthly bleeding, she can have the LNG-IUD inserted any time if it is reasonably certain she is not pregnant. She will need a backup method* for the first 7 days after insertion.
Switching from a hormonal method	• Immediately, if she has been using the method consistently and correctly or if it is otherwise reasonably certain she is not pregnant. No need to wait for her next monthly bleeding. • If she is starting within 7 days after the start of her monthly bleeding, no need for a backup method. • If it is more than 7 days after the start of her monthly bleeding, she will need a backup method* for the first 7 days after insertion. • If she is switching from an injectable, she can have the LNG-IUD inserted when the repeat injection would have been given. No need for a backup method.

* *Backup methods include abstinence, male and female condoms, spermicides, and withdrawal. Tell her that spermicides and withdrawal are the least effective contraceptive methods. If possible, give her condoms.*

Woman's situation	When to start
Soon after childbirth (regardless of breastfeeding status)	• Any time within 48 hours after giving birth (requires a provider with specific training in postpartum insertion by hand or using a ring forceps). • After 48 hours, delay until at least 4 weeks.
Fully or nearly fully breastfeeding Less than 6 months after giving birth	• If the LNG-IUD is not inserted within the first 48 hours and her monthly bleeding has not returned, she can have the LNG-IUD inserted any time between 4 weeks and 6 months. No need for a backup method. • If her monthly bleeding has returned, she can have the LNG-IUD inserted as advised for women having menstrual cycles (see previous page).
More than 6 months since giving birth	• If her monthly bleeding has not returned, she can have the LNG-IUD inserted any time if it is reasonably certain she is not pregnant. She will need a backup method for the first 7 days after insertion. • If her monthly bleeding has returned, she can have the LNG-IUD inserted as advised for women having menstrual cycles (see previous page).
Partially breastfeeding or not breastfeeding	
Less than 4 weeks after giving birth	• If the LNG-IUD is not inserted within the first 48 hours, delay insertion until at least 4 weeks after giving birth.
More than 4 weeks after giving birth	• If her monthly bleeding has not returned, she can have the LNG-IUD inserted any time *if it can be determined that she is not pregnant* (see Ruling Out Pregnancy, p. 439). She will need a backup method for the first 7 days after insertion. • If her monthly bleeding has returned, she can have the LNG-IUD inserted as advised for women having menstrual cycles (see previous page).

Woman's situation	When to start
No monthly bleeding (not related to childbirth or breastfeeding)	• Any time *if it can be determined that she is not pregnant* (see Ruling Out Pregnancy, p. 439). She will need a backup method for the first 7 days after insertion.
After miscarriage or abortion	• Immediately, if the LNG-IUD is inserted within 7 days after first- or second-trimester abortion or miscarriage and if no infection is present. No need for a backup method. • If it is more than 7 days after first- or second-trimester miscarriage or abortion and no infection is present, she can have the LNG-IUD inserted any time if it is reasonably certain she is not pregnant. She will need a backup method for the first 7 days after insertion. • If infection is present, treat or refer and help the client choose another method. If she still wants the LNG-IUD, it can be inserted after the infection has completely cleared. • LNG-IUD insertion after second-trimester abortion or miscarriage requires specific training. If not specifically trained, delay insertion until at least 4 weeks after miscarriage or abortion.
After taking progestin-only, combined, or ulipristal acetate (UPA) emergency contraceptive pills (ECPs)	• She can have the LNG IUD inserted *when it can be determined that she is not pregnant,* for example, after the start of her next monthly bleeding (see Ruling Out Pregnancy, p. 439). Give her a backup method or oral contraceptive pills to use until she can have the IUD inserted. • She should not have the LNG-IUD inserted in the first 6 days after taking UPA-ECPs. These drugs interact. If the LNG-IUD is inserted sooner, and thus both LNG and UPA are present in the body, one or both may be less effective.

Preventing Infection at LNG-IUD Insertion

Proper insertion technique can help prevent many problems, such as infection, expulsion, and perforation.

- Follow proper infection-prevention procedures.
- Use high-level disinfected or sterile instruments. High-level disinfect by boiling, steaming, or soaking instruments in disinfectant chemicals.
- Use a new, presterilized LNG-IUD that is packaged with its inserter.
- The "no-touch" insertion technique is safest. This includes not letting the loaded IUD or uterine sound touch any unsterile surfaces (for example, hands, speculum, vagina, table top). The no-touch technique involves:
  - Cleaning the cervix thoroughly with antiseptic before IUD insertion
  - Being careful not to touch the vaginal wall or speculum blades with the uterine sound or loaded IUD inserter
  - Passing both the uterine sound and the loaded IUD inserter only once each through the cervical canal
- Giving antibiotics routinely is generally not recommended for women at low risk of STIs.

Giving Advice on Side Effects

IMPORTANT: Thorough counseling about bleeding changes must come before IUD insertion. Counseling about bleeding changes may be the most important help a woman needs to keep using the method without concern.

Describe the most common side effects

- Changes in bleeding patterns:
  - Irregular bleeding followed by lighter bleeding, fewer days of bleeding, infrequent bleeding, and then no monthly bleeding.
- Acne, headaches, breast tenderness and pain, and possibly other side effects.

Explain about these side effects

- Bleeding changes usually are not signs of illness. Lack of bleeding does not mean pregnancy.
- Bleeding irregularities usually become less within 3 to 6 months after insertion. Many women have no bleeding at all after using the LNG-IUD for a year or two. Other side effects also become less after the first several months following insertion.
- The client can come back for help if side effects bother her or if she has other concerns.

Inserting the LNG-IUD

Talk with the client before the procedure	• Explain the insertion procedure (see next page). • Show her the speculum, tenaculum, and the IUD and inserter in the package. • Tell her that she will experience some discomfort or cramping during the procedure, and that this is to be expected. • Ask her to tell you any time that she feels discomfort or pain. • Ibuprofen (200–400 mg), paracetamol (325–1000 mg), or other pain reliever may be given 30 minutes before insertion to help reduce cramping and pain. Do not give aspirin, which slows blood clotting.
Talk with the client during the procedure	• Tell her what is happening, step by step, and reassure her. • Alert her before a step that may cause pain or might startle her. • Ask from time to time if she is feeling pain.
Talk with the client after the procedure	• Ask her how she is doing. • Tell her that the procedure was successful and that the IUD is in place. • Tell her that she can rest for a while and then slowly sit up before getting up and dressing. • Remind her that the two of you will be discussing next steps and follow-up.

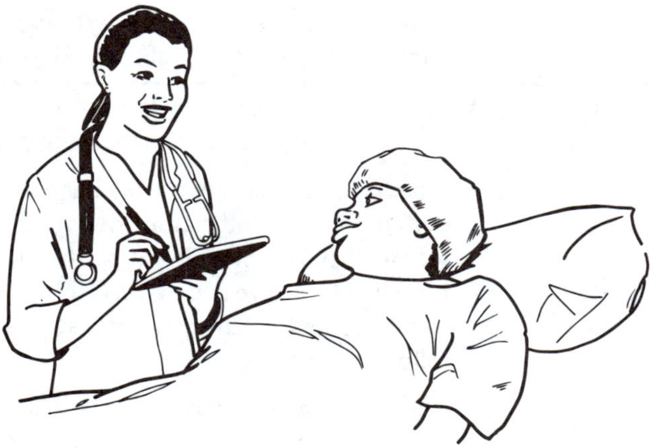

Explaining the Insertion Procedure

A woman who has chosen the LNG-IUD needs to know what will happen during insertion. The following description can help explain the procedure to her. Learning LNG-IUD insertion requires training and practice under direct supervision. Therefore, this description is a summary and not detailed instructions.

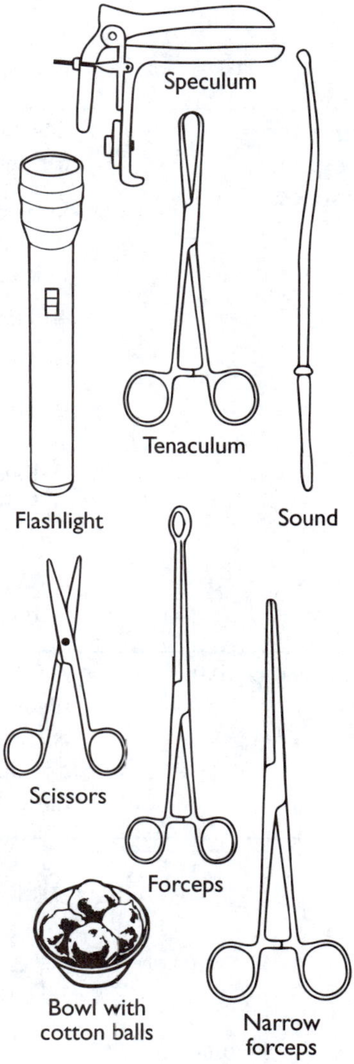

1. The provider uses proper infection-prevention procedures.
2. The provider conducts a pelvic examination to determine the position of the uterus and assess eligibility (see Screening Questions for Pelvic Examination Before IUD Insertion, p. 188). The provider first does the bimanual examination and then inserts a speculum into the vagina to inspect the cervix.
3. The provider cleans the cervix and vagina with appropriate antiseptic.
4. The provider slowly inserts the tenaculum through the speculum and closes the tenaculum just enough to gently hold the cervix and uterus steady.
5. The provider slowly and gently passes the uterine sound through the cervix to measure the depth of the uterus.
6. The provider slowly and gently passes the inserter through the cervix, releases the LNG-IUD inside the uterine cavity, and removes the inserter.
7. The provider cuts the strings on the IUD, leaving about 3 centimeters hanging out of the cervix.
8. After the insertion, the woman rests. She remains on the examination table until she feels ready to get dressed.

Supporting the User

Giving Specific Instructions

Expect cramping and pain

- She can expect some cramping and pain for a few days after insertion.
- Suggest ibuprofen (200–400 mg), paracetamol (325–1000 mg), or other pain reliever as needed.
- Also, she can expect some bleeding or spotting immediately after insertion.

Length of pregnancy protection

- Discuss how to remember the date to return for removal or replacement.
- Give each woman the following information in writing on a reminder card, like the one shown below, if possible, and explain:
  - The type of IUD she has
  - Date of IUD insertion
  - Month and year when IUD will need to be removed or replaced. (For the Mirena and Kyleena LNG-IUDs, 5 years after insertion. For the Liletta, Skyla, and Jaydess LNG-IUDs, 3 years after insertion.)
  - Where to go if she has problems or questions about her IUD.

Follow-up visit

- A follow-up visit after her first monthly bleeding or 3 to 6 weeks after IUD insertion is recommended. No woman should be denied an IUD, however, because follow-up would be difficult or not possible.

IUD Reminder Card

Client's name: ____________________

Type of IUD: ____________________

Date inserted: ____________________

Remove or replace by: Month ______ Year ______

If you have any problems or questions, go to:

(name and location of facility)

How Can a Partner Help?

The client's partner is welcome to participate in counseling and learn about the method and what support he can give to his partner. A male partner can:

- Support a woman's choice of the LNG-IUD
- Show understanding and support if she has side effects
- Use condoms consistently in addition to the IUD if he has an STI/HIV or thinks he may be at risk of an STI/HIV
- Help to remember when the IUD is due for removal

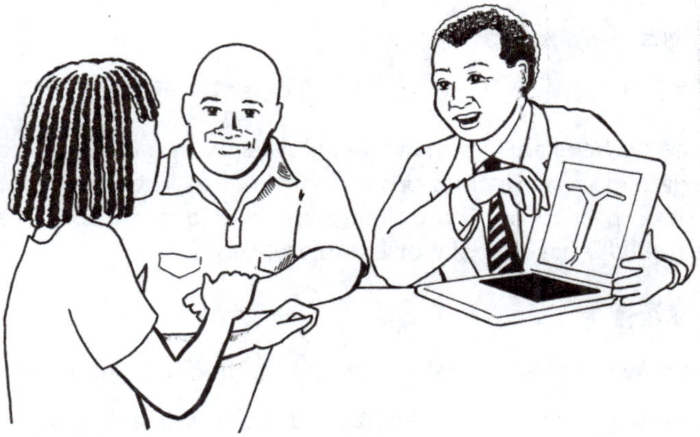

"Come Back Any Time": Reasons to Return

Assure every client that she is welcome to come back any time—for example, if she has problems, questions, or wants another method; or she has a major change in health status. Also if:

- The IUD was expelled or she thinks it may have been expelled from her uterus.
- She has symptoms of pelvic inflammatory disease (increasing or severe pain in the lower abdomen, pain during sex, unusual vaginal discharge, fever, chills, nausea, and/or vomiting), especially in the first 20 days after insertion.
- She thinks she might be pregnant.
- She wants the IUD removed, whatever the reason.

General health advice: Anyone who suddenly feels that something is seriously wrong with her health should immediately seek medical care from a nurse or doctor. Her contraceptive method is most likely not the cause of the condition, but she should tell the nurse or doctor what method she is using.

Helping Continuing Users

Post-Insertion Follow-Up Visit (3 to 6 Weeks)

1. Ask how the client is doing with the method and whether she is satisfied. Ask if she has any questions or anything to discuss.
2. Ask especially if she is concerned about bleeding changes. Give her any information or help that she needs (see Managing Any Problems, p. 202).
3. Ask her if she has:
   - Increasing or severe abdominal pain or pain during sex or urination
   - Unusual vaginal discharge
   - Fever or chills
   - Signs or symptoms of pregnancy
   - Felt the hard plastic of an IUD that has partially come out

A routine pelvic examination at the follow-up visit is not required. It may be appropriate in some settings or for some clients, however. Conduct a pelvic examination particularly if the client's answers lead you to suspect infection or that the IUD has partially or completely come out.

Any Visit

1. Ask how the client is doing with the method and about bleeding changes.
2. Ask a long-term client if she has had any new health problems. Address problems as appropriate. For new health problems that may require switching methods, see p. 208.
3. Ask a long-term client about major life changes that may affect her needs—particularly plans for having children and STI/HIV risk. Follow up as needed.
4. Remind her how much longer the IUD will protect her from pregnancy.

Removing the Intrauterine Device

IMPORTANT: Providers must not refuse or delay when a woman asks to have her IUD removed, whatever her reason, whether it is personal or medical. All staff must understand and agree that she must not be pressured or forced to continue using the IUD.

If a woman is finding side effects difficult to tolerate, first discuss the problems she is having (see Managing Any Problems, p. 202). Ask if she would rather try to manage the problem or to have the IUD removed immediately.

Removing an IUD is usually simple. It can be done any time of the month. Removal may be easier during monthly bleeding, when the cervix is naturally softened. In cases of uterine perforation or if removal is not easy (for example, when IUD strings are missing), refer the woman to an experienced clinician who can use an appropriate removal technique.

Explaining the Removal Procedure

Before removing the IUD, explain to the client what will happen during removal:

1. The provider inserts a speculum to see the cervix and IUD strings and carefully cleans the cervix and vagina with an antiseptic solution, such as iodine.
2. The provider asks the woman to take slow, deep breaths and to relax. The woman should say if she feels pain during the procedure.
3. Using narrow forceps, the provider pulls the IUD strings slowly and gently until the IUD comes completely out of the cervix.

Switching From the LNG-IUD to Another Method

These guidelines ensure that the client is protected from pregnancy without interruption when switching from the LNG-IUD to another method. See also When to Start for each method.

Switching to	When to start
Hormonal methods: combined oral contraceptives (COCs), progestin-only pills (POPs), progestin-only injectables, monthly injectables, combined patch, combined vaginal ring, or implants	• If starting during the first 7 days of monthly bleeding (first 5 days for COCs and POPs), start the hormonal method now and remove the IUD. No need for a backup method.* • If starting after the first 7 days of monthly bleeding (after the first 5 days for COCs and POPs) and she has had sex since her last monthly bleeding, start the hormonal method now. It is recommended that the IUD stay in place until her next monthly bleeding. • If starting after the first 7 days of monthly bleeding (after the first 5 days for COCs and POPs) and she has not had sex since her last monthly bleeding, the IUD can stay in place and be removed during her next monthly bleeding, or the IUD can be removed and she can use a backup method for the next 7 days (2 days for POPs).

* *Backup methods include abstinence, male and female condoms, spermicides, and withdrawal. Tell her that spermicides and withdrawal are the least effective contraceptive methods. If possible, give her condoms.*

Switching to	When to start
Male or female condoms, spermicides, diaphragms, cervical caps, or withdrawal	• The next time she has sex after the IUD is removed.
Fertility awareness methods	• In the cycle that the IUD is removed.
Female sterilization	• If during the first 7 days of monthly bleeding, remove the IUD and perform the female sterilization procedure. No need for a backup method. • If after the first 7 days of monthly bleeding, perform the sterilization procedure. Ideally, the IUD should stay in place until her follow-up visit or her next monthly bleeding. If a follow-up visit is not possible, remove the IUD at the time of sterilization. No need for a backup method.
Vasectomy	• Any time • The woman can keep the IUD until a test of her partner's semen shows that the vasectomy is working, or for 3 months, when the vasectomy will be fully effective.

Managing Any Problems

Problems Reported As Side Effects or Complications

May or may not be due to the method.

- Problems with side effects or complications affect women's satisfaction and use of IUDs. They deserve the provider's attention. If the client reports any side effects or complications, listen to her concerns, give her advice and support, and, if appropriate, treat. Make sure she understands the advice and agrees.
- Offer to help her choose another method—now, if she wishes, or if problems cannot be overcome.

Irregular bleeding or spotting (bleeding at unexpected times that bothers the client)

- Reassure her that some women using LNG-IUDs experience irregular bleeding. It is not harmful and usually becomes less or stops after the first several months of use.
- If irregular bleeding starts after several months of no bleeding, or you suspect that something may be wrong for other reasons, consider underlying conditions unrelated to method use (see Unexplained vaginal bleeding, p. 208).

No monthly bleeding

- Reassure her that many women eventually stop having monthly bleeding when using the LNG-IUD, and this is not harmful. There is no need to lose blood every month. It is similar to not having monthly bleeding during pregnancy. She is not pregnant or infertile. Blood is not building up inside her. (Some women are happy to be free from monthly bleeding.)
- If monthly bleeding stops very soon after insertion of the LNG-IUD, assess for pregnancy or other underlying condition.

Heavier or prolonged bleeding (longer than 8 days)

- Reassure her that some women using LNG-IUDs experience heavier or prolonged bleeding. It is generally not harmful and usually becomes less or stops after the first several months of use.
- Provide iron tablets if possible and tell her it is important for her to eat foods containing iron.
- If heavier or prolonged bleeding continues or starts after several months of no bleeding, or if you suspect that something may be wrong for other reasons, consider underlying conditions unrelated to method use (see Unexplained vaginal bleeding, p. 208).

Cramping and pain

- She can expect some cramping and pain for the first day or 2 after IUD insertion.
  - Suggest aspirin (325–650 mg), ibuprofen (200–400 mg), paracetamol (325–1000 mg), or other pain reliever. If she also has heavy or prolonged bleeding, aspirin should not be used because it may increase bleeding.
- If cramping continues beyond the first 2 days, evaluate for partial expulsion or perforation.

Acne

- If the client wants to stop using the LNG-IUD because of acne, she can consider switching to COCs. Many women's acne improves with COC use.
- Consider locally available remedies.

Ordinary headaches (nonmigrainous)

- Suggest aspirin (325–650 mg), ibuprofen (200–400 mg), paracetamol (325–1000 mg), or other pain reliever.
- Any headaches that get worse or occur more often during LNG-IUD use should be evaluated.

Breast tenderness

- Recommend that she wear a supportive bra (including during strenuous activity and sleep).
- Try hot or cold compresses.
- Suggest aspirin (325–650 mg), ibuprofen (200–400 mg), paracetamol (325–1000 mg), or other pain reliever.
- Consider locally available remedies.

Weight change

- Review diet and counsel as needed.

Nausea or dizziness

- Consider locally available remedies.

Mood changes

- Clients who have serious mood changes such as major depression should be referred for care.
- Consider locally available remedies.

Partner can feel IUD strings during sex

- Explain that this happens sometimes when strings are cut too short.
- If her partner finds the strings bothersome, describe and discuss this option:
  - Strings can be cut even shorter so they are not coming out of the cervical canal. Her partner will not feel the strings, but it will make the removal procedure somewhat more difficult (may require a specially trained provider).

Severe pain in lower abdomen (suspected pelvic inflammatory disease [PID])

- Some common signs and symptoms of PID often also occur with other abdominal conditions, such as ectopic pregnancy. If ectopic pregnancy is ruled out, assess for PID.
- If possible, do abdominal and pelvic examinations (see Signs and Symptoms of Serious Health Conditions, p. 384, for signs from the pelvic examination that would indicate PID).
- If a pelvic examination is not possible, and she has a combination of the following signs and symptoms in addition to lower abdominal pain, suspect PID:
  - Unusual vaginal discharge
  - Fever or chills
  - Pain during sex or urination
  - Bleeding after sex or between monthly bleeding
  - Nausea and vomiting
  - A tender pelvic mass
  - Pain when the abdomen is gently pressed (direct abdominal tenderness) or when gently pressed and then suddenly released (rebound abdominal tenderness)
- Treat PID or immediately refer for treatment:
  - Because of the serious consequences of PID, health care providers should treat all suspected cases, based on the signs and symptoms above. Treatment should be started as soon as possible. Treatment is more effective at preventing long-term complications when appropriate antibiotics are given immediately.
  - Treat for gonorrhea, chlamydia, and anaerobic bacterial infections. Counsel the client about prevention and treatment of STIs and about condom use. If possible, give her condoms.
  - There is no need to remove the IUD if she wants to continue using it. If she wants it removed, take it out after starting antibiotic treatment. (If the IUD is removed, consider emergency contraceptive pills and discuss choosing another method. See Switching from an LNG-IUD to Another Method, p. 201.)
- If the infection does not improve, consider removing the IUD while continuing antibiotics. If the IUD is not removed, antibiotics should still be continued. In both cases the woman's health should be closely monitored.

Severe pain in lower abdomen (suspected ovarian cyst)

- Abdominal pain may be due to various problems, such as enlarged ovarian follicles or cysts.
  - A woman can continue to use the LNG-IUD during evaluation and treatment.
  - There is no need to treat enlarged ovarian follicles or cysts unless they grow abnormally large, twist, or burst. Reassure the client that they usually disappear on their own. To be sure the problem is resolving, see the client again in 6 weeks, if possible.

Severe pain in lower abdomen (suspected ectopic pregnancy)

- Many conditions can cause severe abdominal pain. Be particularly alert for additional signs or symptoms of ectopic pregnancy, which is rare but can be life-threatening. The LNG-IUD reduces the risk of ectopic pregnancy, but it does not eliminate the risk altogether (see Question 10, p. 180).
- In the early stages of ectopic pregnancy, symptoms may be absent or mild, but eventually they will become severe. A combination of these signs or symptoms should increase suspicion of ectopic pregnancy:
  - Unusual abdominal pain or tenderness
  - Abnormal vaginal bleeding or no monthly bleeding—especially if this is a change from her current bleeding pattern
  - Light-headedness or dizziness
  - Fainting
- If ectopic pregnancy or other serious health condition is suspected, refer at once for immediate diagnosis and care. (See Female Sterilization, Managing Ectopic Pregnancy, p. 227, for more on ectopic pregnancies.)
- If the client does not have these additional symptoms or signs, assess for pelvic inflammatory disease (see Severe pain in lower abdomen, previous page).

Suspected uterine puncturing (perforation)

- If puncturing is suspected at the time of insertion or sounding of the uterus, stop the procedure immediately (and remove the IUD if inserted). Observe the client in the clinic carefully:
  - For the first hour, keep the woman at bed rest and check her vital signs (blood pressure, pulse, respiration, and temperature) every 5 to 10 minutes.
  - If the woman remains stable after one hour, check for signs of intra-abdominal bleeding, such as low hematocrit or hemoglobin or rebound

on abdominal examination, if possible, and her vital signs. Observe for several more hours. If she has no signs or symptoms, she can be sent home, but she should avoid sex for 2 weeks. Help her choose another method.

– If she has a rapid pulse and falling blood pressure, or new pain or increasing pain around the uterus, refer her to a higher level of care.

– If uterine perforation is suspected, based on clinical symptoms, within 6 weeks or more after insertion, refer the client for evaluation to a clinician experienced at removing such IUDs (see Question 6, p. 179).

IUD partially comes out (partial expulsion)

- If the IUD partially comes out, remove the IUD. Discuss with the client whether she wants another IUD or a different method. If she wants another IUD, she can have one inserted immediately if it is reasonably certain she is not pregnant. If the client does not want to continue using an IUD, help her choose another method.

IUD completely comes out (complete expulsion)

- If the client reports that the IUD came out, discuss with her whether she wants another IUD or a different method. If she wants another IUD, she can have one inserted at any time if it is reasonably certain she is not pregnant.
- If complete expulsion is suspected (for example, if strings are not found on pelvic exam) and the client does not know whether the IUD came out, refer for ultrasound (or x-ray, if pregnancy can be ruled out) to assess whether the IUD might have moved to the abdominal cavity. Give her a backup method to use in the meantime.

Missing strings (suggesting possible pregnancy, uterine perforation, or expulsion)

- Ask the client:
  - Whether and when she saw the IUD come out
  - When she had her last monthly bleeding
  - If she has any symptoms of pregnancy
  - If she has used a backup method since she noticed that the IUD came out
- Always start with minor and safe procedures and be gentle. Check for the strings in the folds of the cervical canal with forceps. About half of missing IUD strings can be found in the cervical canal.
- If strings cannot be located in the cervical canal, either they have gone up into the uterus or the IUD has been expelled unnoticed. Refer for ultrasound (or x-ray, if pregnancy can be ruled out). Give her a backup method to use in the meantime, in case the IUD came out.

New Problems That May Require Switching Methods

May or may not be due to the method.

Unexplained vaginal bleeding (that suggests a medical condition not related to the method)

- Refer or evaluate by history or pelvic examination. Diagnose and treat as appropriate.
- She can continue using the IUD while her condition is being evaluated.
- If bleeding is caused by sexually transmitted infection or pelvic inflammatory disease, she can continue using the IUD during treatment.

Heart disease due to blocked or narrowed arteries (ischemic heart disease)

- A woman who has this condition can safely start the LNG-IUD. If, however, the condition develops while she is using the LNG-IUD:
  - Remove the IUD or refer for removal.
  - Help her choose a method without hormones.
  - Refer for diagnosis and care if not already under care.

Migraine headaches (see Identifying Migraine Headaches and Auras, p. 436)

- If she has migraine headaches without aura, she can continue to use the LNG-IUD if she wishes.
- If she develops migraine with aura, remove the LNG-IUD. Help her choose a method without hormones.

Certain serious health conditions (blood clots in deep veins of legs or lungs, breast cancer, gestational trophoblast disease, or pelvic tuberculosis). See Signs and Symptoms of Serious Health Conditions, p. 384.

- Remove the IUD or refer for removal.
- Give her a backup method to use until the condition is evaluated.
- Refer for diagnosis and care if not already under care.

Suspected pregnancy

- Assess for pregnancy, including ectopic pregnancy.
- Explain that exposure of the fetus to an LNG-IUD does not increase the risk of birth defects. However, an IUD in the uterus during pregnancy increases the risk of preterm delivery or miscarriage, including infected (septic) miscarriage during the first or second trimester, which can be life-threatening.
- If the woman does not want to continue the pregnancy, counsel her according to program guidelines.
- If she continues the pregnancy:
  - Advise her that it is best to remove the IUD.
  - Explain the risks of pregnancy with an IUD in place. Early removal of the IUD reduces these risks, although the removal procedure itself involves a small risk of miscarriage.
  - If she agrees to removal, gently remove the IUD or refer for removal.
  - Explain that she should return at once if she develops any signs of miscarriage or septic miscarriage (vaginal bleeding, cramping, pain, abnormal vaginal discharge, or fever).
  - If she chooses to keep the IUD, a nurse or doctor should follow her pregnancy closely. She should see a nurse or doctor at once if she develops any signs of septic miscarriage.
- If the IUD strings are not visible and cannot be found in the cervical canal, the IUD cannot be safely retrieved. Refer for ultrasound, if possible, to determine whether the IUD is still in the uterus. If it is, or if ultrasound is not available, her pregnancy should be followed closely. She should seek care at once if she develops any signs of septic miscarriage.

Questions and Answers About the LNG-IUD

See also Questions and Answers About the Copper-Bearing IUD, pp. 178–180.

1. How is the LNG-IUD different from the copper-bearing IUD?

The LNG-IUD and the copper-bearing IUD are very similar, but they have important differences. Both the LNG-IUD and the copper-bearing IUD are very effective, but the LNG-IUD is slightly more effective. The LNG-IUD has different side effects from those of the copper-bearing IUD. LNG-IUD users usually experience lighter bleeding (regular or irregular) or no bleeding at all, while copper-bearing IUD users usually have regular but sometimes heavier or longer bleeding. In addition, LNG-IUD users may experience hormonal side effects (for example, headaches), which are not side effects of copper-bearing IUDs. The duration of use is shorter—3 or 5 years for the LNG-IUD, depending on brand, versus 12 years for the copper-bearing IUD. Also, the LNG-IUD costs more than the copper-bearing IUD. (See Comparing IUDs, p. 430.)

2. How is the LNG-IUD different from other hormonal methods?

The LNG-IUD continuously releases a small amount of hormone into the uterus. Because the hormone is released directly into the uterus, the amount in the bloodstream is lower than with other hormonal methods. Thus, women experience fewer side effects. The LNG-IUD requires no action by the woman once it is inserted, unlike pills that a woman must take every day or injections that a woman must have every one to three months. The LNG-IUD must be inserted into the uterus, while most other hormonal methods come in the form of pills, injections, or implants under the skin.

3. What are the other benefits of the LNG-IUD, besides contraception?

The LNG-IUD is an effective treatment for heavy monthly blood loss. It is the most effective nonsurgical approach for this condition. Also, the LNG-IUD decreases bleeding for women with fibroids. Reduced blood loss can help women with anemia as well. Additionally, the LNG-IUD may help to treat endometriosis, endometrial hyperplasia, endometrial cancer, and perimenopausal menstrual disturbances.

CHAPTER 12

Female Sterilization

Key Points for Providers and Clients

- **Permanent.** Intended to provide life-long, permanent, and very effective protection against pregnancy. Reversal is usually not possible.
- **Involves a physical examination and surgery.** The procedure is done by a specifically trained provider.
- **No long-term side effects.**

What Is Female Sterilization?

- Permanent surgical contraception for women who will not want more children.
- The 2 surgical approaches most often used:
  - Minilaparotomy involves making a small incision in the abdomen. The fallopian tubes are brought to the incision to be cut or blocked.
  - Laparoscopy involves inserting a long, thin tube containing lenses into the abdomen through a small incision. This laparoscope enables the doctor to reach and block or cut the fallopian tubes in the abdomen.
- Also called tubal sterilization, tubal ligation, voluntary surgical contraception, tubectomy, bi-tubal ligation, tying the tubes, minilap, and "the operation."
- Works because the fallopian tubes are blocked or cut. Eggs released from the ovaries cannot move down the tubes, and so they do not meet sperm.

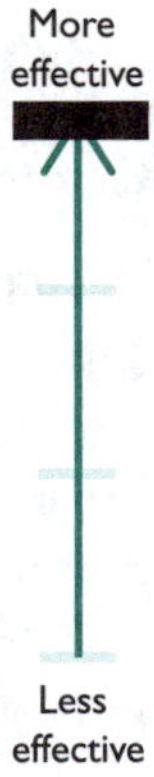

How Effective?

One of the most effective contraceptive methods but carries a small risk of failure:

- Less than 1 pregnancy per 100 women over the first year after having the sterilization procedure (5 per 1,000). This means that 995 of every 1,000 women relying on female sterilization will not become pregnant.

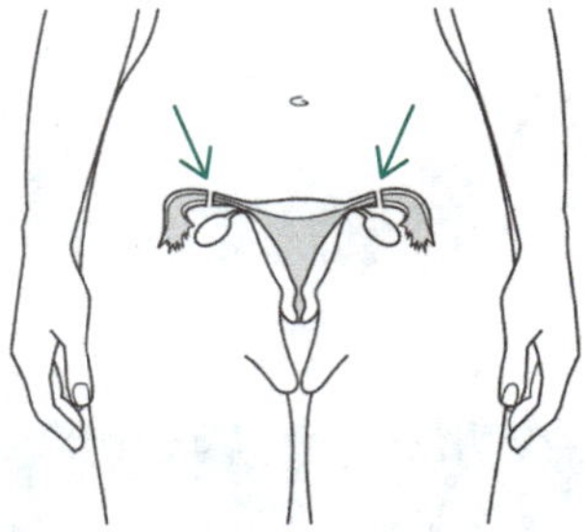

- A small risk of pregnancy remains beyond the first year after the procedure and until the woman reaches menopause.
  - Over 10 years of use: About 2 pregnancies per 100 women (18 to 19 per 1,000 women).
- Effectiveness varies slightly depending on how the tubes are blocked, but pregnancy rates are low with all techniques. One of the most effective techniques is cutting and tying the cut ends of the fallopian tubes after childbirth (postpartum female sterilization).

Fertility does not return because sterilization generally cannot be reversed. The procedure is intended to be permanent. Reversal surgery is difficult, expensive, and not available in most areas. When performed, reversal surgery often does not lead to pregnancy (see Question 7, p. 229).

Protection against sexually transmitted infections (STIs): None

Side Effects, Health Benefits, Health Risks, and Complications

Side Effects

None

Known Health Benefits

Helps protect against:

- Risks of pregnancy
- Pelvic inflammatory disease (PID)

May help protect against:

- Ovarian cancer

Reduces:

- Risk of ectopic pregnancy

Known Health Risks

Uncommon to extremely rare:

- Complications of surgery and anesthesia (see below)

Complications of Surgery (see also Managing Any Problems, p. 226)

Uncommon to extremely rare:

- Female sterilization is a safe method of contraception. It requires surgery and anesthesia, however. Like other minor surgeries, female sterilization carries some risks, such as infection or abscess of the wound. Serious complications are uncommon. Death, due to the procedure or anesthesia, is extremely rare.
- The risk of complications with local anesthesia, with or without sedation and analgesia, is significantly lower than with general anesthesia.

Complications can be kept to a minimum if appropriate techniques are used and if the procedure is performed in an appropriate setting by a skilled provider.

Correcting Misunderstandings (see also Questions and Answers, p. 228)

Female sterilization:

- Does not make women weak.
- Does not cause lasting pain in back, uterus, or abdomen.
- Does not remove a woman's uterus or lead to a need to have it removed.
- Does not cause hormonal imbalances.
- Does not cause heavier bleeding or irregular bleeding or otherwise change women's menstrual cycles.
- Does not cause any changes in weight, appetite, or appearance.
- Does not change women's sexual behavior or sex drive.
- Does not cause ectopic pregnancy. Instead, it substantially reduces the risk of ectopic pregnancy (see Question 11, page 230).

Why Some Women Say They Like Female Sterilization

- Has no side effects
- No need to worry about getting pregnant or about contraception again
- Nothing to do or remember after the procedure

Safe for All Women

With proper counseling and informed consent, any woman can have female sterilization safely, including women who:

- Have no children or few children
- Are married or are not married
- Do not have husband's permission
- Are young
- Just gave birth (within the last 7 days)
- Are breastfeeding
- Are living with HIV, whether or not on antiretroviral therapy (see Female Sterilization for Women With HIV, p. 217)

In some of these situations, especially careful counseling is important to make sure the woman will not regret her decision (see Because Sterilization Is Permanent, p. 220).

Avoid Unnecessary Procedures

(see Importance of Procedures, p. 368)

Women can have female sterilization:

- Without any blood tests or routine laboratory tests
- Without cervical cancer screening
- Without a pregnancy test. A woman can have female sterilization even when she is not having monthly bleeding at the time, if it is reasonably certain she is not pregnant (see Pregnancy Checklist, inside back cover).

For female sterilization a pelvic examination and blood pressure screening are essential. When available, a hemoglobin test can contribute to safe and effective use. (See The Importance of Clinical Assessment, p. 218.)

Medical Eligibility Criteria for

Female Sterilization

All women can have female sterilization. No medical conditions prevent a woman from using female sterilization. This checklist asks the client about known medical conditions that may limit when, where, or how the female sterilization procedure should be performed. Ask the client the questions below. If she answers "no" to all of the questions, then the female sterilization procedure can be performed in a routine setting without delay. If she answers "yes" to a question, follow the instructions, which recommend caution, delay, or special arrangements.

In the checklist below:

- **Caution** means the procedure can be performed in a routine setting but with extra preparation and precautions, depending on the condition.
- **Delay** means postpone female sterilization. These conditions must be treated and resolved before female sterilization can be performed. Help the client choose another method to use until the procedure can be performed.
- **Special** means special arrangements should be made to perform the procedure in a setting with an experienced surgeon and staff, equipment to provide general anesthesia, and other backup medical support. For these conditions, the capacity to decide on the most appropriate procedure and anesthesia regimen also is needed. Help the client choose another method to use until the procedure can be performed.

1. Do you have or have you ever had any female conditions or problems, such as infection or cancer? If so, what problems?

❑ NO ❑ **YES** If she has any of the following, use **caution**:

- Previous abdominal or pelvic surgery
- Past pelvic inflammatory disease since last pregnancy
- Uterine fibroids
- Breast cancer

▶ If she has any of the following, **delay** female sterilization:

Related to pregnancy

- Current pregnancy
- 7–42 days postpartum
- Postpartum after a pregnancy with severe pre-eclampsia or eclampsia
- Serious postpartum or postabortion complications (such as infection, hemorrhage, or trauma) except uterine rupture or perforation (**special**; see below)
- Hematometra (a large collection of blood in the uterus)

Unrelated to pregnancy

- Unexplained vaginal bleeding that suggests an underlying medical condition
- Purulent cervicitis, chlamydia, or gonorrhea
- Pelvic inflammatory disease
- Pelvic cancers (treatment may make her sterile in any case)
- Malignant trophoblast disease

▶ If she has any of the following, make **special** arrangements:

- Fixed uterus due to previous surgery or infection
- Endometriosis
- Hernia (abdominal wall or umbilical)
- Postpartum or postabortion uterine rupture or perforation

(Continued on next page)

2. Do you have any heart problems, stroke, high blood pressure, diabetes, or complications of diabetes? If so, what?

❑ NO ❑ **YES** If she has any of the following, use **caution**:

- Controlled high blood pressure
- Mild high blood pressure (140/90 to 159/99 mm Hg)
- Past stroke or heart disease without complications
- Diabetes without damage to arteries, vision, kidneys, or nervous system

▶ If she has any of the following, **delay** female sterilization:

- Heart disease due to blocked or narrowed arteries
- Blood clots in deep veins of legs or lungs

▶ If she has any of the following, make **special** arrangements:

- Several conditions together that increase chances of heart disease or stroke, such as older age, smoking, high blood pressure, or diabetes
- Moderately high or severely high blood pressure (160/100 mm Hg or higher)
- Diabetes for more than 20 years *or* damage to arteries, vision, kidneys, or nervous system caused by diabetes
- Complicated valvular heart disease

3. Do you have any lingering, long-term diseases or any other conditions? If so, what?

❑ NO ❑ **YES** If she has any of the following, use **caution**:

- Moderate iron-deficiency anemia (hemoglobin 7–10 g/dl)
- Severe lack of nutrition (Is she extremely thin?)
- Sickle cell disease
- Inherited anemia (thalassemia)
- Diaphragmatic hernia
- Epilepsy
- Hypothyroidism
- Mild cirrhosis of the liver, liver tumors, or schistosomiasis with liver fibrosis
- Kidney disease

- Obesity (Is she extremely overweight?)
- Elective abdominal surgery at time sterilization is desired
- Depression
- Young age
- Uncomplicated lupus with negative antiphospholipid antibodies

▶ If she has any of the following, **delay** female sterilization:

- Gallbladder disease with symptoms
- Active viral hepatitis
- Severe iron-deficiency anemia (hemoglobin less than 7 g/dl)
- Lung disease (bronchitis or pneumonia)
- Systemic infection or significant gastroenteritis
- Abdominal skin infection
- Undergoing abdominal surgery for emergency or infection, or major surgery with prolonged immobilization

▶ If she has any of the following, make **special** arrangements:

- Severe cirrhosis of the liver
- Hyperthyroidism
- Coagulation disorders (blood does not clot)
- Chronic lung disease (asthma, bronchitis, emphysema, lung infection)
- Pelvic tuberculosis
- HIV with advanced or severe clinical disease (see Female Sterilization for Women With HIV, below)
- Lupus with positive (or unknown) antiphospholipid antibodies, with severe thrombocytopenia, or on immunosuppressive treatment

Female Sterilization for Women With HIV

- Women who are living with HIV or are on antiretroviral (ARV) therapy can safely undergo female sterilization. Special arrangements are needed to perform female sterilization on a woman with advanced or severe clinical disease. The procedure may need to be delayed if she has an HIV-related illness.
- Urge these women to use condoms in addition to female sterilization. Used consistently and correctly, condoms help prevent transmission of HIV and other STIs.
- *No one should be coerced or pressured into having female sterilization, and that includes women with HIV.*

The Importance of Clinical Assessment

Because female sterilization involves a surgical procedure and the administration of local anesthesia (with or without mild sedation and analgesia), the client must undergo a careful, comprehensive yet focused clinical assessment. This assessment is important in every case, but it is even more important when the procedure is performed in hard-to-reach areas, in an outreach service, or in facilities far from supporting higher-level health services.

The assessment must include review of the Medical Eligibility Criteria (above) and a pelvic/genital examination. See Chapter 25, p. 368, on the Importance of Selected Procedures for Providing Family Planning Methods.

Providing Female Sterilization

When to Perform the Procedure

IMPORTANT: If there is no medical reason to delay, a woman can have the female sterilization procedure any time she wants if it is reasonably certain she is not pregnant and there are no medical conditions that limit when, where, or how the female sterilization procedure should be performed. To be reasonably certain she is not pregnant, use the Pregnancy Checklist (see inside back cover).

Woman's situation	When to perform
Having menstrual cycles or switching from another method	**Any time of the month** • Any time within 7 days after the start of her monthly bleeding. No need to use another method before the procedure. • If it is more than 7 days after the start of her monthly bleeding, she can have the procedure any time it is reasonably certain she is not pregnant. • If she is switching from oral contraceptives, she can continue taking pills until she has finished the pill pack to maintain her regular cycle. • If she is switching from an IUD, she can have the procedure immediately (see Copper-Bearing IUD, Switching From an IUD to Another Method, p. 172).
No monthly bleeding	• Any time if it is reasonably certain she is not pregnant.

After childbirth	• Immediately or within 7 days after giving birth, if she has made a voluntary, informed choice in advance. • Any time 6 weeks or more after childbirth if it is reasonably certain she is not pregnant.
After miscarriage or abortion	• Within 48 hours after uncomplicated abortion, if she has made a voluntary, informed choice in advance.
After using emergency contraceptive pills (ECPs)	• The sterilization procedure can be done within 7 days after the start of her next monthly bleeding or any other time if it is reasonably certain she is not pregnant. Give her a backup method or oral contraceptives to start the day after she finishes taking the ECPs, to use until she can have the procedure.

Ensuring Informed Choice

IMPORTANT: A friendly counselor who listens to a woman's concerns, answers her questions, and gives adequate, clear, and practical information about the procedure—especially its permanence—will help a woman make an informed choice and be a successful and satisfied user, without later regret (see Because Sterilization Is Permanent, next page). Involving her partner in counseling can be helpful but is not necessary or required.

The 7 Points of Informed Consent

Counseling must cover all 7 points of informed consent. In some programs the client and the counselor also sign an informed consent form. To give informed consent to sterilization, the client must understand the following points:

1. Temporary contraceptives also are available to the client, including long-acting reversible contraceptives.
2. Voluntary sterilization is a surgical procedure.
3. There are certain risks of the procedure as well as benefits. (Both risks and benefits must be explained in a way that the client can understand.)
4. If successful, the procedure will prevent the client from ever having any more children.
5. The procedure is considered permanent and probably cannot be reversed.
6. The client can decide against the procedure at any time before it takes place (without losing rights to other medical, health, or other services or benefits).
7. The procedure does not protect against sexually transmitted infections, including HIV.

Because Sterilization Is Permanent

A woman or man considering sterilization should think carefully: "Could I want more children in the future?" Health care providers can help the client think about this question and make an informed choice. If the client is considering having more children, another family planning method would be a better choice.

Asking questions can help. The provider might ask:

- "Do you want to have any more children in the future?"
- "If not, do you think your mind could change later? What might change your mind? For example, suppose one of your children died?"
- "Suppose you lost your spouse, and you married again?"
- "Does your partner want more children in the future?"

Clients who cannot answer these questions may need encouragement to think further about their decisions about sterilization.

In general, people most likely to regret sterilization:

- Are young
- Have few or no children
- Have just lost a child
- Are not married
- Are having marital problems
- Have a partner who opposes sterilization

None of these characteristics rules out sterilization, but health care providers should make especially sure that people with these characteristics make informed, thoughtful choices.

Also, for a woman, just after delivery or abortion is a convenient and safe time for voluntary sterilization, but women sterilized at this time may be more likely to regret it later. Thorough counseling during pregnancy and a decision made before labor and delivery or before abortion care help to avoid regrets.

The Decision About Sterilization Belongs to the Client Alone

A man or woman may consult a partner and others about the decision to have sterilization and may consider their views, but the decision cannot be made for that person by a partner, another family member, a health care provider, a community leader, or anyone else. Family planning providers have a duty to make sure that the decision for or against sterilization is made by the client and is not pressured or forced by anyone.

Performing the Sterilization Procedure

Explaining the Procedure

A woman who has chosen female sterilization needs to know what will happen during the procedure. The following description can help to explain the procedure to her. Learning to perform female sterilization takes training and practice under direct supervision. Therefore, this description is a summary and not detailed instructions.

(The description below is for procedures done more than 6 weeks after childbirth. The procedure used up to 7 days after childbirth is slightly different.)

The Minilaparotomy Procedure

1. The provider uses proper infection-prevention procedures at all times (see Infection Prevention in the Clinic, p. 376).
2. The provider performs a physical examination and a pelvic examination. The pelvic examination is to assess the condition and mobility of the uterus.
3. The provider inserts a special instrument (uterine elevator) into the vagina, through the cervix, and into the uterus to raise each of the 2 fallopian tubes so they are closer to the incision. This may cause discomfort.
4. The woman usually receives light sedation and analgesia to relax her. She stays awake. Local anesthetic is injected above the pubic hair line. She will not experience serious pain.
5. The provider makes a small horizontal incision (2–5 centimeters) in the anesthetized area. This usually causes little pain. (For women who have just given birth, the incision is made at the lower edge of the navel.)
6. Each tube is tied and cut or else closed with a clip or ring.
7. The provider closes the incision with stitches and covers it with an adhesive bandage.
8. The woman receives instructions on what to do after she leaves the clinic or hospital (see Explaining Self-Care for Female Sterilization, p. 224). She usually can leave in a few hours.

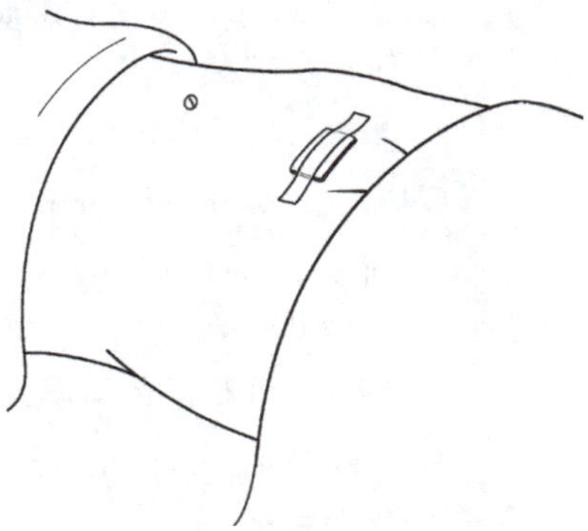

12

Female Sterilization

The Laparoscopy Procedure

1. The provider uses proper infection-prevention procedures at all times (see Infection Prevention in the Clinic, p. 376).
2. The provider performs a physical examination and a pelvic examination. The pelvic examination is to assess condition and mobility of the uterus.
3. The woman usually receives light sedation and analgesia to relax her. She stays awake. Local anesthetic is injected under her navel. She will not experience serious pain.
4. The provider places a special needle into the woman's abdomen and, through the needle, inflates (insufflates) the abdomen with gas or air. This raises the wall of the abdomen away from the pelvic organs.
5. The provider makes a small incision (about one centimeter) in the anesthetized area and inserts a laparoscope. A laparoscope is a long, thin tube containing lenses. Through the lenses the provider can see inside the body and find the 2 fallopian tubes.
6. The provider inserts an instrument through the laparoscope (or, sometimes, through a second incision) to close off the fallopian tubes.
7. Each tube is closed with a clip or a ring, or by electric current applied to block the tube (electrocoagulation).
8. The provider then removes the instrument and laparoscope. The gas or air is let out of the woman's abdomen. The provider closes the incision with stitches and covers it with an adhesive bandage.
9. The woman receives instructions on what to do after she leaves the clinic or hospital (see Explaining Self-Care for Female Sterilization, p. 224). She usually can leave in a few hours.

How Can a Partner Help?

The client's partner is welcome to participate in counseling and learn about the method and what support he can give to his partner. A male partner can:

- Understand that female sterilization is permanent
- Discuss with his partner whether they will want more children
- Support her decision to end her fertility if they will not want more children
- Discuss the alternative of vasectomy
- Show understanding and support her through the procedure and recovery
- Use condoms consistently in addition to female sterilization if he has an STI/HIV or thinks he may be at risk of an STI/HIV

Local Anesthesia Is Best for Female Sterilization

Local anesthesia, used with or without mild sedation and analgesia, is preferable to general anesthesia. Local anesthesia with sedation and analgesia:

- Is safer than general, spinal, or epidural anesthesia
- Lets the woman leave the clinic or hospital sooner
- Allows faster recovery
- Makes it possible to perform female sterilization in more facilities

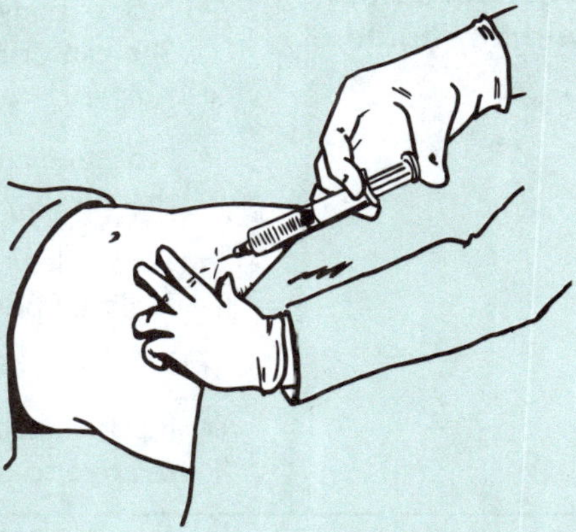

Sterilization under local anesthesia, with or without mild sedation and analgesia, can be done when a member of the surgical team has been trained to provide sedation and analgesia and the surgeon has been trained to provide local anesthesia. The surgical team should be trained to manage emergencies, and the facility should have the basic equipment and drugs to manage any emergencies.

Health care providers should explain to a woman ahead of time that being awake during the procedure is safer for her. During the procedure providers should talk with the woman and help to reassure her if needed.

The most common anesthetic used is lidocaine (lignocaine). Many different sedatives and analgesics may be used. The dosage of drugs must be adjusted to body weight. Oversedation should be avoided because it can reduce the client's ability to stay conscious and could slow or stop her breathing.

In some cases, general anesthesia may be needed. See Medical Eligibility Criteria for Female Sterilization, p. 214, for medical conditions needing special arrangements, which may include general anesthesia.

Supporting the User

Explaining Self-Care for Female Sterilization

Before the procedure the woman should	• Use another contraceptive until the procedure. • Not eat anything for 8 hours before surgery. She can drink clear liquids until 2 hours before surgery. • Not take any medication for 24 hours before the surgery (unless she is told to do so). • Wear clean, loose-fitting clothing to the health facility if possible. • Not wear nail polish or jewelry. • If possible, bring her partner, a friend, or a relative to help her go home afterwards.
After the procedure the woman should	• Rest for 2 days and avoid vigorous work and heavy lifting for a week. • Keep the incision clean and dry for 1 to 2 days. • Avoid rubbing the incision for 1 week. • Not have sex for at least 1 week, and then only when she feels comfortable having sex.
What to do about the most common problems	• She may have some abdominal pain and swelling after the procedure. It usually goes away within a few days. Suggest ibuprofen (200–400 mg), paracetamol (325–1000 mg), or other pain reliever. She should not take aspirin, which slows blood clotting. Stronger pain reliever is rarely needed. If she had laparoscopy, she may have shoulder pain or feel bloated for a few days.
Plan the follow-up visit	• Following up within 7 days or at least within 2 weeks is strongly recommended. No woman should be denied sterilization, however, because follow-up would be difficult or not possible. • A health care provider checks the site of the incision, looks for any signs of infection, and removes any stitches. This can be done in the clinic, in the client's home (by a specifically trained paramedical worker, for example), or at any other health center.

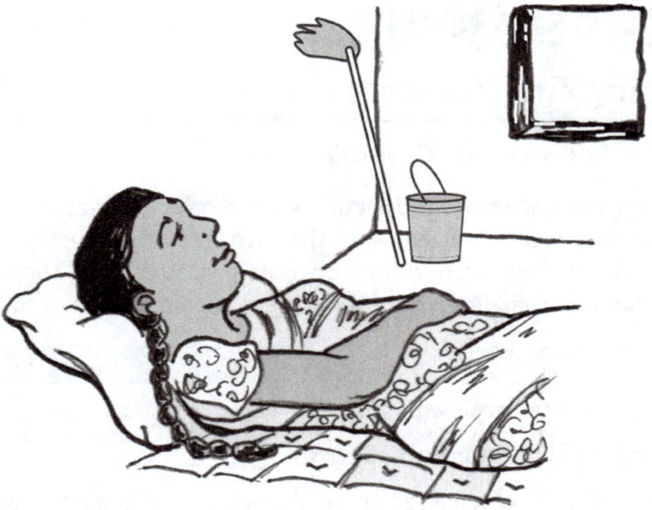

"Come Back Any Time": Reasons to Return

Assure every client that she is welcome to come back any time—for example, if she has problems or questions, or she thinks she might be pregnant. (A few sterilizations fail and the woman becomes pregnant.) Also if:

- She has bleeding, pain, pus, heat, swelling, or redness of the wound that becomes worse or does not go away.
- She develops high fever (greater than 38° C/101° F).
- She experiences fainting, persistent light-headedness, or extreme dizziness in the first 4 weeks and especially in the first week.

General health advice: Anyone who suddenly feels that something is seriously wrong with her health after the female sterilization procedure should immediately seek medical care from a nurse or doctor. After a surgical procedure any health problem must be assessed carefully and considered to be related to the procedure until it is medically demonstrated that it is not.

Helping Users

Managing Any Problems

Problems Reported as Complications

- Problems affect women's satisfaction with female sterilization. They deserve the provider's attention. If the client reports complications of female sterilization, listen to her concerns, give advice and support, and, if appropriate, treat. Make sure she understands the advice and agrees.

Infection at the incision site (redness, heat, pain, pus)

- Clean the infected area with soap and water or antiseptic.
- Give oral antibiotics for 7 to 10 days.
- Ask the client to return after taking all antibiotics if the infection has not cleared.

Abscess (a pocket of pus under the skin caused by infection)

- Clean the area with antiseptic.
- Cut open (incise) and drain the abscess.
- Treat the wound.
- Give oral antibiotics for 7 to 10 days.
- Ask the client to return after taking all antibiotics if she has heat, redness, pain, or drainage of the wound.

Severe pain in lower abdomen

- If the surgical procedure was recently performed, assess for any other problem that may indicate that the condition is related to the surgery, such as bleeding, lack of appetite, lack of bowel transit, lack of urination, or fever. If any of these are present, rapidly refer the client to a higher-level facility with surgical capability.
- If the surgery took place some months or years ago, suspect an ectopic pregnancy.
- See also Managing Ectopic Pregnancy, next page.

Suspected pregnancy

- Assess for pregnancy, including ectopic pregnancy.

Managing Ectopic Pregnancy

- Ectopic pregnancy is any pregnancy that occurs outside the uterine cavity. Early diagnosis is important. Ectopic pregnancy is rare but could be life-threatening (see Question 11, p. 230).
- In the early stages of ectopic pregnancy, symptoms may be absent or mild, but eventually they will become severe. A combination of these signs or symptoms should increase suspicion of ectopic pregnancy:
  - Unusual abdominal pain or tenderness
  - Abnormal vaginal bleeding or no monthly bleeding—especially if this is a change from a woman's usual bleeding pattern
  - Light-headedness or dizziness
  - Fainting
- *Ruptured ectopic pregnancy*: Sudden sharp or stabbing lower abdominal pain, sometimes on one side and sometimes throughout the body, suggests a ruptured ectopic pregnancy (when the fallopian tube breaks due to the pregnancy). Right shoulder pain may develop due to blood from a ruptured ectopic pregnancy pressing on the diaphragm. Usually, within a few hours the abdomen becomes rigid and the woman goes into shock.
- *Care*: Ectopic pregnancy is a life-threatening, emergency condition requiring immediate surgery. If ectopic pregnancy is suspected, perform a pelvic examination only if facilities for immediate surgery are available. Otherwise, immediately refer and/or transport the woman to a facility where definitive diagnosis and surgical care can be provided.

Questions and Answers About Female Sterilization

1. Will sterilization change a woman's monthly bleeding or make monthly bleeding stop?

No. Most research finds no major changes in bleeding patterns after female sterilization. If a woman was using a hormonal method or IUD before sterilization, her bleeding pattern will return to the way it was before she used these methods. For example, women switching from combined oral contraceptives to female sterilization may notice heavier bleeding as their monthly bleeding returns to usual patterns. Note, however, that a woman's monthly bleeding usually becomes less regular as she approaches menopause.

2. Will sterilization make a woman lose her sexual desire? Will it make her fat?

No. After sterilization a woman will look and feel the same as before. She can have sex the same as before. She may find that she enjoys sex more because she does not have to worry about getting pregnant. She will not gain weight because of the sterilization procedure.

3. Should sterilization be offered only to women who have had a certain number of children, who have reached a certain age, or who are married?

No. There is no justification for denying sterilization to a woman just because of her age, the number or sex of her living children, or her marital status. Health care providers must not impose rigid rules about age, number of children, age of last child, or marital status. Each woman must be allowed to decide for herself whether or not she will want more children and whether or not to have sterilization.

4. Is it not easier for the woman and the health care provider to use general anesthesia? Why use local anesthesia?

Local anesthesia is safer. General anesthesia is more risky than the sterilization procedure itself. Correct use of local anesthesia removes the single greatest source of risk in female sterilization procedures—general anesthesia. Also, after general anesthesia, women usually feel nauseous. This does not happen as often after local anesthesia.

When using local anesthesia with sedation and analgesia, however, providers must take care not to overdose the woman with the sedative. They also must handle the woman gently and talk with her throughout the procedure. This helps her to stay calm. With many clients, sedatives can be avoided, especially with good counseling and a skilled provider.

5. **Does a woman who has had a sterilization procedure ever have to worry about getting pregnant again?**

Generally, no. Female sterilization is very effective at preventing pregnancy and is intended to be permanent. It is not 100% effective, however. Women who have been sterilized have a slight risk of becoming pregnant: About 5 of every 1,000 women become pregnant within a year after the procedure. The small risk of pregnancy remains beyond the first year and until the woman reaches menopause.

6. **Pregnancy after female sterilization is rare, but why does it happen at all?**

Most often it is because the woman was already pregnant at the time of sterilization. In some cases an opening in the fallopian tube develops. Pregnancy also can occur if the provider makes a cut in the wrong place instead of the fallopian tubes.

7. **Can sterilization be reversed if the woman decides she wants another child?**

Generally, no. Sterilization is intended to be permanent. People who may want more children should choose a different family planning method. Surgery to reverse sterilization is possible for only some women—those who have enough fallopian tube left. Even among these women, reversal often does not lead to pregnancy. The procedure is difficult and expensive, and providers who are able to perform such surgery are hard to find. When pregnancy does occur after reversal, the risk that the pregnancy will be ectopic is greater than usual. Thus, sterilization should be considered irreversible.

8. **Is it better for the woman to have female sterilization or for the man to have a vasectomy?**

Each couple must decide for themselves which method is best for them. Both are very effective, safe, permanent methods for couples who know that they will not want more children. Ideally, a couple should consider both methods. If both are acceptable to the couple, vasectomy would be preferable because it is simpler, safer, easier, and less expensive than female sterilization.

9. **Will the female sterilization procedure hurt?**

Yes, a little. Women receive local anesthetic to stop pain, and, except in special cases, they remain awake. A woman can feel the health care provider moving her uterus and fallopian tubes. This can be uncomfortable. If a trained anesthetist or anesthesiologist and suitable equipment are available, general anesthesia may be chosen for women who are very frightened of pain. A woman may feel sore and weak for several days or even a few weeks after surgery, but she will soon regain her strength.

10. How can health care providers help a woman decide about female sterilization?

Provide clear, balanced information about female sterilization and other family planning methods, and help a woman think through her decision fully. Thoroughly discuss her feelings about having children and ending her fertility. For example, a provider can help a woman think how she would feel about possible life changes such as a change of partner or a child's death. Review The 7 Points of Informed Consent to be sure the woman understands the sterilization procedure (see p. 219).

11. Does female sterilization increase the risk of ectopic pregnancy?

No. On the contrary, female sterilization greatly reduces the risk of ectopic pregnancy. Ectopic pregnancies are very rare among women who have had a sterilization procedure. The rate of ectopic pregnancy among women after female sterilization is 6 per 10,000 women per year. The rate of ectopic pregnancy among women in the United States using no contraceptive method is 65 per 10,000 women per year.

On the rare occasions that sterilization fails and pregnancy occurs, 33 of every 100 (1 of every 3) of these pregnancies are ectopic. Thus, most pregnancies after sterilization failure are not ectopic. Still, ectopic pregnancy can be life-threatening, so a provider should be aware that ectopic pregnancy is possible if sterilization fails.

12. Where can female sterilization be performed?

If no pre-existing medical conditions require special arrangements:

- Minilaparotomy can be provided in maternity centers and basic health facilities where surgery can be done. These include both permanent and temporary facilities that can refer the woman to a higher level of care in case of emergency.
- Laparoscopy requires a better-equipped center, where the procedure is performed regularly and an anesthetist is available.

CHAPTER 13

Vasectomy

Key Points for Providers and Clients

- **Permanent.** Intended to provide life-long, permanent, and very effective protection against pregnancy. Reversal is usually not possible.
- **Involves a safe, simple surgical procedure.**
- **3-month delay in taking effect.** The man or couple must use condoms or another contraceptive method for 3 months after the vasectomy.
- **Does not affect male sexual performance.**

What Is Vasectomy?

- Permanent contraception for men who will not want more children.
- Through a puncture or small incision in the scrotum, the provider locates each of the 2 tubes that carries sperm to the penis (vas deferens) and cuts or blocks them by cutting and tying them closed or by applying heat or electricity (cautery).
- Also called male sterilization and male surgical contraception.
- Works by closing off each vas deferens, keeping sperm out of semen. Semen is ejaculated, but it cannot cause pregnancy.

How Effective?

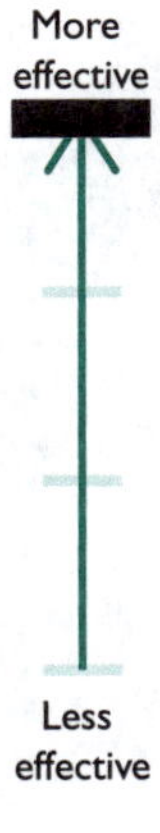

One of the most effective methods but carries a small risk of failure:

- Among the partners of men who have vasectomies, far less than 1 in every 100 will become pregnant in the first year of use of the method. In fact, less than 2 women in every 1,000 will become pregnant. This means that 998 or 999 of 1,000 women whose partners have had vasectomy will not become pregnant.
- Sometimes men can have their semen examined at 3 months after the procedure to see if it still contains sperm. If no sperm is found, 1 woman in every 1,000 of these men's partners will become pregnant in the first year.

- Among partners of men who do not have their semen examined, pregnancies are slightly more common, but still less than 2 per 1,000 women.
- Vasectomy is not fully effective for 3 months after the procedure.
  - Some pregnancies occur within the first year because the couple does not use condoms or another effective method consistently and correctly in the first 3 months, before the vasectomy is fully effective.

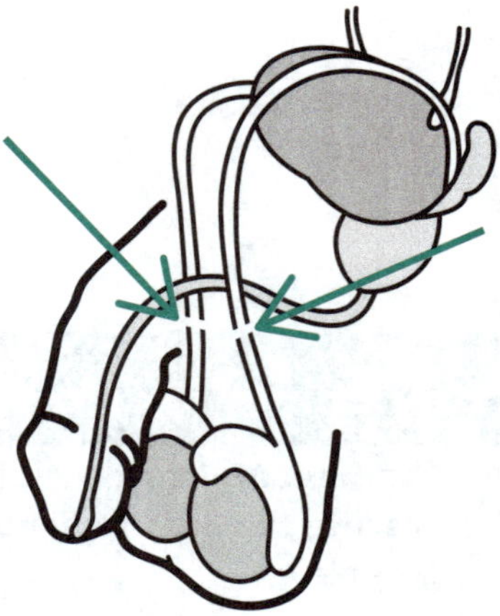

- A small risk of pregnancy remains beyond the first year after the vasectomy and until the man's partner reaches menopause.
  - Over 3 years of use: About 4 pregnancies per 1,000 women
- If the partner of a man who has had a vasectomy becomes pregnant, it may be because:
  - The couple did not always use another method during the first 3 months after the procedure
  - The provider made a mistake
  - The cut ends of the vas deferens grew back together

Fertility does not return because vasectomy generally cannot be stopped or reversed. The procedure is intended to be permanent. Reversal surgery is difficult, expensive, and not available in most areas. When performed, reversal surgery often does not lead to pregnancy (see Question 7, p. 244).

Protection against sexually transmitted infections (STIs): None

Why Some Men Say They Like Vasectomy

- Is safe, permanent, and convenient
- Has fewer side effects and complications than many methods for women
- The man takes responsibility for contraception—takes burden off the woman
- Increases enjoyment and frequency of sex

Side Effects, Health Benefits, Health Risks, and Complications

Side Effects

None

Known Health Benefits

- Helps protect against risks of pregnancy in a partner

Known Health Risks

None

Complications (see also Managing Any Problems, p. 242)

Uncommon to rare:

- Severe scrotal or testicular pain that lasts for months or years (see Question 2, p. 243).

Uncommon to very rare:

- Infection at the incision site or inside the incision (uncommon with conventional incision technique; very rare with no-scalpel technique; see Vasectomy Techniques, p. 238).

Rare:

- Bleeding under the skin that may cause swelling or bruising (hematoma).

Correcting Misunderstandings (see also Questions and Answers, p. 243)

Vasectomy:

- Does not remove the testicles. In vasectomy the tubes carrying sperm from the testicles are blocked. The testicles remain in place.
- Does not decrease sex drive.
- Does not affect sexual function. A man's erection is as hard, it lasts as long, and he ejaculates the same as before.
- Does not cause a man to grow fat or become weak, less masculine, or less productive.
- Does not cause any diseases later in life.
- Does not prevent transmission of sexually transmitted infections, including HIV.

Who Can Have a Vasectomy

Safe for All Men

With proper counseling and informed consent, any man can have a vasectomy safely, including men who:

- Have no children or few children
- Are married or are not married
- Do not have wife's permission
- Are young
- Have sickle cell disease
- Are at high risk of infection with HIV or another STI
- Are living with HIV, whether or not on antiretroviral therapy (see Vasectomy for Men with HIV, p. 236).

In some of these situations, especially careful counseling is important to make sure the man will not regret his decision (see Female Sterilization, Because Sterilization Is Permanent, p. 220).

Avoid Unnecessary Procedures

(see Importance of Procedures, p. 368)

Men can have vasectomy:

- Without any blood tests or routine laboratory tests
- Without a blood pressure check
- Without a hemoglobin test
- Without a cholesterol or liver function check
- Even if the semen cannot be examined by microscope later to see if it still contains sperm.

A genital examination should be conducted before performing vasectomy.

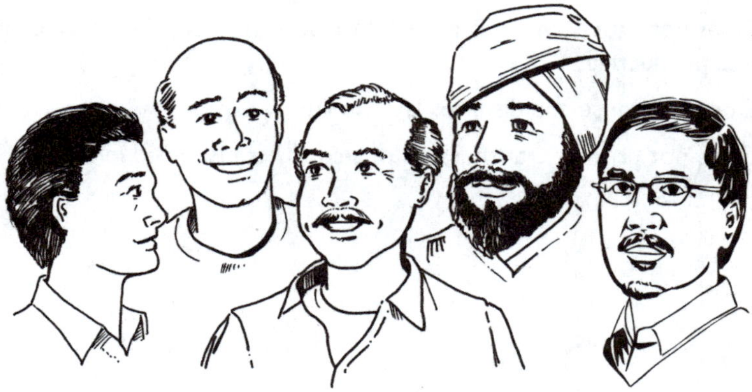

Medical Eligibility Criteria for

Vasectomy

All men can have vasectomy. No medical conditions prevent a man from using vasectomy. This checklist asks the client about known medical conditions that may limit when, where, or how the vasectomy procedure should be performed. Ask the client the questions below. If he answers "no" to all of the questions, then the vasectomy procedure can be performed in a routine setting without delay. If he answers "yes" to a question below, follow the instructions, which recommend caution, delay, or special arrangements.

In the checklist below:

- **Caution** means the procedure can be performed in a routine setting but with extra preparation and precautions, depending on the condition.
- **Delay** means postpone vasectomy. These conditions must be treated and resolved before vasectomy can be performed. Give the client another method to use until the procedure can be performed.
- **Special** means special arrangements should be made to perform the procedure in a setting with an experienced surgeon and staff, equipment to provide general anesthesia, and other backup medical support. For these conditions, the capacity to decide on the most appropriate procedure and anesthesia regimen also is needed. Help the client choose another method* to use until the procedure can be performed.

1. Do you have any problems with your genitals, such as infections, swelling, injuries, or lumps on your penis or scrotum? If so, what problems?

❑ NO ❑ **YES** If he has any of the following, use **caution**:

- Previous scrotal injury
- Swollen scrotum due to swollen veins or membranes in the spermatic cord or testes (large varicocele or hydrocele)
- Undescended testicle—one side only. (Vasectomy is performed only on the normal side. Then, if any sperm are present in a semen sample after 3 months, the other side must be done, too.)

(Continued on next page)

* *Backup methods include abstinence, male and female condoms, spermicides, and withdrawal. Tell him that spermicides and withdrawal are the least effective contraceptive methods. If possible, give him condoms.*

▶ If he has any of the following, **delay** vasectomy:
- Active sexually transmitted infection
- Swollen, tender (inflamed) tip of the penis, sperm ducts (epididymis), or testicles
- Scrotal skin infection or a mass in the scrotum

▶ If he has any of the following, make **special** arrangements:
- Hernia in the groin. (If able, the provider can perform the vasectomy at the same time as repairing the hernia. If this is not possible, the hernia should be repaired first.)
- Undescended testicles—both sides

2. Do you have any other conditions or infections? If so, what?

❑ NO ❑ **YES** If he has the following, use **caution**:
- Diabetes
- Depression
- Young age
- Lupus with positive (or unknown) antiphospholipid antibodies or on immunosuppressive treatment

▶ If he has any of the following, **delay** vasectomy:
- Systemic infection or gastroenteritis
- Filariasis or elephantiasis

▶ If he has any of the following, make **special** arrangements:
- HIV with advanced or severe clinical disease (see Vasectomy for Men With HIV, below)
- Blood fails to clot (coagulation disorders)
- Lupus with severe thrombocytopenia

Vasectomy for Men With HIV

- Men who are living with HIV or are on antiretroviral (ARV) therapy can safely have a vasectomy. Special arrangements are needed to perform vasectomy on a man who has advanced or severe clinical disease.
- Vasectomy does not prevent transmission of HIV.
- Urge these men to use condoms in addition to vasectomy. Used consistently and correctly, condoms help prevent transmission of HIV and other STIs.
- No one should be coerced or pressured into getting a vasectomy, and that includes men with HIV.

Providing Vasectomy

When to Perform the Procedure

- Any time a man requests it (if there is no medical reason to delay).

Ensuring Informed Choice

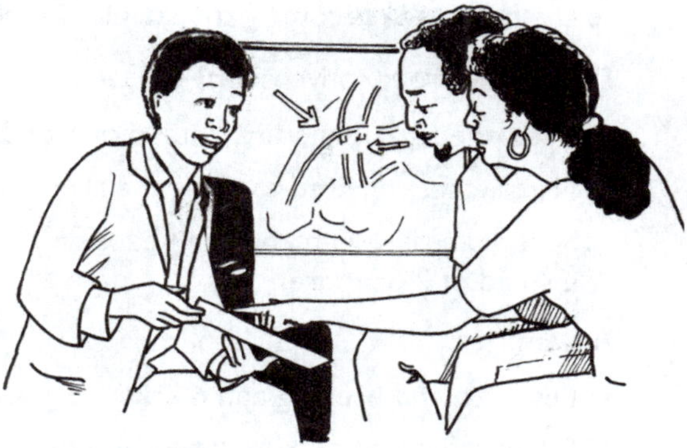

IMPORTANT: A friendly counselor who listens to a man's concerns, answers his questions, and gives adequate, clear and practical information about the procedure—especially its permanence—will help a man make an informed choice and be a successful and satisfied user, without later regret (see Female Sterilization, Because Sterilization Is Permanent, p. 220). Involving his partner in counseling can be helpful but is not necessary or required.

The 7 Points of Informed Consent

Counseling must cover all 7 points of informed consent. In some programs the client and the counselor sign an informed consent form. To give informed consent to vasectomy, the client must understand the following points:

1. Temporary contraceptives also are available to the client.
2. Voluntary vasectomy is a surgical procedure.
3. There are certain risks of the procedure as well as benefits. (Both risks and benefits must be explained in a way that the client can understand.)
4. If successful, the procedure will prevent the client from ever having any more children.
5. The procedure is considered permanent and probably cannot be reversed.
6. The client can decide against the procedure at any time before it takes place (without losing rights to other medical, health, or other services or benefits).
7. The procedure does not protect against sexually transmitted infections, including HIV.

Vasectomy Techniques

Reaching the Vas: No-Scalpel Vasectomy

No-scalpel vasectomy is the recommended technique for reaching each of the 2 tubes in the scrotum (vas deferens) that carries sperm to the penis. It is becoming the standard around the world.

Differences from conventional procedure using incisions:

- Uses one small puncture instead of 1 or 2 incisions in the scrotum.
- No stitches required to close the skin.
- Special anesthesia technique needs only one needle puncture instead of 2 or more.

Advantages:

- Less pain and bruising and quicker recovery.
- Fewer infections and less collection of blood in the tissue (hematoma).
- Total time for the vasectomy has been shorter when skilled providers use the no-scalpel approach.

Both no-scalpel and conventional incision procedures are quick, safe, and effective.

Blocking the Vas

For most vasectomies ligation and excision is used. This entails cutting and removing a short piece of each tube and then tying both remaining cut ends of the vas. This procedure has a low failure rate. Applying heat or electricity to the ends of each vas (cauterizing) has an even lower failure rate than ligation and excision. The chances that vasectomy will fail can be reduced further by enclosing a cut end of the vas, after the ends have been tied or cauterized, in the thin layer of tissue that surrounds the vas (fascial interposition). If training and equipment are available, cautery and/or fascial interposition are recommended. Blocking the vas with clips is not recommended because of higher pregnancy rates.

Performing the Vasectomy Procedure

Explaining the Procedure

A man who has chosen a vasectomy needs to know what will happen during the procedure. The following description can help to explain the procedure to him. Learning to perform a vasectomy takes training and practice under direct supervision. Therefore, this description is a summary and not detailed instructions.

1. The provider uses proper infection-prevention procedures at all times (see Infection Prevention in the Clinic, p. 376).
2. The man receives an injection of local anesthetic in his scrotum to prevent pain. He stays awake throughout the procedure.
3. The provider feels the skin of the scrotum to find each vas deferens—the 2 tubes in the scrotum that carry sperm.
4. The provider makes a puncture or incision in the skin:
   - Using the no-scalpel vasectomy technique, the provider grasps the tube with specially designed forceps and makes a tiny puncture in the skin at the midline of the scrotum with a special sharp surgical instrument.
   - Using the conventional procedure, the provider makes 1 or 2 small incisions in the skin with a scalpel.

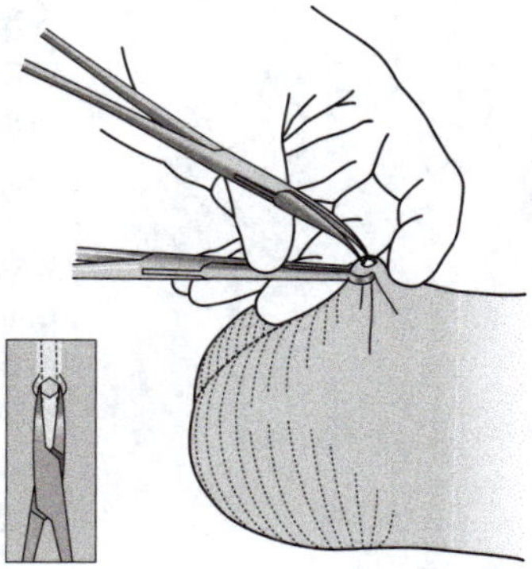

5. The provider lifts out a small loop of each vas from the puncture or incision. Most providers then cut each tube and tie one or both cut ends closed with thread. Some close off the tubes with heat or electricity. They may also enclose one end of the vas in the thin layer of tissue that surrounds the vas (see Vasectomy Techniques, previous page).
6. The puncture is covered with an adhesive bandage, or the incision may be closed with stitches.
7. The man receives instructions on what to do after he leaves the clinic or hospital (see Explaining Self-Care for Vasectomy, next page). The man may feel faint briefly after the procedure. He should stand first with help, and he should rest for 15 to 30 minutes. He usually can leave within an hour.

Supporting the User

Explaining Self-Care for Vasectomy

Before the procedure the man should	• Wear clean, loose-fitting clothing to the health facility.
After the procedure the man should	• Rest for 2 days if possible. • If possible, put cold compresses on the scrotum for the first 4 hours, which may decrease pain and bleeding. He will have some discomfort, swelling, and bruising. These should go away within 2 to 3 days. • Wear snug underwear or pants for 2 to 3 days to help support the scrotum. This will lessen swelling, bleeding, and pain. • Keep the puncture/incision site clean and dry for 2 to 3 days. He can use a towel to wipe his body clean but should not soak in water. • Not have sex for at least 2 to 3 days. • Use condoms or another effective family planning method for 3 months after the procedure. (The previously recommended alternative, to wait for 20 ejaculations, has proved less reliable than waiting 3 months and is no longer recommended.)
What to do about the most common problems	• Discomfort in the scrotum usually lasts 2 to 3 days. Suggest ibuprofen (200–400 mg), paracetamol (325–1000 mg), or other pain reliever. He should not take aspirin, which slows blood clotting.
Plan the follow-up visit	• Ask him to return in 3 months for semen analysis, if available (see Question 4, p. 244). • No man should be denied a vasectomy, however, because follow-up would be difficult or not possible.

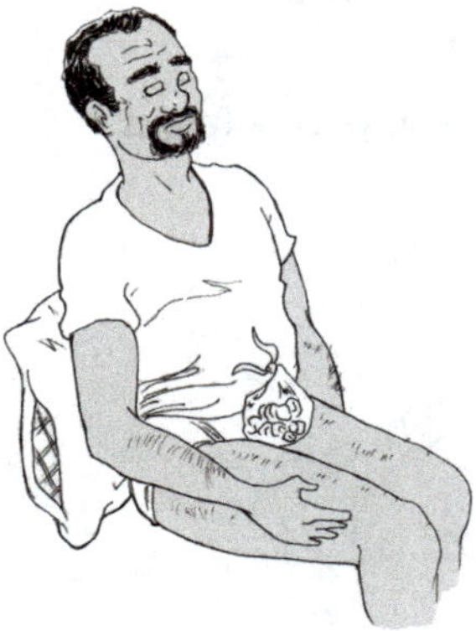

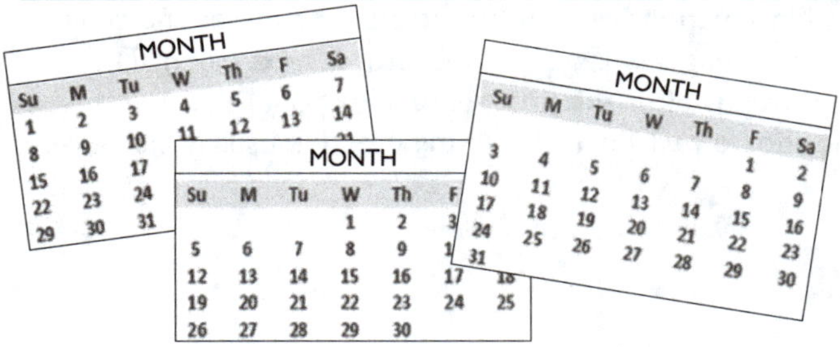

Use another effective family planning method for 3 months after the vasectomy procedure.

How Can a Partner Help?

The client's partner is welcome to participate in counseling and learn about the method and what support she can give to her partner. A female partner can:

- Understand that vasectomy is permanent
- Discuss as a couple whether they will want more children
- If they will not want more children, support his decision to end his fertility
- Discuss the alternative of female sterilization
- Discuss how they are going to prevent pregnancy during the first 3 months after the procedure, while waiting for vasectomy to become effective: Either use condoms or another method during this time.
- Show understanding and support him through the procedure and recovery
- Use female condoms consistently or encourage him to use male condoms consistently in addition to vasectomy if either partner has an STI/HIV or may be at risk of an STI/HIV

"Come Back Any Time": Reasons to Return

Assure every client that he is welcome to come back any time—for example, if he has problems or questions, or his partner thinks she might be pregnant. (A few vasectomies fail and the men's partners become pregnant.) Also if:

- He has bleeding, pain, pus, heat, swelling, or redness in the genital area that becomes worse or does not go away.

General health advice: Anyone who suddenly feels that something is seriously wrong with his health after a vasectomy procedure should immediately seek medical care from a nurse or doctor. After a surgical procedure any health problem must be assessed carefully and considered to be related to the procedure until it is medically demonstrated that it is not.

Helping Users

Managing Any Problems

Problems Reported as Complications

- Problems affect men's satisfaction with vasectomy. They deserve the provider's attention. If the client reports complications of vasectomy, listen to his concerns, give advice and support, and, if appropriate, treat. Make sure he understands the advice and agrees.

Bleeding or blood clots after the procedure

- Reassure him that minor bleeding and small uninfected blood clots usually go away without treatment within a couple of weeks.
- Large blood clots may need to be surgically drained.
- Infected blood clots require antibiotics and hospitalization.

Infection at the puncture or incision site (redness, heat, pain, pus)

- Clean the infected area with soap and water or antiseptic.
- Give oral antibiotics for 7 to 10 days.
- Ask the client to return after taking all antibiotics if the infection has not cleared.

Abscess (a pocket of pus under the skin caused by infection)

- Clean the area with antiseptic.
- Cut open (incise) and drain the abscess.
- Treat the wound.
- Give oral antibiotics for 7 to 10 days.
- Ask the client to return after taking all antibiotics if he has heat, redness, pain, or drainage of the wound.

Pain lasting for months

- Suggest elevating the scrotum with snug underwear or pants or an athletic supporter.
- Suggest soaking in warm water.
- Suggest aspirin (325–650 mg), ibuprofen (200–400 mg), paracetamol (325–1000 mg), or other pain reliever.
- Provide antibiotics if infection is suspected.
- If pain persists and cannot be tolerated, refer for further care (see Question 2, next page).

Questions and Answers About Vasectomy

1. Will vasectomy make a man lose his sexual ability? Will it make him weak or fat?

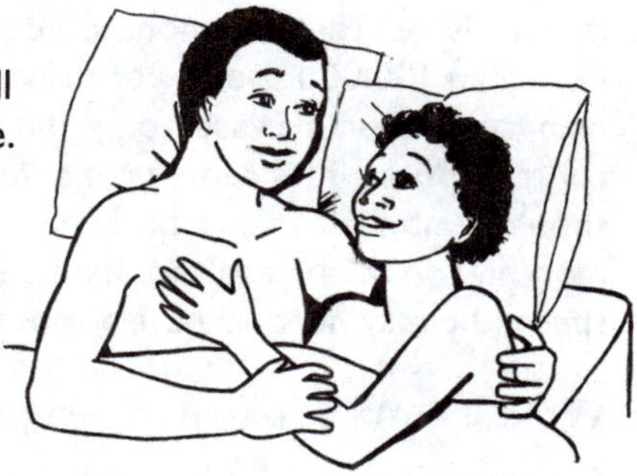

No. After vasectomy, a man will look and feel the same as before. He can have sex the same as before. His erections will be as hard and last as long as before, and ejaculations of semen will be the same. He can work as hard as before, and he will not gain weight because of the vasectomy.

2. Will there be any long-lasting pain from vasectomy?

Some men report having chronic pain or discomfort in the scrotum or testicles that can last from 1 to 5 years or more after a vasectomy. In the largest studies, involving several thousand men, less than 1% reported pain in the scrotum or testicles that had to be treated with surgery. In smaller studies, of about 200 men, as many as 6% reported severe pain in the scrotum or testicles more than 3 years after the vasectomy. In a similar group of men who did not have vasectomies, however, 2% reported similar pain. Few men with severe pain say that they regret having the vasectomy. The cause of the pain is unknown. It may result from pressure caused by the build-up of sperm that has leaked from an improperly sealed or tied vas deferens, or from nerve damage. Treatment includes elevating the scrotum and taking pain relievers. An anesthetic can be injected into the spermatic cord to numb the nerves to the testicles. Some providers report that surgery to remove the painful site or reversing the vasectomy relieves the pain. Severe, long-lasting pain following vasectomy is uncommon, but all men considering a vasectomy should be told about this risk.

3. Does a man need to use another contraceptive method after a vasectomy?

Yes, for the first 3 months. If his partner has been using a contraceptive method, she can continue to use it during this time. Not using another method in the first 3 months is the main cause of pregnancies among couples relying on vasectomy.

4. Is it possible to check if a vasectomy is working?

Yes. A provider can examine a semen sample under a microscope to see if it still contains sperm. If the provider sees no moving (motile) sperm, the vasectomy is working. A semen examination is recommended at any time after 3 months following the procedure, but it is not essential.

If there is less than one nonmotile sperm per 10 high-power fields (less than 100,000 sperm per milliliter) in the fresh sample, then the man can rely on his vasectomy and stop using a backup method for contraception. If his semen contains more moving sperm, the man should continue to use a backup method and return to the clinic monthly for semen analysis. If his semen continues to have moving sperm, he may need to have a repeat vasectomy.

5. What if a man's partner gets pregnant?

Every man having a vasectomy should know that vasectomies sometimes fail and his partner could become pregnant as a result. He should not make the assumption that his partner was unfaithful if she becomes pregnant. If a man's partner becomes pregnant during the first 3 months after his vasectomy, remind the man that for the first 3 months they needed to use another contraceptive method. If possible, offer a semen analysis and, if sperm are found, a repeat vasectomy.

6. Will the vasectomy stop working after a time?

Generally, no. Vasectomy is intended to be permanent. In rare cases, however, the tubes that carry sperm grow back together and the man will require a repeat vasectomy.

7. Can a man have his vasectomy reversed if he decides that he wants another child?

Generally, no. Vasectomy is intended to be permanent. People who may want more children should choose a different family planning method. Surgery to reverse vasectomy is possible for only some men, and reversal often does not lead to pregnancy. The procedure is difficult and expensive, and providers who are able to perform such surgery are hard to find. Thus, vasectomy should be considered irreversible.

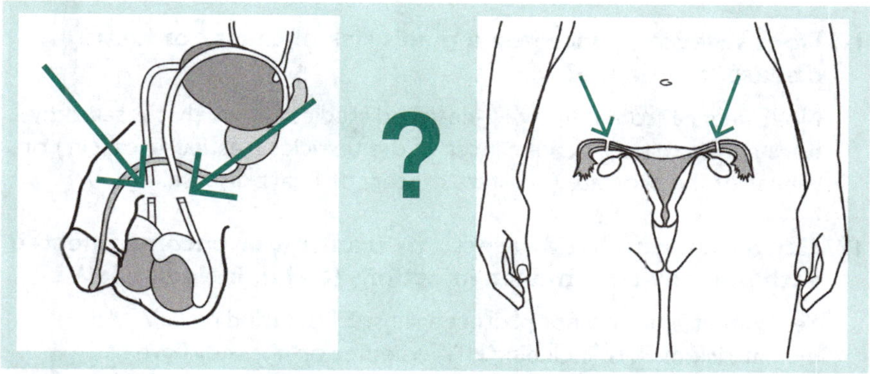

8. Is it better for the man to have a vasectomy or for the woman to have female sterilization?

Each couple must decide for themselves which method is best for them. Both are very effective, safe, permanent methods for couples who know that they will not want more children. Ideally, a couple should consider both methods. If both are acceptable to the couple, vasectomy would be preferable because it is simpler, safer, easier, and less expensive than female sterilization.

9. How can health care providers help a man decide about vasectomy?

Provide clear, balanced information about vasectomy and other family planning methods, and help a man think through his decision fully. Thoroughly discuss his feelings about having children and ending his fertility. For example, a provider can help a man think how he would feel about possible life changes such as a change of partner or a child's death. Review The 7 Points of Informed Consent to be sure the man understands the vasectomy procedure (see p. 237).

10. Should vasectomy be offered only to men who have reached a certain age or have a certain number of children?

No. There is no justification for denying vasectomy to a man just because of his age, the number of his living children, or his marital status. Health care providers must not impose rigid rules about age, number of children, age of last child, or marital status. Each man must be allowed to decide for himself whether or not he will want more children and whether or not to have a vasectomy.

11. Does vasectomy increase a man's risk of cancer or heart disease later in life?

No. Evidence from large, well-designed studies shows that vasectomy does not increase risks of cancer of the testicles (testicular cancer) or cancer of the prostate (prostate cancer) or heart disease.

12. Can a man who has a vasectomy transmit or become infected with sexually transmitted infections (STIs), including HIV?

Yes. Vasectomies do not protect against STIs, including HIV. All men at risk of STIs, including HIV, whether or not they have had vasectomies, need to use condoms to protect themselves and their partners from infection.

13. Where can vasectomies be performed?

If no pre-existing medical conditions require special arrangements, vasectomy can be performed in almost any health facility, including health care centers, family planning clinics, and the treatment rooms of private doctors. Where other vasectomy services are not available, mobile teams can perform vasectomies and any follow-up examinations in basic health facilities and specially equipped vehicles, so long as basic medications, supplies, instruments, and equipment can be made available.

CHAPTER 14

Male Condoms

This chapter describes male latex condoms. Female condoms, which are inserted into a woman's vagina, are available in some areas (see Female Condoms, p. 261, and Comparing Condoms, p. 428).

Key Points for Providers and Clients

- **Male condoms help protect against sexually transmitted infections, including HIV.** Condoms are the only contraceptive method that can protect against both pregnancy and sexually transmitted infections.
- **Require correct use with every act of sex for greatest effectiveness.**
- **Require both male and female partner's cooperation.** Talking about condom use before sex can improve the chances one will be used.
- **May dull the sensation of sex for some men.** Discussion between partners sometimes can help overcome this objection.

What Are Male Condoms?

- Sheaths, or coverings, that fit over a man's erect penis.
- Also called rubbers, "raincoats," "umbrellas," skins, prophylactics and preservativos; known by many different brand names.
- Most are made of thin latex rubber. Male condoms also are made from other materials, including polyurethane, polyisoprene, lambskin, and nitrile.
- Work by forming a barrier that keeps sperm out of the vagina, preventing pregnancy. Also keep infections in semen, on the penis, or in the vagina from infecting the other partner.

How Effective?

Effectiveness depends on the user: Risk of pregnancy or sexually transmitted infection (STI) is greatest when condoms are not used with every act of sex. Very few pregnancies or infections occur due to incorrect use, slips, or breaks.

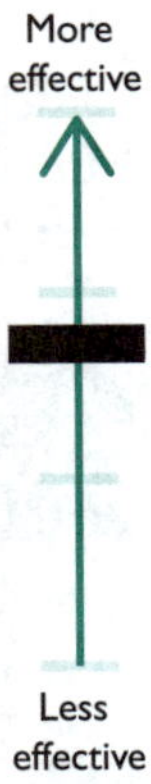

Protection against pregnancy:

- As commonly used, about 13 pregnancies per 100 women whose partners use male condoms over the first year. This means that 87 of every 100 women whose partners use male condoms will not become pregnant.
- When used correctly with every act of sex, about 2 pregnancies per 100 women whose partners use male condoms over the first year.

Return of fertility after use of condoms is stopped: No delay

Protection against HIV and other STIs:

- Male condoms significantly reduce the risk of becoming infected with HIV when used correctly with every act of vaginal or anal sex.
- When used consistently and correctly, condom use prevents 80% to 95% of HIV transmission that would have occurred without condoms (see Question 2, p. 257).
- Condoms reduce the risk of becoming infected with many STIs when used consistently and correctly during vaginal or anal sex.
  - Protect best against STIs spread by discharge, such as HIV, gonorrhea, and chlamydia.
  - Also protect against STIs spread by skin-to-skin contact, such as herpes and human papillomavirus.

Side Effects, Health Benefits, and Health Risks

Side Effects

None

Known Health Benefits

Help protect against:

- Risks of pregnancy
- STIs, including HIV

May help protect against:

- Conditions caused by STIs:
  - Recurring pelvic inflammatory disease and chronic pelvic pain
  - Cervical cancer
  - Infertility (male and female)

Known Health Risks

Extremely rare:

- Severe allergic reaction (among people with latex allergy)

Why Some Men and Women Say They Like Condoms

- Have no hormonal side effects
- Can be used as a regular, temporary or backup method
- Can be used without seeing a health care provider
- Are sold in many places and generally easy to obtain
- Help protect against both pregnancy and STIs, including HIV
- Can make sex last longer

Bringing Up Condom Use

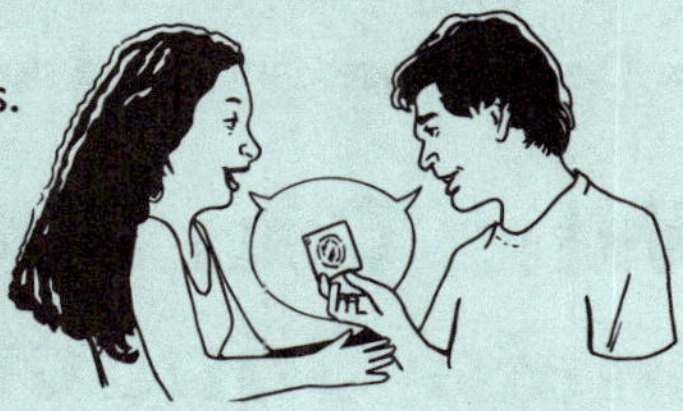

Some women find it hard to discuss their desire to use condoms with their partners. Others have difficulty persuading their partners to use condoms every time they have sex. Men give different reasons for not using condoms. Some do not like the way condoms can dull the sensation of sex. Sometimes men's reasons are based on rumors or misunderstanding. Having the facts can help a woman respond to her partner's objections (see Correcting Misunderstandings, next page).

Talking first can help. Woman who talk to their partners about using condoms before they begin to have sex can improve the chances that condoms are used. Women can try the approaches they think are best, depending on the partner and the circumstances. Some points that have been persuasive in different situations include:

- Emphasizing use of condoms for pregnancy prevention rather than STI protection.
- Appealing to concern for each other—for example: "Many people in the community have HIV infection, so we need to be careful."
- Suggesting that condom use can make sex more pleasurable for both of you.
- Taking an uncompromising stance—for example: "I cannot have sex with you unless you use a condom."
- Suggesting to try a female condom, if available. Some men prefer them to male condoms.
- For pregnant women, discussing the risks that STIs pose to the health of the baby and stressing how condoms can help protect the baby.

Also, a woman can suggest that her partner or the couple together come to the clinic for counseling on the importance of condom use.

Correcting Misunderstandings (see also Questions and Answers, p. 257)

Male condoms:

- Do not make men sterile, impotent, or weak.
- Do not decrease men's sex drive.
- Cannot get lost in the woman's body.
- Do not have holes that HIV can pass through.
- Are not laced with HIV.
- Do not cause illness in a woman. Exposure to semen or sperm is not needed for a woman's good health.
- Do not cause illness in men by making sperm "back up".
- Not only for use outside marriage. They are also used by married couples.
- Do not cause cancer and do not contain cancer-causing chemicals.

Who Can and Cannot Use Male Condoms

Medical Eligibility Criteria for

Male Condoms

All men and women can safely use latex male condoms except those with:

- Severe allergic reaction to latex rubber

In special circumstances, such as high risk of STIs or HIV, if non-latex condoms are not available, a qualified provider who can carefully assess the man's or woman's condition and situation may decide that he or she can use latex condoms.

Male condoms made from materials other than latex do not cause allergic reactions.

For more information on latex allergy, see Mild irritation in or around the vagina or penis or mild allergic reaction to condom, p. 256; Severe allergic reaction to condom, p. 256; and Question 11, p. 260.

Providing Male Condoms

When to Start

- Any time, whenever a man or a couple wants protection from pregnancy or STIs.

Explaining How to Use

IMPORTANT: Whenever possible, show clients how to put on a condom. Use a model of a penis, if available, or other item, like a banana, to demonstrate.

Explain the 5 Basic Steps of Using a Male Condom

Basic Steps	Important Details
1. Use a new condom for each act of sex	• Check the condom package. Do not use if torn or damaged. Avoid using a condom past the expiration date. Do so only if a newer condom is not available. • Tear open the package carefully. Do not use fingernails, teeth, or anything that can damage the condom. 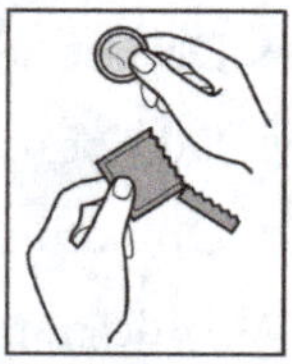
2. Before any physical contact, place the condom on the tip of the erect penis with the rolled side out	• For the most protection, put the condom on before the penis makes any genital, oral, or anal contact. 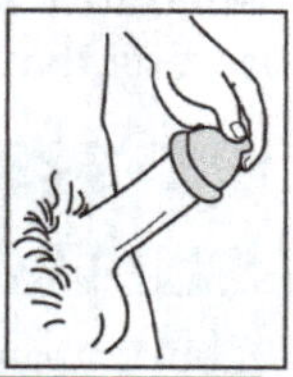
3. Unroll the condom all the way to the base of the erect penis	• The condom should unroll easily. Forcing it on could cause it to break during use. • If the condom does not unroll easily, it may be on backwards, damaged, or too old. Throw it away and use a new condom. 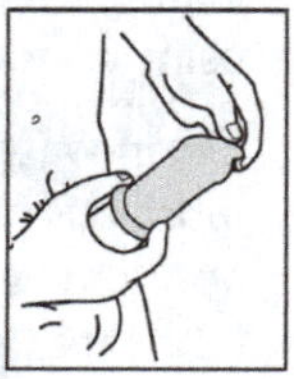 • If the condom is on backwards and another one is not available, turn it over and unroll it onto the penis.
4. Immediately after ejaculation, hold the rim of the condom in place and withdraw the penis while it is still erect	• Withdraw the penis. • Slide the condom off, avoiding spilling semen. • If having sex again or switching from one sex act to another, use a new condom. 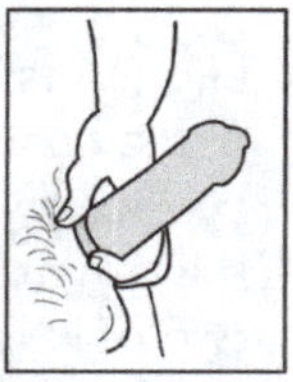
5. Dispose of the used condom safely	• Wrap the condom in its package and put it in the rubbish bin or latrine. Do not put the condom into a flush toilet, as it can cause problems with plumbing. 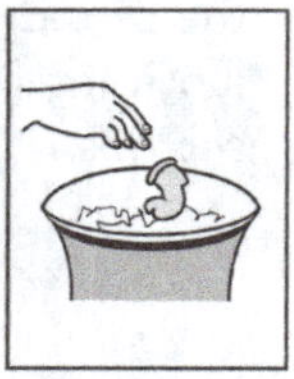

What Condom Users Should Not Do

Some practices can increase the risk that the condom will break and should be avoided.

- Do not unroll the condom first and then try to put it on the penis.
- Do not use lubricants with an oil base. These lubricants can damage latex.
- Do not use a condom if the color is uneven or changed.
- Do not use a condom that feels brittle, dried out, or very sticky.
- Do not reuse condoms.
- Do not have dry sex.
- Do not use more than one condom at the same time.
- Do not use a male and female condom at the same time.

Also, do not use the same condom when switching between different penetrative sex acts, such as from anal to vaginal sex. This can transfer bacteria that can cause infection.

Lubricants for Latex Condoms

Lubrication helps encourage condom use and avoid condom breakage. There are 3 ways to provide lubrication—natural vaginal secretions, adding a lubricant safe for use with condoms, or using condoms packaged with lubricant on them.

Clean water and saliva can be used for lubrication. The lubricants packaged with condoms are usually made of silicone. Silicone lubricants are also packaged separately. Lubricants made with water or glycol also are available and may be less expensive. They, too, are safe to use with condoms.

Lubricants should be applied on the outside of the condom, in the vagina, or in the anus. Lubricants should not be put on the penis, as this can make the condom slip off. A drop or two of lubricant on the inside of the tip of the condom before it is unrolled can help increase the sensation of sex for some men. Too much lubricant inside, however, can make the condom slip off.

Do not use products made with oil as lubricants for latex condoms. They can damage latex.

Materials that should *not* be used with latex condoms include:

- any oils (cooking, baby, coconut, mineral) or products made with oil
- petroleum jelly
- lotions
- cold creams
- butter
- cocoa butter
- margarine

Supporting the User

Ensure client understands correct use	• Ask the client to explain the 5 basic steps of using a condom by putting it on a model or other object and then taking it off. When counseling, you can show the pictures on p. 251.
Ask clients how many condoms they will need until they can return	• Give plenty of condoms and, if available, a water- or silicone-based lubricant. Oil-based lubricants should not be used with latex condoms. See box on previous page. • Tell clients where they can buy condoms, if needed.
Explain why using a condom with every act of sex is important	• Just one unprotected act of sex can lead to pregnancy or STI—or both. • If a condom is not used for one act of sex, try to use one the next time. A mistake once or twice does not mean that it is pointless to use condoms in the future.
Explain about emergency contraceptive pills (ECPs)	• Explain ECP use in case of errors in condom use—including not using a condom—to help prevent pregnancy (see Emergency Contraceptive Pills, p. 49). Give ECPs, if available.
Discuss ways to talk about using condoms	• Discuss skills and techniques for negotiating condom use with partners (see Bringing Up Condom Use, p. 249).

How Can a Partner Help?

The client's partner is welcome to participate in counseling and learn about the method and what support she can give to her partner. A female partner can:

- Support a man's choice of male condoms
- Discuss and agree to use the male condom with a full understanding of how to use it
- Help him remember to use a condom every time
- Help him to use the condom correctly
- Help to keep a supply on hand
- Make sure she has ECPs on hand in case the condom slips or breaks, or if they forget to use it

"Come Back Any Time": Reasons to Return

Assure every client that she or he is welcome to come back any time—for example, if he or she has problems, questions, or wants another method or she thinks she might be pregnant. Also if:

- Client has difficulty using condoms correctly or every time he or she has sex.
- Client has signs or symptoms of severe allergic reaction to latex condom (see Severe allergic reaction to condom, p. 256).
- Woman recently had unprotected sex and wants to avoid pregnancy. She may be able to use ECPs (see Emergency Contraceptive Pills, p. 49).

Helping Continuing Users

1. Ask clients how they are doing with the method and whether they are satisfied. Ask if they have any questions or anything to discuss.
2. Ask especially if they are having any trouble using condoms correctly and every time they have sex. Give clients any information or help that they need (see Managing Any Problems, below).
3. Give clients more condoms and encourage them to come back for more before their supply runs out. Remind them where else they can obtain condoms.
4. Ask a long-term client about major life changes that may affect her or his needs—particularly plans for having children and STI/HIV risk. Follow up as needed.

Managing Any Problems

Problems With Use

May or may not be due to the method.

- Problems with condoms affect clients' satisfaction and use of the method. They deserve the provider's attention. If the client reports any problems, listen to the client's concerns and give advice and support. Make sure he understands the advice and agrees.
- Offer to help the client choose another method—now, if he or she wishes, or if problems cannot be overcome—unless condoms are needed for protection from STIs, including HIV.

Condom breaks, slips off the penis, or is not used

- ECPs can help prevent pregnancy in such cases (see Emergency Contraceptive Pills, p. 49). If a man notices a break or slip, he should tell his partner so that she can use ECPs if she wants.
- If a client reports that a condom broke, slipped off, or was not used, refer for possible post-exposure prophylaxis against HIV and possible presumptive treatment against other STIs (see Question 7, p. 259). If the client has signs or symptoms of STIs after having unprotected sex, assess or refer.
- If a client reports breaks or slips:
  - Ask clients to show how they are opening the condom package and putting the condom on, using a model or other item. Correct any errors.
  - Ask if any lubricants are being used. The wrong lubricant or too little lubricant can increase breakage (see Lubricants for Latex Condoms, p. 252). Too much lubricant can cause the condom to slip off.
  - Ask when the man withdraws his penis. Waiting too long to withdraw, when the erection begins to subside, can increase the chance of slips.

Difficulty putting on the condom

- Ask clients to show how they put the condom on, using a model or other item. Correct any errors.

Difficulty persuading partner to use condoms or not able to use a condom every time

- Discuss ways to talk about condoms with partner (see Bringing Up Condom Use, p. 249) and also dual protection rationales (see Choosing a Dual Protection Strategy, p. 335).
- Consider combining condoms with:
  - Another effective contraceptive method for better pregnancy protection.
  - If no risk of STIs, a fertility awareness method, and using condoms only during the fertile time (see Fertility Awareness Methods, p. 291).
- Especially if the client or partner is at risk for STIs, encourage continued condom use while working out problems. If neither partner has an infection, a mutually faithful sexual relationship provides STI protection without requiring condom use but does not protect against pregnancy.

Mild irritation in or around the vagina or penis or mild allergic reaction to condom (itching, redness, rash, and/or swelling of genitals, groin, or thighs during or after condom use)

- Suggest trying another brand of condoms. A person may be more sensitive to one brand of condoms than to others.
- Suggest putting lubricant or water on the condom to reduce rubbing that may cause irritation.
- If symptoms persist, assess or refer for possible vaginal infection or STI as appropriate.
  - If there is no infection and irritation continues or recurs, the client may have an allergy to latex.
  - If not at risk of STIs, including HIV, help the client choose another method.
  - If the client or partner is at risk for STIs, suggest using female condoms or plastic male condoms, if available. If not available, urge continued use of latex condoms. Tell the client to stop using latex condoms if symptoms become severe (see Severe allergic reaction to condom, below).
  - If neither partner has an infection, a mutually faithful sexual relationship provides STI protection without requiring condom use but does not protect against pregnancy.

New Problems That May Require Switching Methods

May or may not be due to the method.

Female partner is using miconazole or econazole (for treatment of vaginal infections)

- A woman should not rely on latex condoms during vaginal use of miconazole or econazole. They can damage latex. (Oral treatment will not harm condoms.)
- She should use female condoms or plastic male condoms, another contraceptive method, or abstain from sex until treatment is completed.

Severe allergic reaction to condom (hives or rash over much of body, dizziness, difficulty breathing, or loss of consciousness during or after condom use). See Signs and Symptoms of Serious Health Conditions, p. 384.

- Tell the client to stop using latex condoms.
- Refer for care, if necessary. Severe allergic reaction to latex could lead to life-threatening anaphylactic shock. Help the client choose another method.
- If the client or partner cannot avoid risk of STIs, suggest they use female condoms or plastic male condoms, if available. If neither partner has an infection, a mutually faithful sexual relationship provides STI protection without requiring condom use but does not protect against pregnancy.

Questions and Answers About Male Condoms

1. Are condoms effective at preventing pregnancy?

Yes, male condoms are effective, but only if used correctly with every act of sex. When used consistently and correctly, only 2 of every 100 women whose partners use condoms become pregnant over the first year of use. Many people, however, do not use condoms every time they have sex or do not use them correctly. This reduces protection from pregnancy.

2. How well do condoms help protect against HIV infection?

On average, condoms are 80% to 95% effective in protecting people from HIV infection when used correctly with every act of sex. This means that condom use prevents 80% to 95% of HIV transmissions that would have occurred without condoms. (It does *not* mean that 5% to 20% of condom users will become infected with HIV.) For example, among 10,000 uninfected women whose partners have HIV, if each couple has vaginal sex just once and has no additional risk factors for infection, on average:

- If all 10,000 did not use condoms, about 10 women would likely become infected with HIV.
- If all 10,000 used condoms correctly, 1 or 2 women would likely become infected with HIV.

The chances that a person who is exposed to HIV will become infected can vary greatly. These chances depend on the partner's stage of HIV infection (early and late stages are more infectious), whether the person exposed has other STIs (increases susceptibility), male circumcision status (uncircumcised men are more likely to become infected with HIV), and pregnancy (women who are pregnant may be at higher risk of infection), among other factors. On average, women face twice the risk of infection, if exposed, that men do.

3. **Does using a condom only some of the time offer any protection from STIs, including HIV?**

   For best protection, a condom should be used with every act of sex. In some cases, however, occasional use can be protective. For example, if a person has a regular, faithful partner and has one act of sex outside of the relationship, using a condom for that one act can be very protective. For people who are exposed frequently to STIs, including HIV, however, using a condom only some of the time will offer limited protection.

4. **Will using condoms reduce the risk of STI transmission during anal sex?**

   Yes. STIs can be passed from one person to another during any sex act that inserts the penis into any part of another person's body (penetration). Some sex acts are riskier than others. For example, the risk of becoming infected with HIV is 5 times higher with unprotected receptive anal sex than with unprotected receptive vaginal sex. When using a latex condom for anal sex, a water- or silicone-based lubricant is essential to help keep the condom from breaking.

5. **Are plastic (synthetic) condoms effective for preventing STIs, including HIV?**

   Yes. Plastic condoms are expected to provide the same protection as latex condoms, but they have not been studied as thoroughly. Condoms made of animal membrane such as lambskin condoms (also called natural skin condoms) are not effective for preventing STIs, including HIV.

6. **Do condoms often break or slip off during sex?**

   No. On average, about 2% of condoms break, tear, or slip off completely during sex, primarily because they are used incorrectly. Used properly, condoms seldom break. In some studies with higher breakage rates, often a few users experienced most of the breakage in the entire study. Other studies also suggest that, while most people use condoms correctly, there are a few who consistently misuse condoms, which leads to breaks or slips. Thus, it is important to teach people the right way to open, put on, and take off condoms (see p. 251) and also to avoid practices that increase the risk of breakage (see What Condom Users Should Not Do, p. 252).

7. **What can men and women do to reduce the risk of pregnancy and STIs if a condom slips or breaks during sex?**

If a condom slips or breaks, taking emergency contraceptive pills can reduce the risk that a woman will become pregnant (see Emergency Contraceptive Pills, p. 49). If exposure to HIV is likely, treatment with antiretroviral medications (post-exposure prophylaxis), where available, can help reduce HIV transmission. If exposure to other STIs is likely, a provider can treat presumptively for those STIs—that is, treat the client as if he or she were infected.

Washing the penis does not help prevent STIs. Vaginal douching is not very effective in preventing pregnancy, and it increases a woman's risk of acquiring STIs, including HIV, and pelvic inflammatory disease.

8. **Can a man put 2 or 3 condoms on at once for more protection?**

There is little evidence for the benefits of using 2 or more condoms. It is generally not recommended because of concerns that friction between the condoms could increase the chance of breakage.

9. **Will condoms make a man unable to have an erection (impotent)?**

No, not for most men. Impotence has many causes. Some causes are physical, some are emotional. Condoms themselves do not cause impotence. A few men may have problems keeping an erection when using condoms, however. Other men—especially older men—may have difficulty keeping an erection because condoms can dull the sensation of having sex. Using more lubrication may help increase sensation for men using condoms.

10. **Aren't condoms used mainly in casual relationships or by people who have sex for money?**

No. While many casual partners rely on condoms for STI protection, married couples all over the world use condoms for pregnancy protection, too. In Japan, for example, about 40% of married couples use condoms—more than any other family planning method.

11. Is allergy to latex common?

No. Allergy to latex is uncommon in the general population, and reports of mild allergic reactions to condoms are very rare. Severe allergic reactions to condoms are extremely rare.

People who have an allergic reaction to rubber gloves or balloons may have a similar reaction to latex condoms. A mild reaction involves redness, itching, rash, or swelling of the skin that comes in contact with latex rubber. A severe reaction involves hives or rash over much of the body, dizziness, difficulty breathing, or loss of consciousness after coming in contact with latex. Both men and women can be allergic to latex and latex condoms.

CHAPTER 15

Female Condoms

Key Points for Providers and Clients

- **Female condoms help protect against sexually transmitted infections, including HIV.** Condoms are the only contraceptive method that can protect against both pregnancy and sexually transmitted infections.
- **Require correct use with every act of sex for greatest effectiveness.**
- **A woman can initiate female condom use,** but the method requires her partner's cooperation.
- **May require some practice.** Inserting and removing the female condom from the vagina becomes easier with experience.

What Are Female Condoms?

- Sheaths, or linings, that fit loosely inside a woman's vagina, made of thin, transparent, soft film.
  - Have flexible rings at both ends
  - One ring at the closed end helps to insert the condom
  - The ring at the open end holds part of the condom outside the vagina
- Female condoms are made of various materials, such as latex, polyurethane, and nitrile.
- Work by forming a barrier that keeps sperm out of the vagina, preventing pregnancy. Also helps to keep infections in semen, on the penis, or in the vagina from infecting the other partner.

How Effective?

Effectiveness depends on the user: Risk of pregnancy or sexually transmitted infection (STI) is greatest when female condoms are not used with every act of sex. Few pregnancies or infections occur due to incorrect use, slips, or breaks.

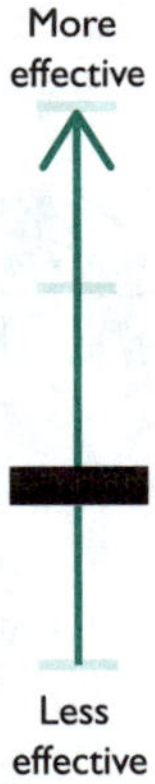

Protection against pregnancy:

- As commonly used, about 21 pregnancies per 100 women using female condoms over the first year. This means that 79 of every 100 women using female condoms will not become pregnant.
- When used correctly with every act of sex, about 5 pregnancies per 100 women using female condoms over the first year.

Return of fertility after use of female condom is stopped: No delay

Protection against HIV and other STIs:

- Female condoms reduce the risk of infection with STIs, including HIV, when used correctly with every act of sex.

Why Some Women Say They Like Female Condoms

- Women can initiate their use
- Have a soft, moist texture that feels more natural than male latex condoms during sex
- Help protect against both pregnancy and STIs, including HIV
- Outer ring provides added sexual stimulation for some women
- Can be used without seeing a health care provider

Why Some Men Say They Like Female Condoms

- Can be inserted ahead of time so do not interrupt sex
- Are not tight or constricting like male condoms
- Do not dull the sensation of sex like male condoms
- Do not have to be removed immediately after ejaculation

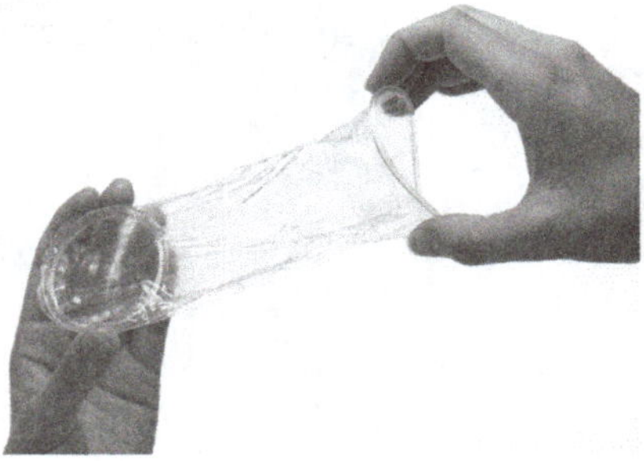

Side Effects, Health Benefits, and Health Risks

Side Effects

None

Known Health Benefits

Help protect against:

- Risks of pregnancy
- STIs, including HIV

Known Health Risks

None

Correcting Misunderstandings (see also Questions and Answers, p. 269)

Female condoms:

- Cannot get lost in the woman's body.
- Are not difficult to use, but correct use needs to be learned.
- Do not have holes that HIV can pass through.
- Are used by married couples. They are not only for use outside marriage.
- Do not cause illness in a woman because they prevent semen or sperm from entering her body.

Who Can Use Female Condoms

Medical Eligibility Criteria for

Female Condoms

All women and men can use female condoms, except those with severe allergic reaction to latex should not use latex female condoms.

In special circumstances, such as high risk of STIs or HIV, if non-latex condoms are not available, a qualified provider who can carefully assess the woman's or man's condition and situation may decide that she or he can use latex condoms.

Condoms made from materials other than latex do not cause allergic reactions.

For information on managing clients with latex allergy, see Male Condoms, Mild irritation in or around the vagina and penis or mild allergic reaction to condom, p. 256, and Severe allergic reaction to condom, p. 256.

Providing Female Condoms

When to Start

- Any time, whenever a woman or a couple wants protection from pregnancy or STIs.

Explaining How to Use

IMPORTANT: Whenever possible, show the client how to insert the female condom. Use a model or picture, if available, or your hands to demonstrate. You can create an opening similar to a vagina with one hand and show how to insert the female condom with the other hand.

Explain the 5 Basic Steps of Using a Female Condom

Basic Steps	Important Details
1. Use a new female condom for each act of sex	• Check the condom package. Do not use if torn or damaged. Avoid using a condom past its expiration date. Do so only if newer condoms are not available. • If possible, wash your hands with mild soap and clean water before inserting the condom.
2. Before any physical contact, insert the condom into the vagina	• For the most protection, insert the condom before the penis comes in contact with the vagina. Can be inserted up to 8 hours before sex. • Choose a position that is comfortable for insertion—squat, raise one leg, sit, or lie down. • Rub the sides of the female condom together to spread the lubricant evenly. • Grasp the ring at the closed end, and squeeze it so it becomes long and narrow. • With the other hand, separate the outer lips (labia) and locate the opening of the vagina. • Gently push the inner ring into the vagina as far up as it will go. Insert a finger into the condom to push it into place. About 2 to 3 centimeters of the condom and the outer ring remain outside the vagina.

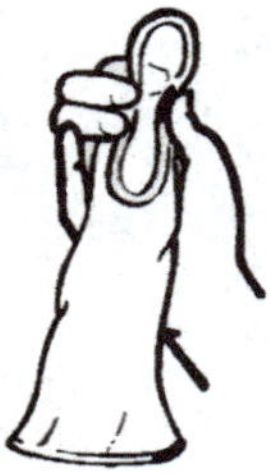

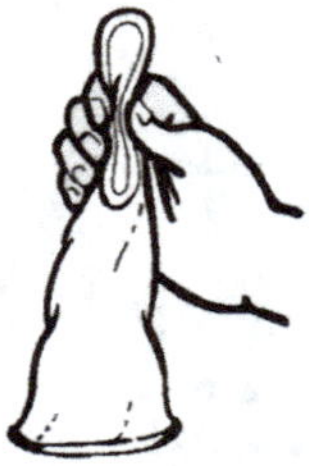

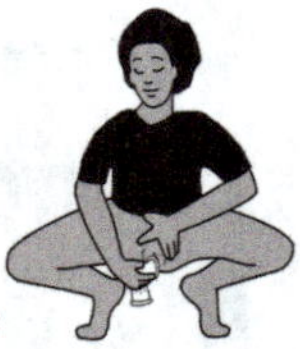

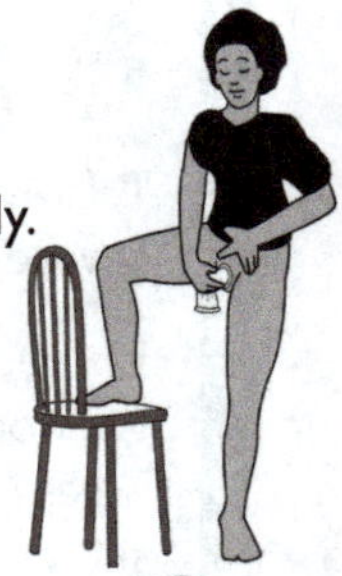

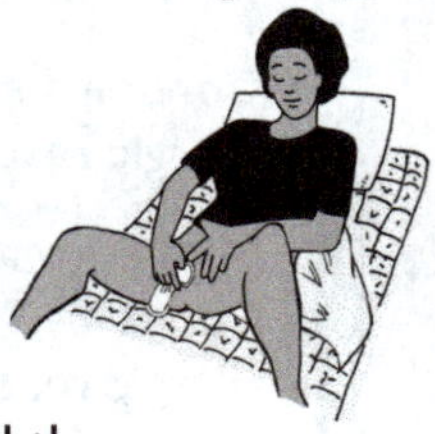

Basic Steps	Important Details
3. Ensure that the penis enters the condom and stays inside the condom	• The man or woman should carefully guide the tip of his penis inside the condom—not between the condom and the wall of the vagina. If his penis goes outside the condom, withdraw and try again. • If the condom is accidentally pulled out of the vagina or the outer ring is pushed into it during sex, put the condom back in place.

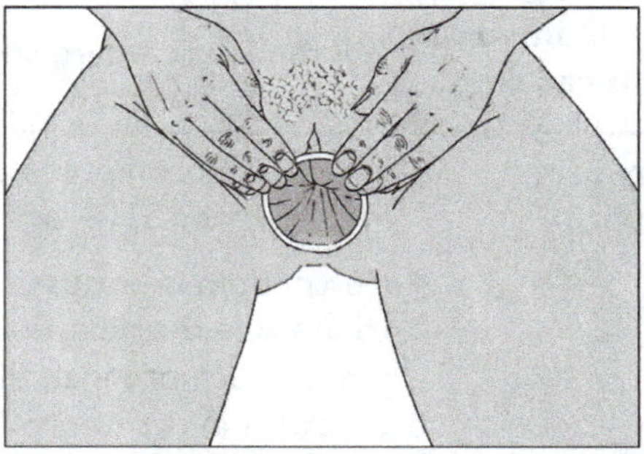

4. After the man withdraws his penis, hold the outer ring of the condom, twist to seal in fluids, and gently pull it out of the vagina	• The female condom does not need to be removed immediately after sex. • Remove the condom before standing up, to avoid spilling semen. • If the couple has sex again, they should use a new condom. • Reuse of female condoms is not recommended (see Question 5, p. 270).

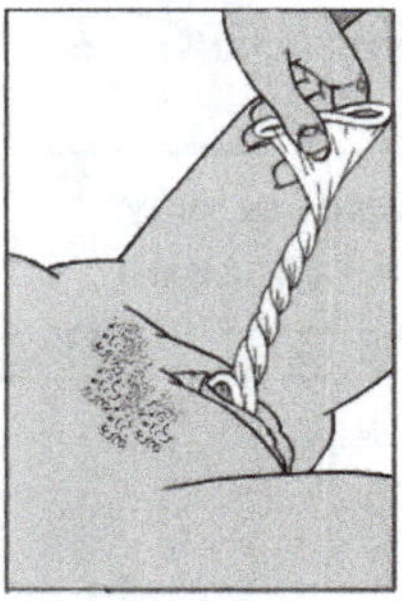

5. Dispose of the used condom safely	• Wrap the condom in its package and put it in the rubbish bin or latrine. Do not put the condom into a flush toilet, as it can cause problems with plumbing.

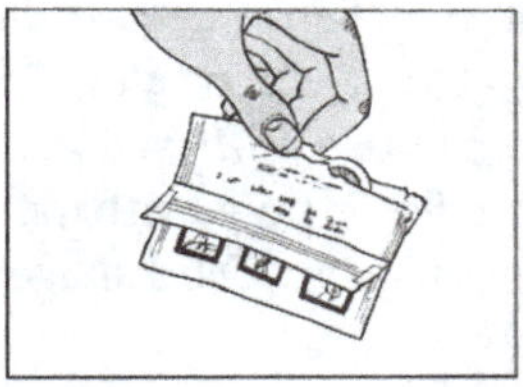

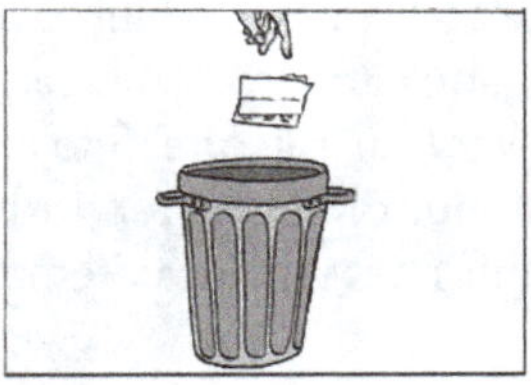

Supporting the User

Ensure client understands correct use	• Ask the client to explain the 5 basic steps of using the female condom while handling one. • If a model is available, the client can practice inserting the condom in the model and then taking it out.
Ask the client how many condoms she thinks she will need until she can return	• Give plenty of condoms and, if available, lubricant. • Tell the client where she can buy female condoms, if needed.
Explain why using a condom with every act of sex is important	• Just one unprotected act of sex can lead to pregnancy or STI—or both. • If a condom is not used for one act of sex, try to use one the next time. A mistake once or twice does not mean that it is pointless to use condoms in the future.
Explain about emergency contraceptive pills (ECPs)	• Explain ECP use in case of errors in condom use—including not using a condom—to help prevent pregnancy (see Emergency Contraceptive Pills, p. 49). Give ECPs if available.
Discuss ways to talk about using condoms	• Discuss skills and techniques for negotiating condom use with partners (see Bringing Up Condom Use, p. 249).

Lubricants for Female Condoms

Some female condoms come pre-lubricated, and others come with a separately packaged lubricant. If a client needs additional lubrication, she can also use clean water, saliva, or a lubricant made of water, glycol, or silicone. She also can use oil-based products such as coconut oil or butter with nitrile or polyurethane female condoms, but not with latex female condoms. Oil damages latex.

Tips for New Users

- Suggest to a new user that she practice putting in and taking out the condom before the next time she has sex. Reassure her that correct use becomes easier with practice. A woman may need to use the female condom several times before she is comfortable with it.
- Suggest she try different positions to see which way insertion is easiest for her.
- The female condom is slippery. Some women find insertion easier if they put it in slowly, especially the first few times.
- If a client is switching from another method to the female condom, suggest that she continue with the previous method until she can use the female condom with confidence.

"Come Back Any Time": Reasons to Return

Assure every client that she is welcome to come back any time—for example, if she has problems, questions, or wants another method; she has any major change in health status; or she thinks she might be pregnant. Also if:

- She has difficulty using female condoms correctly or every time she has sex.
- She recently had unprotected sex and wants to avoid pregnancy. She may be able to use ECPs (see Emergency Contraceptive Pills, p. 49).

How Can a Partner Help?

The client's partner is welcome to participate in counseling and learn about the method and what support he can give to his partner. A male partner can:

- Support a woman's choice of the female condom
- Discuss and agree to use the female condom with a full understanding of how to use it
- Ensure that they use it every time, and correctly (for example, making sure that he inserts penis inside the condom and not between the condom and vaginal wall)
- Help to keep a supply on hand
- Help to make sure she has ECPs on hand in case the condom is not used or is used incorrectly

Helping Continuing Users

1. Ask how the client is doing with the method and whether she is satisfied. Ask if she has any questions or anything to discuss.
2. Ask especially if she has any trouble using female condoms correctly and every time she has sex. Give her any information or help that she needs (see Managing Any Problems, below).
3. Give her more female condoms and encourage her to come back for more before her supply runs out. Remind her where else she can obtain female condoms.
4. Ask a long-term client about major life changes that may affect her needs—particularly plans for having children and STI/HIV risk. Follow up as needed.

Managing Any Problems

Problems With Use

May or may not be due to the method.

- Problems with condoms affect clients' satisfaction and use of the method. They deserve the provider's attention. If the client reports any problems, listen to her concerns and give advice and support. Make sure she understands the advice and agrees.
- Offer to help the client choose another method—now, if she wishes, or if problems cannot be overcome—unless condoms are needed for protection from STIs, including HIV.

Difficulty inserting the female condom

- Ask the client how she inserts a female condom. If a model is available, ask her to demonstrate and let her practice with the model. If not, ask her to demonstrate using her hands. Correct any errors.

Inner ring uncomfortable or painful

- Suggest that she reinsert or reposition the condom so that the inner ring is tucked back behind the pubic bone and out of the way.

Condom squeaks or makes noise during sex

- Suggest adding more lubricant to the inside of the condom or onto the penis.

Condom slips, is not used, or is used incorrectly

- ECPs can help prevent pregnancy (see Emergency Contraceptive Pills, p. 49).

- Refer for possible post-exposure prophylaxis against HIV and possible presumptive treatment against other STIs (see Male Condoms, Question 7, p. 259). If the client has signs or symptoms of STIs after having unprotected sex, assess or refer.
- If a client reports slips, she may be inserting the female condom incorrectly. Ask her to show how she is inserting the condom, using a model or demonstrating with her hands. Correct any errors.

Difficulty persuading partner to use condoms or not able to use a condom every time

- Discuss ways to talk with her partner about the importance of condom use for protection from pregnancy and STIs. (See Male Condoms, Difficulty persuading partner to use condoms or not able to use a condom every time, p. 255.)

Mild irritation in or around the vagina or penis (itching, redness, or rash)

- Usually goes away on its own without treatment.
- Suggest adding lubricant to the inside of the condom or onto the penis to reduce rubbing that may cause irritation.
- If symptoms persist, assess and treat for possible vaginal infection or STI, as appropriate.
  - If there is no infection, help the client choose another method unless the client is at risk for STIs, including HIV.
  - For clients at risk of STIs, including HIV, suggest using male condoms. If using male condoms is not possible, urge continued use of female condoms despite discomfort.
  - If neither partner has an infection, a mutually faithful sexual relationship provides STI protection without requiring condom use but does not protect against pregnancy.

Suspected pregnancy

- Assess for pregnancy.
- A woman can safely use female condoms during pregnancy for continued STI protection.

Questions and Answers About Female Condoms

1. Is the female condom difficult to use?

No, but it does require practice and patience. See Tips for New Users, p. 267.

2. **Can female condoms effectively prevent both pregnancy and STIs, including HIV?**

   Yes. Female condoms offer dual protection, against both pregnancy and STIs, including HIV, if used consistently and correctly. Many people, however, do not use condoms every time they have sex, or do not use them correctly. This reduces protection from both pregnancy and STIs.

3. **Can a female condom and a male condom be used at the same time?**

   No. Male and female condoms should not be used together. This can cause friction that may lead to slipping or tearing of the condoms.

4. **What is the best way to make sure the penis goes into the condom and not outside the condom?**

   To avoid incorrect use, the man or the woman should carefully guide his penis and place the tip inside the outer ring of the condom. If the penis goes between the wall of the vagina and the condom, the man should withdraw and try again.

5. **Can the female condom be used more than once?**

   Reuse of the female condom is not recommended. Reuse of currently available female condoms has not been sufficiently tested.

6. **Can the female condom be used while a woman is having her monthly bleeding?**

   Women can use the female condom during their monthly bleeding. The female condom cannot be used at the same time as a tampon, however. The tampon must be removed before inserting a female condom.

7. **Isn't the female condom too big to be comfortable?**

   No. Female condoms are the same length as male condoms, but wider. They are very flexible and fit to the shape of the vagina. Female condoms have been carefully designed and tested to fit any woman, whatever the size of her vagina, and any man, whatever the size of his penis.

8. **Can a female condom get lost inside a woman's body?**

   No. The female condom remains in a woman's vagina until she takes it out. It cannot go past a woman's cervix and into the womb (uterus) because it is too large for that.

9. **Can the female condom be used in different sexual positions?**

   Yes. The female condom can be used in any sexual position.

CHAPTER 16

Spermicides and Diaphragms

Spermicides

Key Points for Providers and Clients

- **Spermicides are placed deep in the vagina shortly before sex.**
- **Require correct use with every act of sex for greatest effectiveness.**
- **One of the least effective contraceptive methods.**
- **Can be used as a primary method or as a backup method.**

What Are Spermicides?

- Sperm-killing substances inserted deep in the vagina, near the cervix, before sex.
  - Nonoxynol-9 is most widely used.
  - Others include benzalkonium chloride, chlorhexidine, menfegol, octoxynol-9, and sodium docusate.
- Available in foaming tablets, melting or foaming suppositories, cans of pressurized foam, melting film, jelly, and cream.
  - Jellies, creams, and foam from cans can be used alone, with a diaphragm, or with condoms.
  - Films, suppositories, foaming tablets, or foaming suppositories can be used alone or with condoms.
- Work by causing the membrane of sperm cells to break, killing them or slowing their movement. This keeps sperm from meeting an egg.

How Effective?

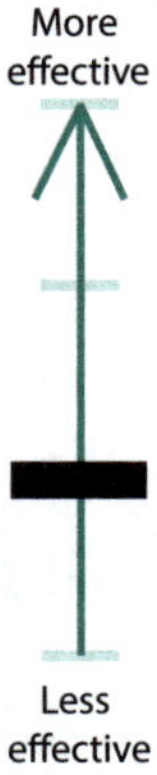

Effectiveness depends on the user: Risk of pregnancy is greatest when spermicides are not used with every act of sex.

- One of the least effective family planning methods.
- As commonly used, about 21 pregnancies per 100 women using spermicides over the first year. This means that 79 of every 100 women using spermicides will not become pregnant.
- When used correctly with every act of sex, about 16 pregnancies per 100 women using spermicides over the first year.

Return of fertility after spermicides are stopped: No delay

Protection against sexually transmitted infections (STIs): None. Frequent use of nonoxynol-9 may increase risk of HIV infection (see Question 3, p. 286).

Side Effects, Health Benefits, and Health Risks

Side Effects (see also Managing Any Problems, p. 283)

Some users report the following:

- Irritation in or around the vagina or penis

Other possible physical changes:

- Vaginal lesions

Known Health Benefits

Help protect against:

- Risks of pregnancy

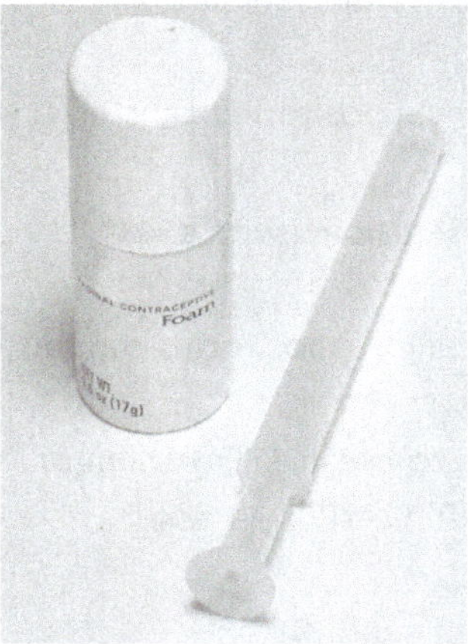

Known Health Risks

Uncommon:

- Urinary tract infection, especially when using spermicides 2 or more times a day

Rare:

- Frequent use of nonoxynol-9 may increase risk of HIV infection (see Question 3, p. 286)

Correcting Misunderstandings (see also Questions and Answers, p. 286)

Spermicides:

- Do not reduce vaginal secretions or make women bleed during sex.
- Do not cause cervical cancer or birth defects.
- Do not protect against STIs.
- Do not change men's or women's sex drive or reduce sexual pleasure for most men.
- Do not stop women's monthly bleeding.

Why Some Women Say They Like Spermicides

- Are controlled by the woman
- Have no hormonal side effects
- Increase vaginal lubrication
- Can be used without seeing a health care provider
- Can be inserted ahead of time and so do not interrupt sex

Who Can and Cannot Use Spermicides

Safe and Suitable for Nearly All Women

Medical Eligibility Criteria for

Spermicides

All women can safely use spermicides except those who:

- Are at high risk for HIV infection
- Have HIV infection

Women who are at high risk for HIV infection or who have HIV should use another method.

Providing Spermicides

When to Start

- Any time the client wants.

Explaining How to Use Spermicides

Give spermicide	• Give as much spermicide as possible—even as much as a year's supply, if available.
Explain how to insert spermicide into the vagina	**1.** Check the expiration date and avoid using spermicide past its expiration date. – Wash hands with mild soap and clean water, if possible. **2.** Foam or cream: Shake cans of foam hard. Squeeze spermicide from the can or tube into a plastic applicator. Insert the applicator deep into the vagina, near the cervix, and push the plunger. Tablets, suppositories, jellies: Insert the spermicide deep into the vagina, near the cervix, with an applicator or with fingers. Film: Fold film in half and insert with fingers that are dry (or else the film will stick to the fingers and not the cervix).
Explain when to insert spermicide into the vagina	• Foam or cream: Any time less than one hour before sex. • Tablets, suppositories, jellies, film: Between 10 minutes and one hour before sex, depending on type.
Explain about multiple acts of sex	• Insert additional spermicide before each act of vaginal sex.
Do not wash the vagina (douche) after sex	• Douching is not recommended because it will wash away the spermicide and also increase the risk of sexually transmitted infections. • If you must douche, wait for at least 6 hours after sex before doing so.

Supporting the Spermicide User

Ensure client understands correct use	• Ask the client to repeat how and when to insert her spermicide.
Describe the most common side effects	• Itching and irritation in or around the vagina or penis.
Explain about emergency contraceptive pills (ECPs)	• Explain ECP use in case the spermicide is not used at all or is not used properly (see Emergency Contraceptive Pills, p. 49). Give her ECPs, if available.
Explain about storage	• Spermicides should be stored in a cool, dry place, if possible, out of the sun. Suppositories may melt in hot weather. If kept dry, foaming tablets are not as likely to melt in hot weather.

How Can a Partner Help?

The client's partner is welcome to participate in counseling and learn about the method and what support he can give to his partner. A male partner can:

- Support a woman's choice of spermicides or diaphragm with spermicide
- Discuss and agree to use spermicides with a full understanding of how to use them
- Help her to remember to use spermicides or diaphragm with spermicide every time
- Help to keep a supply of spermicide on hand
- Help to make sure the woman has ECPs on hand in case the spermicide or the diaphragm is not used or the diaphragm got dislodged
- Use condoms consistently in addition to spermicides or diaphragm with spermicide if he has an STI/HIV or thinks he may be at risk of an STI/HIV

Diaphragms

Key Points for Providers and Clients

- **The diaphragm is placed deep in the vagina before sex.** It covers the cervix. Spermicide provides additional contraceptive protection.
- **A pelvic examination may be needed before starting use.** The provider must select a diaphragm that fits properly.
- **Require correct use with every act of sex for greatest effectiveness.**

What Is the Diaphragm?

- A soft latex cup that covers the cervix. Plastic and silicone diaphragms may also be available.
- The rim contains a firm, flexible spring that keeps the diaphragm in place.
- Used with spermicidal cream, jelly, or foam to improve effectiveness.
- Most diaphragms come in different sizes and require fitting by a specifically trained provider. A one-size-fits-all diaphragm is becoming available. It does not require seeing a provider for fitting. (See Question 9, p. 287.)
- Works by blocking sperm from entering the cervix; spermicide kills or disables sperm. Both keep sperm from meeting an egg.

How Effective?

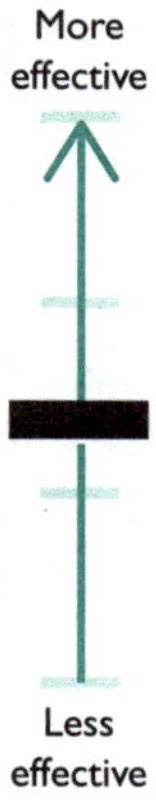

Effectiveness depends on the user: Risk of pregnancy is greatest when the diaphragm with spermicide is not used with every act of sex.

- As commonly used, about 17 pregnancies per 100 women using the diaphragm with spermicide over the first year. This means that 83 of every 100 women using the diaphragm will not become pregnant.
- When used correctly with every act of sex, about 16 pregnancies per 100 women using the diaphragm with spermicide over the first year.

Return of fertility after use of the diaphragm is stopped: No delay

Protection against STIs: May provide some protection against certain STIs but should not be relied on for STI prevention (see Question 8, p. 287).

Side Effects, Health Benefits, and Health Risks

Side Effects (see also Managing Any Problems, p. 283)

Some users report the following:

- Irritation in or around the vagina or penis

Other possible physical changes:

- Vaginal lesions

Known Health Benefits

Help protect against:

- Risks of pregnancy

May help protect against:

- Certain STIs (chlamydia, gonorrhea, pelvic inflammatory disease, trichomoniasis)
- Cervical precancer and cancer

Known Health Risks

Common to uncommon:

- Urinary tract infection

Uncommon:

- Bacterial vaginosis
- Candidiasis

Rare:

- Frequent use of nonoxynol-9 may increase risk of HIV infection (see Question 3, p. 286)

Extremely rare:

- Toxic shock syndrome

Correcting Misunderstandings (see also Questions and Answers, p. 286)

Diaphragms:

- Do not affect the feeling of sex. A few men report feeling the diaphragm during sex, but most do not.
- Cannot pass through the cervix. They cannot go into the uterus or otherwise get lost in the woman's body.
- Do not cause cervical cancer.

Why Some Women Say They Like the Diaphragm

- Is controlled by the woman
- Has no hormonal side effects
- Can be inserted ahead of time and so does not interrupt sex

Who Can and Cannot Use Diaphragms

Safe and Suitable for Nearly All Women

Nearly all women can use the diaphragm safely and effectively.

Medical Eligibility Criteria for

Diaphragms

Ask the client the questions below about known medical conditions. Examinations and tests are not necessary. If she answers "no" to all of the questions, then she can start using the diaphragm if she wants. If she answers "yes" to a question, follow the instructions. In some cases she can still start using the diaphragm. These questions also apply to the cervical cap (see p. 289).

1. Have you recently had a baby or second-trimester spontaneous or induced abortion? If so, when?

❑ NO ❑ **YES** The diaphragm should not be fitted until 6 weeks after childbirth or second-trimester abortion, when the uterus and cervix have returned to normal size. Give her a backup method* to use until then.

2. Are you allergic to latex rubber?

❑ NO ❑ **YES** She should not use a latex diaphragm. She can use a diaphragm made of plastic.

3. Do you have HIV infection? Do you think you are at high risk of HIV infection? (Discuss what places a woman at high risk for HIV—for example, her partner has HIV. [See Sexually Transmitted Infections, Including HIV, Who Is At Risk?, p. 330].)

❑ NO ❑ **YES** Do not provide a diaphragm. For HIV protection, recommend using condoms alone or with another method.

For complete classifications, see Medical Eligibility Criteria for Contraceptive Use, p. 388.

Be sure to explain the health benefits and risks and the side effects of the method that the client will use. Also, point out any conditions that would make the method inadvisable, when relevant to the client.

Using Clinical Judgment in Special Cases of Diaphragm Use

Usually, a woman with any of the conditions listed below should not use the diaphragm. In special circumstances, however, when other, more appropriate methods are not available or acceptable to her, a qualified provider who can carefully assess a specific woman's condition and situation may decide that she can use the diaphragm with spermicide. The provider needs to consider the severity of her condition and, for most conditions, whether she will have access to follow-up.

- History of toxic shock syndrome
- Allergy to latex, especially if the allergic reaction is mild (see Mild irritation in or around the vagina or penis or mild allergic reaction to condom, p. 256)
- HIV infection

Providing Diaphragms

When to Start

Woman's situation	When to start
Any time	**At any time** • If she has had a full-term delivery or second-trimester spontaneous or induced abortion less than 6 weeks ago, give her a backup method* to use, if needed, until 6 weeks have passed.
Special advice for women switching from another method	• Suggest that she try the diaphragm for a time while still using her other method. This way she can safely gain confidence that she can use the diaphragm correctly.

* *Backup methods include abstinence, male and female condoms, spermicides, and withdrawal. Tell her that spermicides and withdrawal are the least effective contraceptive methods. If possible, give her condoms.*

Explaining the Fitting Procedure

Learning to fit women for a diaphragm requires training and practice. Therefore, this is a summary and not detailed instructions.

1. The provider uses proper infection-prevention procedures (see Infection Prevention in the Clinic, p. 376).
2. The woman lies down as for a pelvic examination.
3. The provider checks for conditions that may make it impossible to use the diaphragm, such as uterine prolapse.
4. The provider inserts the index and middle fingers into the vagina to determine the correct diaphragm size.
5. The provider inserts a special fitting diaphragm into the client's vagina so that it covers the cervix. The provider then checks the location of the cervix and makes sure that the diaphragm fits properly and does not come out easily.
6. The provider gives the woman a properly fitting diaphragm and plenty of spermicide to use with it, and teaches her to use it properly (see Explaining How to Use the Diaphragm, below).

With a properly fitted diaphragm in place, the client should not be able to feel anything inside her vagina, even when she walks or during sex.

Explaining How to Use the Diaphragm

IMPORTANT: Whenever possible, show the woman the location of the pubic bone and cervix with a model or a picture. Explain that the diaphragm is inserted behind the pubic bone and covers the cervix.

Explain the 5 Basic Steps to Using a Diaphragm

Basic Steps	Important Details
1. Squeeze a spoonful of spermicidal cream, jelly, or foam into the diaphragm and around the rim	• Wash hands with mild soap and clean water, if possible. • Check the diaphragm for holes, cracks, or tears by holding it up to the light. • Check the expiration date of the spermicide and avoid using any beyond its expiration date.
2. Press the rim together; push into the vagina as far as it goes	• Insert the diaphragm less than 6 hours before having sex. • Choose a position that is comfortable for insertion—squatting, raising one leg, sitting, or lying down.

3. Feel diaphragm to make sure it covers the cervix

- Through the dome of the diaphragm, the cervix feels like the tip of the nose.
- If the diaphragm feels uncomfortable, take it out and insert it again.

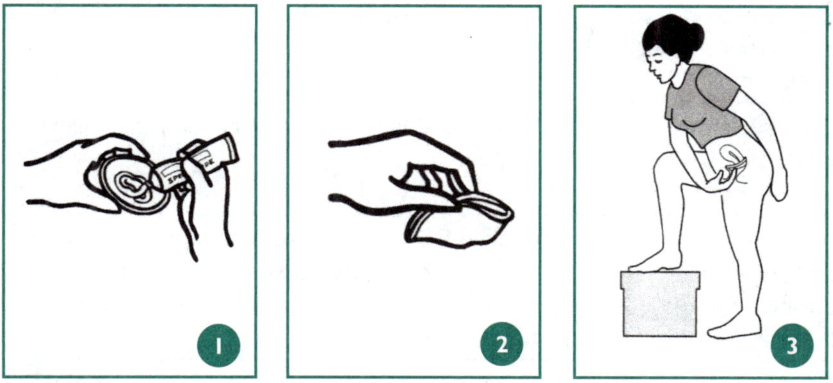

4. Leave in place for at least 6 hours after sex

- Leave the diaphragm in place at least 6 hours after having sex but no longer than 24 hours.
- *Leaving the diaphragm in place for more than one day may increase the risk of toxic shock syndrome.* It can also cause a bad odor and vaginal discharge. (Odor and discharge go away on their own after the diaphragm is removed.)
- For multiple acts of sex, make sure that the diaphragm is in the correct position and also insert additional spermicide in front of the diaphragm before each act of sex.

5. To remove, slide a finger under the rim of the diaphragm and pull it down and out

- Wash hands with mild soap and clean water, if possible.
- Insert a finger into the vagina until the rim of the diaphragm is felt.
- Gently slide a finger under the rim and pull the diaphragm down and out. Use care not to tear the diaphragm with a fingernail.
- Wash the diaphragm with mild soap and clean water and dry it after each use.

Supporting the Diaphragm User

Ensure client understands correct use	• Ask the client to repeat how and when to insert and remove the diaphragm.
Explain that use becomes easier with time	• Inserting and removing the diaphragm becomes easier with practice.
Describe the most common side effects	• Itching and irritation in or around the vagina or penis.
Explain about emergency contraceptive pills (ECPs)	• Explain ECP use in case the diaphragm moves out of place or is not used properly (see Emergency Contraceptive Pills, p. 49). Give her ECPs, if available.
Explain about replacement	• When a diaphragm gets thin, develops holes, or becomes stiff, it should not be used and needs to be replaced. She should obtain a new diaphragm about every 2 years.

Tips for Users of Spermicides or the Diaphragm With Spermicide

- Spermicides should be stored in a cool, dry place, if possible, out of the sun. Suppositories may melt in hot weather. If kept dry, foaming tablets are not as likely to melt in hot weather.
- The diaphragm should be stored in a cool, dry place, if possible.
- She needs a new diaphragm fitted if she has had a baby or a second-trimester miscarriage or abortion.

"Come Back Any Time": Reasons to Return

Assure every client that she is welcome to come back any time—for example, if she has problems, questions, or wants another method; she has any major change in health status; or she thinks she might be pregnant.

General health advice: Anyone who suddenly feels that something is seriously wrong with her health should immediately seek medical care from a nurse or doctor. Her contraceptive method is most likely not the cause of the condition, but she should tell the nurse or doctor what method she is using.

Helping Continuing Users

1. Ask how the client is doing with the method and whether she is satisfied. Ask if she has any questions or anything to discuss.
2. Ask especially if she has any problems using the method correctly and every time she has sex. Give her any information or help she needs (see Managing Any Problems, below).
3. Give her more supplies and encourage her to come back for more before she runs out. Remind her where else she can obtain more spermicides when needed.
4. Ask a long-term client if she has had any new health problems since her last visit. Address problems as appropriate. For new health problems that may require switching methods, see p. 285.
5. Ask a long-term client about major life changes that may affect her needs—particularly plans for having children and STI/HIV risk. Follow up as needed.

Managing Any Problems

Problems Reported as Side Effects or Problems With Use

May or may not be due to the method.

- Side effects or problems with spermicides or diaphragms affect women's satisfaction and use of the method. They deserve the provider's attention. If the client reports side effects or problems, listen to her concerns, give her advice and support, and, if appropriate, treat. Make sure she understands the advice and agrees.
- Offer to help the client choose another method—now, if she wishes, or if problems cannot be overcome.

Difficulty inserting or removing diaphragm

- Give advice on insertion and removal. Ask her to insert and remove the diaphragm in the clinic. Check its placement after she inserts it. Correct any errors.

Discomfort or pain with diaphragm use

- A diaphragm that is too large can cause discomfort. Check if it fits well.
  - Fit her with a smaller diaphragm if it is too large.
  - If fit appears proper and different kinds of diaphragms are available, try a different diaphragm.
- Ask her to insert and remove the diaphragm in the clinic. Check the diaphragm's placement after she inserts it. Give further advice as needed.

- Check for vaginal lesions:
  - If vaginal lesions or sores exist, suggest she use another method temporarily (condoms or oral contraceptives) and give her supplies. Lesions will go away on their own if she switches to another method.
  - Assess for vaginal infection or sexually transmitted infection (STI). Treat or refer for treatment as appropriate.

Irritation in or around the vagina or penis (she or her partner has itching, rash, or irritation that lasts for a day or more)

- Check for vaginal infection or STI. Treat or refer for treatment as appropriate.
- If no infection, suggest trying a different type or brand of spermicide.

Urinary tract infection (burning or pain with urination, frequent urination in small amounts, blood in the urine, back pain)

- Treat with cotrimoxazole 240 mg orally once a day for 3 days, or trimethoprim 100 mg orally once a day for 3 days, or nitrofurantoin 50 mg orally twice a day for 3 days.
- If infection recurs, consider refitting the client with a smaller diaphragm.

Bacterial vaginosis (abnormal white or gray vaginal discharge with unpleasant odor; may also have burning during urination and/or itching around the vagina)

- Treat with metronidazole 2 g orally in a single dose or metronidazole 400–500 mg orally twice a day for 7 days.

Candidiasis (abnormal white vaginal discharge that can be watery or thick and chunky; may also have burning during urination and/or redness and itching around the vagina)

- Treat with fluconazole 150 mg orally in a single dose, miconazole 200 mg vaginal suppository once a day for 3 days, or clotrimazole 100 mg vaginal tablets twice a day for 3 days.
- Miconazole suppositories are oil-based and can weaken a latex diaphragm. Women using miconazole vaginally should not use latex diaphragms or condoms during treatment. They can use a plastic female or male condom or another method until all medication is taken. (Oral treatment will not harm latex.)

Suspected pregnancy

- Assess for pregnancy.
- There are no known risks to a fetus conceived while a woman is using spermicides.

New Problems That May Require Switching Methods

May or may not be due to the method.

Recurring urinary tract infections or vaginal infections (such as bacterial vaginosis or candidiasis)

- Consider refitting the client with a smaller diaphragm.

Latex allergy (redness, itching, rash, and/or swelling of genitals, groin, or thighs [mild reaction]; or hives or rash over much of the body, dizziness, difficulty breathing, loss of consciousness [severe reaction])

- Tell the client to stop using a latex diaphragm. Give her a plastic diaphragm, if available, or help her choose another method, but not latex condoms.

Toxic shock syndrome (sudden high fever, body rash, vomiting, diarrhea, dizziness, sore throat, and muscle aches). See Signs and Symptoms of Serious Health Conditions, p. 384.

- Treat or refer for immediate diagnosis and care. Toxic shock syndrome can be life-threatening.
- Tell the client to stop using the diaphragm. Help her choose another method but not the cervical cap.

Questions and Answers About Spermicides and Diaphragms

1. **Do spermicides cause birth defects? Will the fetus be harmed if a woman accidentally uses spermicides while she is pregnant?**

   No. Good evidence shows that spermicides will not cause birth defects or otherwise harm the fetus if a woman becomes pregnant while using spermicides or accidentally uses spermicides when she is already pregnant.

2. **Do spermicides cause cancer?**

   No, spermicides do not cause cancer.

3. **Do spermicides increase the risk of becoming infected with HIV?**

   Women who use nonoxynol-9 several times a day may face an increased risk of infection with HIV. Spermicides can cause vaginal irritation, which may cause small lesions to form on the lining of the vagina or on the external genitals. These lesions may make it easier for a woman to become infected with HIV. Studies that suggest spermicide use increases HIV risk have involved women who used spermicides several times a day. Women who have multiple daily acts of sex should use another contraceptive method. A study among women using nonoxynol-9 an average of 3 times a week, however, found no increased risk of HIV infection for spermicide users compared with women not using spermicides. New spermicides that are less irritating may become available.

4. **Is the diaphragm uncomfortable for the woman?**

   No, not if it is fitted and inserted correctly. The woman and her partner usually cannot feel the diaphragm during sex. The provider selects the properly sized diaphragm for each woman so that it fits her and does not hurt. If it is uncomfortable, she should come back to have the fit checked and to make sure that she is inserting and removing the diaphragm properly.

5. **If a woman uses the diaphragm without spermicides, will it still prevent pregnancy?**

   There is not enough evidence to be certain. A few studies find that diaphragm users have higher pregnancy rates when they do not use a spermicide with the diaphragm. Thus, using a diaphragm without spermicide is not recommended.

6. Could a woman leave a diaphragm in all day?

Yes, although doing so is usually not recommended. A woman could leave a diaphragm in all day if she cannot put it in shortly before having sex. She should not leave the diaphragm in for more than 24 hours, however. This can increase the risk of toxic shock syndrome.

7. Can a woman use lubricants with a diaphragm?

Yes, but only water- or silicone-based lubricants if the diaphragm is made of latex. Products made with oil cannot be used as lubricants because they damage latex. Materials that should not be used with latex diaphragms include any oils (cooking, baby, coconut, mineral), petroleum jelly, lotions, cold creams, butter, cocoa butter, and margarine. Oil-based lubricants will not harm a plastic diaphragm. Spermicides usually provide enough lubrication for diaphragm users.

8. Do diaphragms help protect women from STIs, including HIV?

Research suggests that the diaphragm may help protect somewhat against infections of the cervix such as gonorrhea and chlamydia. Some studies have also found that it also may help protect against pelvic inflammatory disease and trichomoniasis. Studies are underway to assess whether incorporating a microbicide into the diaphragm would help to prevent HIV and other STIs. Currently, only male and female condoms are recommended for protection from HIV and other STIs.

9. Is there a new diaphragm that does not require fitting?

Yes. The one-size SILCS diaphragm has been developed to fit most women without the need for a provider specifically trained to fit the diaphragm. Made of silicone, it can be easier to handle and more comfortable than conventional latex diaphragms. It is registered under the brand name Caya in 3 dozen countries. Used with a spermicidal gel, it offers similar protection to conventional diaphragms.

10. What is the vaginal sponge, and how effective is it?

The vaginal sponge is made of plastic and contains spermicides. It is moistened with water and inserted into the vagina so that it rests against the cervix. Each sponge can be used only once. It is not widely available.

Effectiveness depends on the user: Risk of pregnancy is greatest when a woman does not use the sponge with every act of sex.

Women who have given birth:

- One of the least effective methods, as commonly used.
- As commonly used, about 32 pregnancies per 100 women using the sponge over the first year.
- When used correctly with every act of sex, about 20 pregnancies per 100 women over the first year.

More effective among women who have not given birth:

- As commonly used, about 16 pregnancies per 100 women using the sponge over the first year.
- When used correctly with every act of sex, about 9 pregnancies per 100 women over the first year.

Only the Essentials CHAPTER 17

Cervical Caps

Key Points for Providers and Clients

- **The cervical cap is placed deep in the vagina before sex.** It covers the cervix.
- **Requires correct use with every act of sex for greatest effectiveness.**
- **Used together with spermicide to improve effectiveness.**

What Is the Cervical Cap?

- A soft, deep, latex or plastic rubber cup that snugly covers the cervix.
- Comes in different sizes; requires fitting by a specifically trained provider.

How Effective?

Effectiveness depends on the user: Risk of pregnancy is greatest when the cervical cap with spermicide is not used with every act of sex.

Women who have given birth:

- One of the least effective methods, as commonly used.
- As commonly used, about 32 pregnancies per 100 women using the cervical cap with spermicide over the first year. This means that 68 of every 100 women using the cervical cap will not become pregnant.
- When used correctly with every act of sex, about 26 pregnancies per 100 women using the cervical cap over the first year.

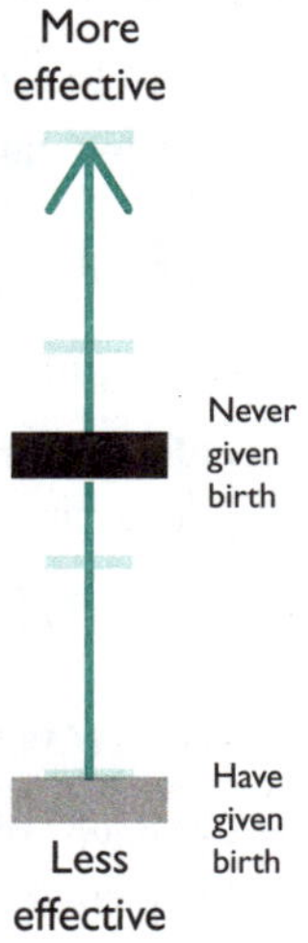

More effective among women who have not given birth:

- As commonly used, about 16 pregnancies per 100 women using the cervical cap with spermicide over the first year. This means that 84 of every 100 women using the cervical cap will not become pregnant.
- When used correctly with every act of sex, about 9 pregnancies per 100 women using the cervical cap over the first year.

Return of fertility after use of cervical cap is stopped: No delay
Protection against sexually transmitted infections: None

Side Effects, Health Benefits, and Health Risks

Same as for diaphragms (see Diaphragms, Side Effects, Health Benefits, and Health Risks, p. 277).

Medical Eligibility Criteria for

Cervical Caps

Ask the client the Medical Eligibility Criteria questions for diaphragms (see p. 278). Also ask the question below about known medical conditions. Examinations and tests are not necessary. If she answers "no" to all of the questions here and for the diaphragm, then she can start the cervical cap if she wants. If she answers "yes" to a question, follow the instructions. In some cases she can still start the cervical cap.

1. Have you been treated or are you going to be treated for cervical precancer (cervical intraepithelial neoplasia [CIN]) or cervical cancer?

❑ NO ❑ **YES** Do not provide the cervical cap.

For complete classifications, see Medical Eligibility Criteria for Contraceptive Use, p. 388.

Be sure to explain the health benefits and risks and the side effects of the method that the client will use. Also, point out any conditions that would make the method inadvisable, when relevant to the client.

Providing Cervical Caps

Providing the cervical cap is similar to providing diaphragms (see p. 279) and helping diaphragm users (see p. 283). Differences include:

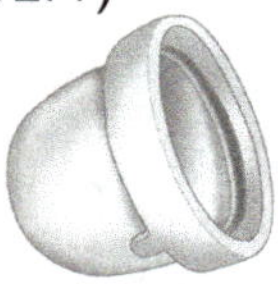

Inserting

- Fill one-third of the cap with spermicidal cream, jelly, or foam.
- Press the rim of the cap around the cervix until it is completely covered, pressing gently on the dome to apply suction and seal the cap.
- Insert the cervical cap any time up to 42 hours before having sex.

Removing

- Leave the cervical cap in for at least 6 hours after her partner's last ejaculation, but not more than 48 hours from the time it was put in.
- Leaving the cap in place for more than 48 hours may increase the risk of toxic shock syndrome and can cause a bad odor and vaginal discharge.
- Tip the cap rim sideways to break the seal against the cervix, and then gently pull the cap down and out of the vagina.

CHAPTER 18

Fertility Awareness Methods

Key Points for Providers and Clients

- **Fertility awareness methods require partners' cooperation.** Couple must be committed to abstaining or using another method on fertile days.
- **Must stay aware of body changes or keep track of days, according to rules of the specific method.**
- **No side effects or health risks.**

What Are Fertility Awareness Methods?

- "Fertility awareness" means that a woman knows how to tell when the fertile time of her menstrual cycle starts and ends. (The fertile time is when she can become pregnant.)
- Sometimes called periodic abstinence or natural family planning.
- A woman can use several ways, alone or in combination, to tell when her fertile time begins and ends.
- *Calendar-based methods* involve keeping track of days of the menstrual cycle to identify the start and end of the fertile time.
  - Examples: Standard Days Method, which avoids unprotected vaginal sex on days 8 through 19 of the menstrual cycle, and calendar rhythm method.
- *Symptoms-based methods* depend on observing signs of fertility.
  - Cervical secretions: When a woman sees or feels cervical secretions, she may be fertile. She may feel just a little vaginal wetness.
  - Basal body temperature (BBT): A woman's resting body temperature goes up slightly after the release of an egg (ovulation). She is not likely to become pregnant from 3 days after this temperature rise through the start of her next monthly bleeding. Her temperature stays higher until the beginning of her next monthly bleeding.
  - Examples: TwoDay Method, BBT method, ovulation method (also known as Billings method or cervical mucus method), and symptothermal method.

- Work primarily by helping a woman know when she could become pregnant. The couple prevents pregnancy by avoiding unprotected vaginal sex during these fertile days—usually by abstaining or by using condoms or a diaphragm. Some couples use spermicides or withdrawal, but these are among the least effective methods.

How Effective?

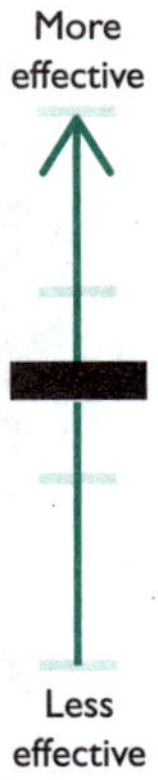

Effectiveness depends on the user: Risk of pregnancy is greatest when couples have sex on the fertile days without using another method.

- As commonly used, in the first year about 15 pregnancies per 100 women using periodic abstinence. This means that 85 of every 100 women relying on periodic abstinence will not become pregnant. Most of the couples in this study were using the calendar rhythm method.
- Pregnancy rates with consistent and correct use vary for different types of fertility awareness methods (see table below). These rates reflect the experience of couples who volunteered to use these methods in research projects (see Question 3, p. 306). Reliable effectiveness rates are not available for the calendar rhythm method or the basal body temperature method.
- In general, abstaining during fertile times is more effective than using another method during fertile times.

	Pregnancies per 100 Women Over the First Year of Use	
Method	**Consistent and correct use**	**As commonly used**
Calendar-based methods		
Standard Days Method	5	12
Symptoms-based methods		
TwoDay Method	4	14
Ovulation method	3	23
Symptothermal method	<1	2

Return of fertility after fertility awareness methods are stopped: No delay

Protection against sexually transmitted infections (STIs): None

Side Effects, Health Benefits, and Health Risks

Side Effects

None

Known Health Benefits

Help protect against:

- Risks of pregnancy

Known Health Risks

None

Why Some Women Say They Like Fertility Awareness Methods

- Have no side effects
- Do not require procedures and usually do not require supplies
- Help women learn about their bodies and fertility
- Allow some couples to adhere to their religious or cultural norms about contraception
- Can be used to identify fertile days by both women who want to become pregnant and women who want to avoid pregnancy

Correcting Misunderstandings (see also Questions and Answers, p. 305)

Fertility awareness methods:

- Can be effective if used consistently and correctly.
- Do not require literacy or advanced education.
- Do not harm men who abstain from sex.
- Do not work when a couple is mistaken about when the fertile time occurs, such as thinking it occurs during monthly bleeding.

Fertility Awareness Methods for Women With HIV

- Women who are living with HIV or are on antiretroviral (ARV) therapy can safely use fertility awareness methods.
- Urge these women to use condoms along with fertility awareness methods. Used consistently and correctly, condoms help prevent transmission of HIV and other STIs.

Who Can Use Calendar-Based Methods

Medical Eligibility Criteria for
Calendar-Based Methods

All women can use calendar-based methods. No medical conditions prevent the use of these methods, but some conditions can make them harder to use effectively.

Caution means that additional or special counseling may be needed to ensure correct use of the method.

Delay means that use of a particular fertility awareness method should be delayed until the condition is evaluated or corrected. Give the client another method to use until she can start the calendar-based method.

In the following situation, use **caution** with calendar-based methods:

- Menstrual cycles are irregular. (For example, menstrual cycle irregularities are common in young women in the first several years after their first monthly bleeding and in older women who are approaching menopause. Identifying the fertile time may be difficult.)

In the following situations, **delay** starting calendar-based methods:

- Recently gave birth or is breastfeeding, (**Delay** until she has had at least 3 menstrual cycles and her cycles are regular again. For several months after regular cycles have returned, use with **caution**.)
- Recently had an abortion or miscarriage (**Delay** until the start of her next monthly bleeding.)
- Irregular vaginal bleeding (**Delay** until cycles have become more regular.)

In the following situation, **delay** or use **caution** with calendar-based methods:

- Taking drugs that can make the menstrual cycle irregular (for example, certain antidepressants, thyroid medications, long-term use of certain antibiotics, or long-term use of any nonsteroidal anti-inflammatory drug, such as aspirin or ibuprofen).

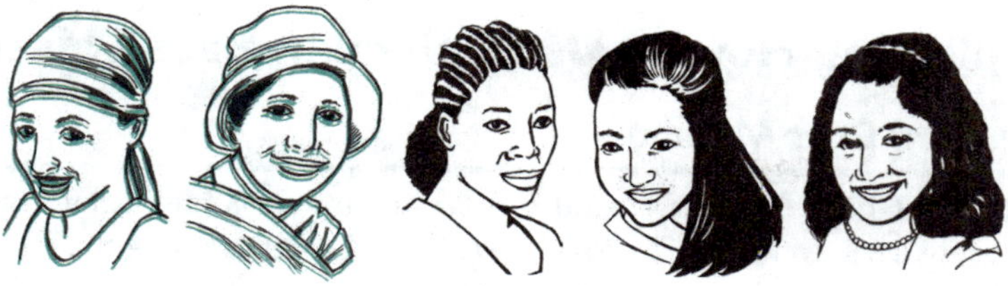

Providing Calendar-Based Methods

When to Start

Once trained, a woman or couple usually can begin using calendar-based methods at any time. Give clients who cannot start immediately another method to use until they can start.

Woman's situation	When to start
Having regular menstrual cycles	**Any time of the month** • No need to wait until the start of next monthly bleeding.
No monthly bleeding	• Delay calendar-based methods until monthly bleeding returns.
After childbirth (whether or not breastfeeding)	• Delay the Standard Days Method until she has had 4 menstrual cycles and the last one was 26–32 days long. • Regular cycles will return later in breastfeeding women than in women who are not breastfeeding.
After miscarriage or abortion	• Delay the Standard Days Method until the start of her next monthly bleeding, when she can start if she has no bleeding due to injury to the genital tract.
Switching from a hormonal method	• Delay starting the Standard Days Method until the start of her next monthly bleeding. • If she is switching from injectables, delay the Standard Days Method at least until her repeat injection would have been given, and then start it at the beginning of her next monthly bleeding.
After taking emergency contraceptive pills	• Delay the Standard Days Method until the start of her next monthly bleeding.

Explaining How to Use Calendar-Based Methods

Standard Days Method

IMPORTANT: A woman can use the Standard Days Method if most of her menstrual cycles are 26 to 32 days long. If she has more than 2 longer or shorter cycles within a year, the Standard Days Method will be less effective and she may want to choose another method.

Keep track of the days of the menstrual cycle	• A woman keeps track of the days of her menstrual cycle, counting the first day of monthly bleeding as day 1.
Avoid unprotected sex on days 8–19	• Days 8 through 19 of every cycle are considered fertile days for all users of the Standard Days Method. • The couple avoids vaginal sex or uses condoms or a diaphragm during days 8 through 19. They can also use withdrawal or spermicides, but these are less effective. • The couple can have unprotected sex on all the other days of the cycle—days 1 through 7 at the beginning of the cycle and from day 20 until her next monthly bleeding begins.
Use memory aids if needed	• The couple can use CycleBeads, a color-coded string of beads that indicates fertile and nonfertile days of a cycle (see diagram below), or they can mark a calendar or use some other memory aid.

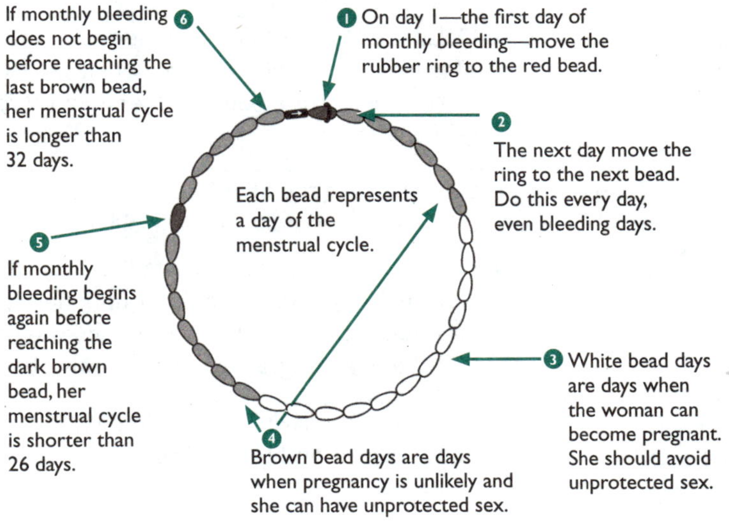

Calendar Rhythm Method

Keep track of the days of the menstrual cycle	• Before relying on this method, a woman records the number of days in each menstrual cycle for at least 6 months. The first day of monthly bleeding is always counted as day 1.
Estimate the fertile time	• The woman subtracts 18 from the length of her shortest recorded cycle. This tells her the estimated first day of her fertile time. Then she subtracts 11 days from the length of her longest recorded cycle. This tells her the estimated last day of her fertile time.
Avoid unprotected sex during fertile time	• The couple avoids vaginal sex, or uses condoms or a diaphragm, during the fertile time. They can also use withdrawal or spermicides, but these are less effective.
Update calculations monthly	• She updates these calculations each month, always using the 6 most recent cycles. Example: – If the shortest of her last 6 cycles was 27 days, 27 – 18 = 9. She starts avoiding unprotected sex on day 9. – If the longest of her last 6 cycles was 31 days, 31 – 11 = 20. She can have unprotected sex again on day 21. – Thus, she must avoid unprotected sex from day 9 through day 20 of her cycle.

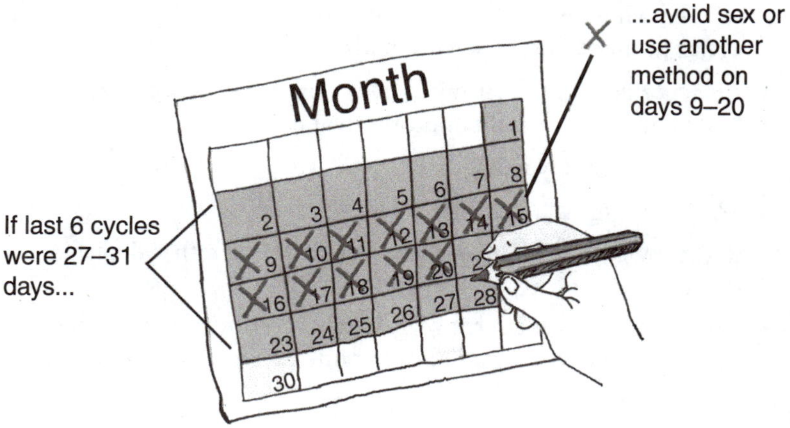

Who Can Use Symptoms-Based Methods

Medical Eligibility Criteria for

Symptoms-Based Methods

All women can use symptoms-based methods. No medical conditions prevent the use of these methods, but some conditions can make them harder to use effectively.

Caution means that additional or special counseling may be needed to ensure correct use of the method.

Delay means that use of a particular fertility awareness method should be delayed until the condition is evaluated or corrected. Give the client another method to use until she can start the symptoms-based method.

In the following situations, use **caution** with symptoms-based methods:

- Recently had an abortion or miscarriage
- Menstrual cycles have just started or have become less frequent or stopped due to older age. (Menstrual cycle irregularities are common in young women in the first several years after their first monthly bleeding and in older women who are approaching menopause. Identifying the fertile time may be difficult.)
- A chronic condition that raises her body temperature (for basal body temperature and symptothermal methods)

In the following situations, **delay** starting symptoms-based methods:

- Recently gave birth or is breastfeeding. (**Delay** until normal secretions have returned—usually at least 6 months after childbirth for breastfeeding women and at least 4 weeks after childbirth for women who are not breastfeeding. For several months after regular cycles have returned, use with **caution**.)
- An acute condition that raises her body temperature (for basal body temperature and symptothermal methods)
- Irregular vaginal bleeding
- Abnormal vaginal discharge

In the following situation, **delay** or use **caution** with symptoms-based methods:

- Taking any drugs that change cervical secretions, for example, antihistimines, or drugs that raise body temperature, for example, antibiotics.

Providing Symptoms-Based Methods

When to Start

Once trained, a woman or couple usually can begin using symptoms-based methods at any time. Women not using a hormonal method can practice monitoring their fertility signs before they start using symptoms-based methods. Give clients who cannot start immediately another method to use until they can start.

Woman's situation	When to start
Having regular menstrual cycles	**Any time of the month** • No need to wait until the start of next monthly bleeding.
No monthly bleeding	• Delay symptoms-based methods until monthly bleeding returns.
After childbirth (whether or not breastfeeding)	• She can start symptoms-based methods once normal secretions have returned. • Normal secretions will return later in breast-feeding women than in women who are not breastfeeding.
After miscarriage or abortion	• She can start symptoms-based methods immediately with special counseling and support, if she has no infection-related secretions or bleeding due to injury to the genital tract.
Switching from a hormonal method	• She can start symptoms-based methods in the next menstrual cycle after stopping a hormonal method.
After taking emergency contraceptive pills	• She can start symptoms-based methods once normal secretions have returned.

Explaining How to Use Symptoms-Based Methods

TwoDay Method

IMPORTANT: If a woman has a vaginal infection or another condition that changes cervical mucus, the TwoDay Method will be difficult to use.

Check for secretions

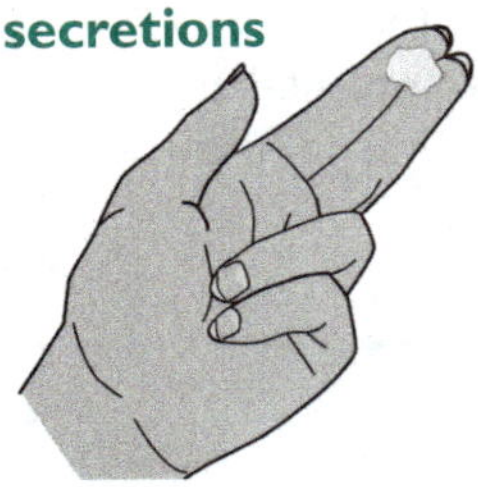

- The woman checks for cervical secretions every afternoon and/or evening, on fingers, underwear, or tissue paper or by sensation in or around the vagina.
- As soon as she notices any secretions of any type, color, or consistency, she considers herself fertile that day and the following day.

Avoid sex or use another method on fertile days

- The couple avoids vaginal sex or uses condoms or a diaphragm on each day with secretions and on each day following a day with secretions. They can also use withdrawal or spermicides, but these are less effective.

Resume unprotected sex after 2 dry days

- The couple can have unprotected sex again after the woman has had 2 dry days (days without secretions of any type) in a row.

Basal Body Temperature (BBT) Method

IMPORTANT: If a woman has a fever or other changes in body temperature, the BBT method will be difficult to use.

Take body temperature daily

- The woman takes her body temperature at the same time each morning before she gets out of bed and before she eats anything. She records her temperature on a special graph.
- She watches for her temperature to rise slightly—0.2° to 0.5°C (0.4° to 1.0°F)—just after ovulation (usually about midway through the menstrual cycle).

Avoid sex or use another method until 3 days after the temperature rise

- The couple avoids vaginal sex, or uses condoms or a diaphragm from the first day of monthly bleeding until 3 days after the woman's temperature has risen above her regular temperature. They can also use withdrawal or spermicides, but these are less effective.

Resume unprotected sex until next monthly bleeding begins	• When the woman's temperature has risen above her regular temperature and stayed higher for 3 full days, ovulation has occurred and the fertile period has passed. • The couple can have unprotected sex on the 4th day and until her next monthly bleeding begins.

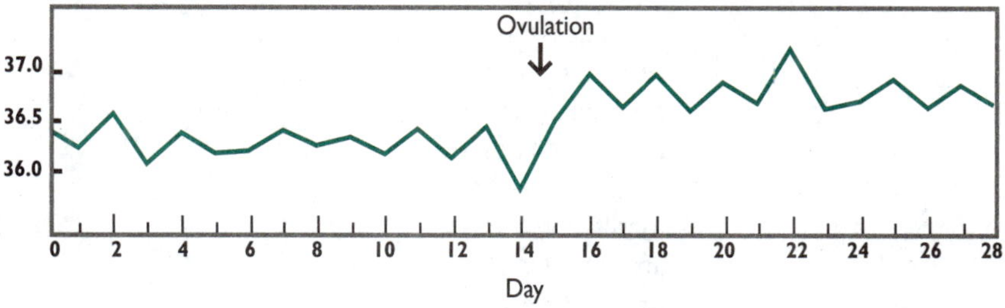

Ovulation Method

IMPORTANT: If a woman has a vaginal infection or another condition that changes cervical mucus, this method may be difficult to use.

Check cervical secretions daily	• The woman checks every day for any cervical secretions on fingers, underwear, or tissue paper or by sensation in or around the vagina.
Avoid unprotected sex on days of heavy monthly bleeding	• Ovulation might occur early in the cycle, during the last days of monthly bleeding. Heavy bleeding could make mucus difficult to observe.
Resume unprotected sex until secretions begin	• Between the end of monthly bleeding and the start of secretions, the couple can have unprotected sex, but not on 2 days in a row. (Avoiding sex on the second day allows time for semen to disappear and for cervical mucus to be observed.) • It is recommended that they have sex in the evenings, after the woman has been in an upright position for at least a few hours and has been able to check for cervical mucus.

(Continued on next page)

Avoid unprotected sex when secretions begin and until 4 days after "peak day"	• As soon as she notices any secretions, she considers herself fertile and avoids unprotected sex. • She continues to check her cervical secretions each day. The secretions have a "peak day"—the last day that they are clear, slippery, stretchy, and wet. She will know this has passed when, on the next day, her secretions are sticky or dry, or she has no secretions at all. She continues to consider herself fertile for 3 days after that peak day and avoids unprotected sex.
Resume unprotected sex	• The couple can have unprotected sex on the 4th day after her peak day and until her next monthly bleeding begins.

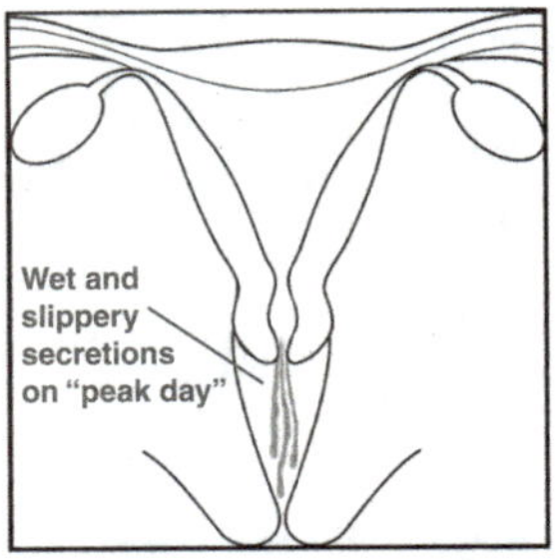

Symptothermal Method (basal body temperature + cervical secretions + other fertility signs)

Avoid unprotected sex on fertile days	• Users identify fertile and nonfertile days by combining BBT and ovulation method instructions. • Women may also identify the fertile time by other signs such as breast tenderness and ovulatory pain (lower abdominal pain or cramping around the time of ovulation). • The couple avoids unprotected sex between the first day of monthly bleeding and either the fourth day after peak cervical secretions or the third full day after the rise in temperature (BBT), whichever happens later. • Some women who use this method have unprotected sex between the end of monthly bleeding and the beginning of secretions, but not on 2 days in a row.

How Can a Partner Help?

The client's partner is welcome to participate in counseling and learn about the method and what support he can give to his partner. A male partner can:

- Support a woman's choice of a fertility awareness method
- Discuss and agree to use a fertility awareness method with a full understanding of how to use it
- Share responsibility for keeping track of cycles and knowing when is the fertile period
- Not insist on sex without contraception during the fertile period
- Agree in advance how to avoid pregnancy if they are going to have sex in the fertile period (for example, use of another method)
- Help to make sure she has ECPs on hand in case they have unprotected sex during the fertile period
- Use condoms consistently in addition to a fertility awareness method if he has an STI/HIV or thinks he may be at risk of an STI/HIV

Supporting the User

"Come Back Any Time": Reasons to Return

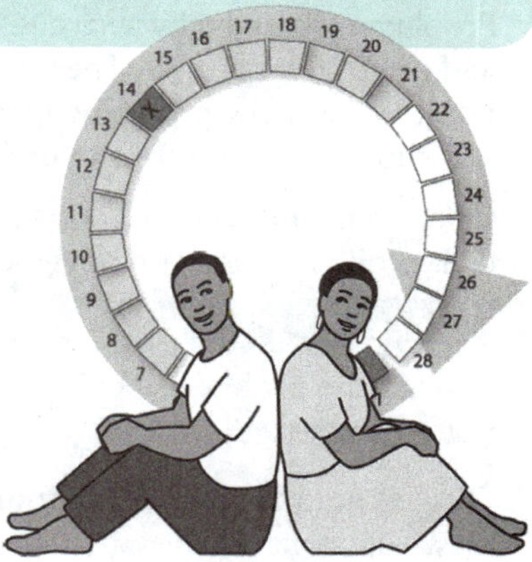

No routine return visit is required. Providers should invite a woman or couple to meet with them a few times during the first few cycles if they want more help. Assure every client that she is welcome to come back any time—for example, if she has problems, questions, or wants another method; she has any major change in health status; or thinks she might be pregnant. Also if:

- She is having difficulty identifying her fertile days.
- She is having trouble avoiding sex or using another method on the fertile days. For example, her partner does not cooperate.

Helping Continuing Users

Helping Clients at Any Visit

1. Ask clients how they are doing with the method and whether they are satisfied. Ask if they have any questions or anything to discuss.
2. Ask especially if they are having difficulty identifying her fertile days or trouble avoiding unprotected sex on the fertile days.
3. Check whether the couple is using the method correctly. Review observations or records of fertility signs. If needed, plan for another visit.
4. Ask a long-term client if she has had any new health problems since her last visit. Address problems as appropriate.
5. Ask a long-term client about major life changes that may affect her needs—particularly plans for having children and STI/HIV risk. Follow up as needed.

Managing Any Problems

Problems With Use

- Problems with fertility awareness methods affect women's satisfaction and use of the method. They deserve the provider's attention. If the client reports any problems, listen to her concerns and give her advice and support. Make sure she understands the advice and agrees.
- Offer to help the client choose another method—now, if she wishes, or if problems cannot be overcome.

Inability to abstain from sex during the fertile time

- Discuss the problem openly with the couple and help them feel at ease, not embarrassed.
- Discuss possible use of condoms, diaphragm, withdrawal, or spermicides or sexual contact without vaginal sex during the fertile time.
- If she has had unprotected sex in the past 5 days, she can consider ECPs (see Emergency Contraceptive Pills, p. 49).

Calendar-Based Methods

Cycles are outside the 26–32 day range for Standard Days Method

- If she has 2 or more cycles outside the 26–32 day range within any 12 months, suggest she use the calendar rhythm method or a symptoms-based method instead.

Very irregular menstrual cycles among users of calendar-based methods

- Suggest use of a symptoms-based method instead.

Symptoms-Based Methods

Difficulty recognizing different types of secretions for the ovulation method

- Counsel the client and help her learn how to interpret cervical secretions.
- Suggest she use the TwoDay Method, which does not require the user to tell the difference among types of secretions.

Difficulty recognizing the presence of secretions for the ovulation method or the TwoDay Method

- Provide additional guidance on how to recognize secretions.
- Suggest she use a calendar-based method instead.

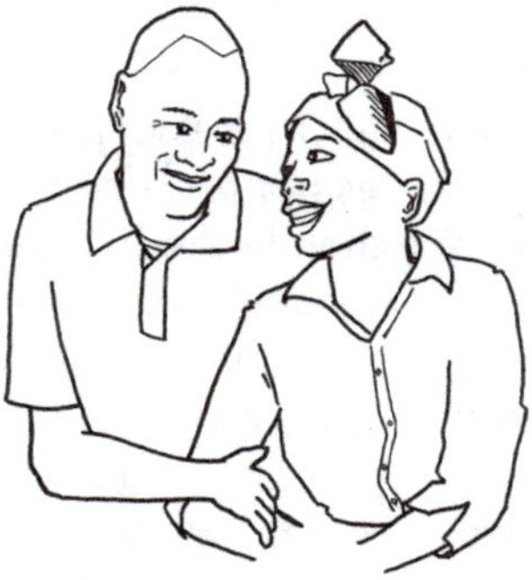

Questions and Answers About Fertility Awareness Methods

1. Can only well-educated couples use fertility awareness methods?

No. Couples with little or no formal schooling can and do use fertility awareness methods effectively. Couples must be highly motivated, well-trained in their method, and committed to avoiding unprotected sex during the fertile time.

2. Are fertility awareness methods reliable?

For many couples, these methods provide reliable information about the fertile days. If the couple avoids vaginal sex, or uses condoms or a diaphragm during the woman's fertile time, fertility awareness methods can be effective. Using withdrawal or spermicides during the fertile time is less effective.

3. What is different about the newer fertility awareness methods, the Standard Days Method and the TwoDay Method?

These fertility awareness methods are easier to use correctly than some of the older ones. Thus, they could appeal to more couples and be more effective for some people. They are like older methods, however, in that they rely on the same ways of judging when a woman might be fertile—by keeping track of the days of the cycle for the Standard Days Method and by cervical secretions for the TwoDay Method. So far, there are few studies of these methods. A clinical trial found that, as the Standard Days Method was commonly used by women who had most cycles between 26 and 32 days long, there were 12 pregnancies per 100 women over the first year of use. In a clinical trial of the TwoDay Method as it was commonly used, there were 14 pregnancies per 100 women over the first year of use. This rate is based on those who remained in the study. Women who detected secretions on fewer than 5 days or more than 14 days in each cycle were excluded.

4. How likely is a woman to become pregnant if she has sex during monthly bleeding?

During monthly bleeding the chances of pregnancy are low but not zero. Bleeding itself does not prevent pregnancy, and it does not promote pregnancy, either. In the first several days of monthly bleeding, the chances of pregnancy are lowest. For example, on day 2 of the cycle (counting from the first day of bleeding as day 1), the chance of getting pregnant is extremely low (less than 1%). As the days pass, the chances of pregnancy increase, whether or not she is still bleeding. The risk of pregnancy rises until ovulation. The day after ovulation the chances of pregnancy begin to drop steadily. Some fertility awareness methods that depend on cervical secretions advise avoiding unprotected sex during monthly bleeding because cervical secretions cannot be detected during bleeding and there is a small risk of ovulation at this time.

5. How many days of abstinence or use of another method might be required for each of the fertility awareness methods?

The number of days varies based on the woman's cycle length. The average number of days a woman would be considered fertile—and would need to abstain or use another method—with each method is: Standard Days Method, 12 days; TwoDay Method, 13 days; symptothermal method, 17 days; ovulation method, 18 days.

Withdrawal

Key Points for Providers and Clients

- **One of the least effective contraceptive methods.** Some men use this method effectively, however. Offers better pregnancy protection than no method at all.
- **Always available in every situation.** Can be used as a primary method or as a backup method.
- **Requires no supplies and no clinic or pharmacy visit.**
- **Promotes male involvement and couple communication.**

What Is Withdrawal?

- Just before ejaculation, the man withdraws his penis from his partner's vagina and ejaculates outside the vagina, keeping his semen away from her external genitalia.
- Also known as coitus interruptus and "pulling out."
- Works by keeping sperm out of the woman's body.

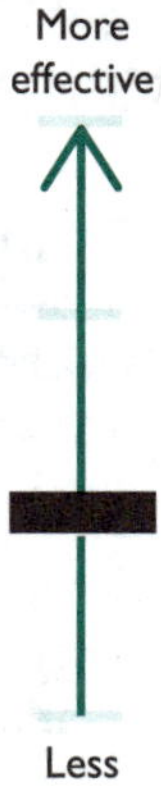

How Effective?

Effectiveness depends on the user: Risk of pregnancy is greatest when the man does not withdraw his penis from the vagina before he ejaculates with every act of sex.

- One of the least effective methods, as commonly used.
- As commonly used, about 20 pregnancies per 100 women whose partners use withdrawal over the first year. This means that 80 of every 100 women whose partners use withdrawal will not become pregnant.
- When used correctly with every act of sex, about 4 pregnancies per 100 women whose partners use withdrawal over the first year.

Return of fertility after use of withdrawal is stopped: No delay

Protection against sexually transmitted infections: None

Side Effects, Health Benefits, and Health Risks

None

19 Withdrawal

Who Can and Cannot Use Withdrawal

- **All men can use withdrawal.** No medical conditions prevent its use.
- Withdrawal may be especially appropriate for couples who:
  - have no other method available at the time
  - are waiting to start another method
  - have sex infrequently
  - have objections to using other methods

Using Withdrawal

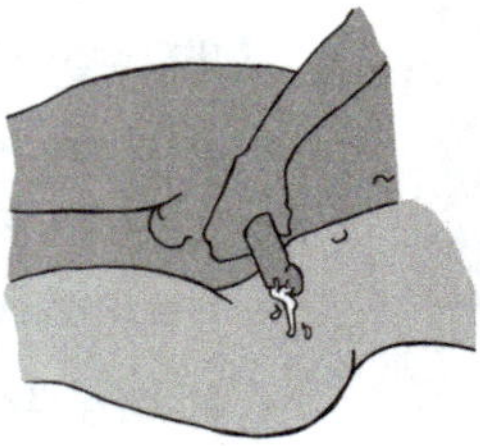

- Can be used at any time.
- Effectiveness depends on the willingness and ability of the couple to use withdrawal with every act of intercourse.

Explaining How to Use

When the man feels close to ejaculating	• He should withdraw his penis from the woman's vagina and ejaculate outside the vagina, keeping his semen away from her external genitalia.
If the man has ejaculated recently	• Before sex he should urinate and wipe the tip of his penis to remove any semen remaining.

Giving Advice on Use

Learning proper use can take time	• Suggest the couple also use another method until the man feels that he can use withdrawal correctly with every act of sex.
Greater protection from pregnancy is available	• Suggest an additional or alternative family planning method. (Couples who have been using withdrawal effectively should not be discouraged from continuing.)
Some men may have difficulty using withdrawal	• Men who cannot sense consistently when ejaculation is about to occur. • Men who ejaculate prematurely.
Can use emergency contraceptive pills (ECPs)	• Explain ECP use in case a man ejaculates before withdrawing (see Emergency Contraceptive Pills, p. 49). Give ECPs if available.

CHAPTER 20

Lactational Amenorrhea Method

Key Points for Providers and Clients

- **A family planning method based on breastfeeding.** Provides contraception for the mother and best feeding for the baby.
- **Can be effective for up to 6 months after childbirth,** as long as monthly bleeding has not returned and the woman is fully or nearly fully breastfeeding.
- **Requires breastfeeding often, day and night.** Almost all of the baby's feedings should be breast milk.
- **Provides an opportunity to offer a woman an ongoing method that she can continue to use after 6 months.**

What Is the Lactational Amenorrhea Method?

- A temporary family planning method based on the natural effect of breastfeeding on fertility. ("Lactational" means related to breastfeeding. "Amenorrhea" means not having monthly bleeding.)
- The lactational amenorrhea method (LAM) requires 3 conditions. All 3 must be met:
    1. The mother's monthly bleeding has not returned.
    2. The baby is fully or nearly fully breastfed and is fed often, day and night.
    3. The baby is less than 6 months old.
- "Fully breastfeeding" includes both exclusive breastfeeding (the infant receives no other liquid or food, not even water, in addition to breast milk) and almost-exclusive breastfeeding (the infant receives vitamins, water, juice, or other nutrients once in a while in addition to breast milk).
- "Nearly fully breastfeeding" means that the infant receives some liquid or food in addition to breast milk, but the majority of feedings (more than three-fourths of all feeds) are breast milk.

- Works primarily by preventing the release of eggs from the ovaries (ovulation). Frequent breastfeeding temporarily prevents the release of the natural hormones that cause ovulation.

How Effective?

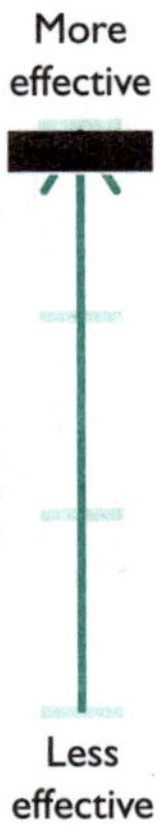

Effectiveness depends on the user: Risk of pregnancy is greatest when a woman cannot fully or nearly fully breastfeed her infant.

- As commonly used, about 2 pregnancies per 100 women using LAM in the first 6 months after childbirth. This means that 98 of every 100 women relying on LAM will not become pregnant.
- When used correctly, less than 1 pregnancy per 100 women using LAM in the first 6 months after childbirth.

Return of fertility after LAM is stopped: Depends on how much the woman continues to breastfeed

Protection against sexually transmitted infections: None

Side Effects, Health Benefits, and Health Risks

Side Effects

None. Any problems are the same as for other breastfeeding women.

Known Health Benefits

Helps protect against:

- Risks of pregnancy

Encourages:

- The best breastfeeding patterns, with health benefits for both mother and baby

Known Health Risks

None

Correcting Misunderstandings (see also Questions and Answers, p. 318)

The lactational amenorrhea method:

- Is highly effective when a woman meets all 3 LAM criteria.
- Is just as effective among fat or thin women.
- Can be used by women with normal nutrition. No special foods are required.
- Can be used for a full 6 months without the need for supplementary foods. Mother's milk alone can fully nourish a baby for the first 6 months of life. In fact, it is the ideal food for this time in a baby's life.
- Can be used for 6 months without worry that the woman will run out of milk. Milk will continue to be produced through 6 months and longer in response to the baby's suckling or the mother's expression of her milk.

Who Can Use the Lactational Amenorrhea Method

Medical Eligibility Criteria for the

Lactational Amenorrhea Method

All breastfeeding women can safely use LAM, but a woman in the following circumstances may want to consider other contraceptive methods:

- Has HIV infection (see The Lactational Amenorrhea Method for Women With HIV, next page)
- Is using certain medications during breastfeeding (including mood-altering drugs, reserpine, ergotamine, anti-metabolites, cyclosporine, high doses of corticosteroids, bromocriptine, radioactive drugs, lithium, and certain anticoagulants)
- The newborn has a condition that makes it difficult to breastfeed (including being small-for-date or premature and needing intensive neonatal care, unable to digest food normally, or having deformities of the mouth, jaw, or palate)

Why Some Women Say They Like the Lactational Amenorrhea Method

- It is a natural family planning method
- It supports optimal breastfeeding, providing health benefits for the baby and the mother
- It has no direct cost for family planning or for feeding the baby

The Lactational Amenorrhea Method for Women With HIV

- Women who are living with HIV can use LAM. Breastfeeding will not make their condition worse. There is a chance, however, that mothers living with HIV, if they are not taking antiretroviral therapy (ART), will transmit HIV to their infants through breastfeeding.
- Women taking ART can use LAM. Giving ART to an HIV-infected mother or an HIV-exposed infant very significantly reduces the risk of HIV transmission through breastfeeding. Among women who are not taking ART, 14% of their babies will be infected after 2 years of breastfeeding. Among women taking ART, less than 1% of their babies will be infected.
- Exclusive breastfeeding reduces the risk of death from common childhood illness and improves the health and development of the child and also the health of the mother.
- If national policy supports breastfeeding by women with HIV, they should receive the appropriate ART interventions and should exclusively breastfeed their infants for the first 6 months of life, introduce appropriate complementary foods at 6 months, and continue breastfeeding for the first 12 months. Breastfeeding should then stop only once a nutritionally adequate and safe diet without breast milk can be provided.
- Urge women with HIV to use condoms along with LAM. Used consistently and correctly, condoms help prevent transmission of HIV and other STIs.
- At 6 months—or earlier if her monthly bleeding has returned or she stops exclusive breastfeeding—a woman should begin to use another contraceptive method in place of LAM.

(For further guidance on infant feeding for women with HIV, see Maternal and Newborn Health, Preventing Mother-to-Child Transmission of HIV, p. 352.)

Providing the Lactational Amenorrhea Method

When to Start

Woman's situation	When to start
Within 6 months after childbirth	• Start breastfeeding immediately (within one hour) or as soon as possible after the baby is born. In the first few days after childbirth, the yellowish fluid produced by the mother's breasts (colostrum) contains substances very important to the baby's health. • Any time, if she has been fully or nearly breastfeeding her baby since birth and her monthly bleeding has not returned.

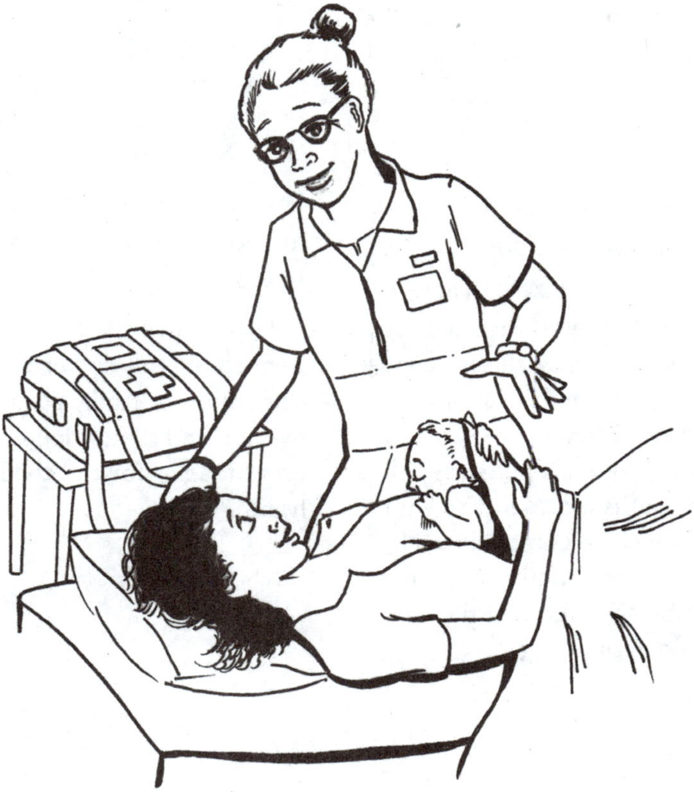

When Can a Woman Use LAM?

A breastfeeding woman can use LAM to space her next birth and as a transition to another contraceptive method. She may start LAM at any time if she meets all 3 criteria required for using the method.

Ask the mother these 3 questions:

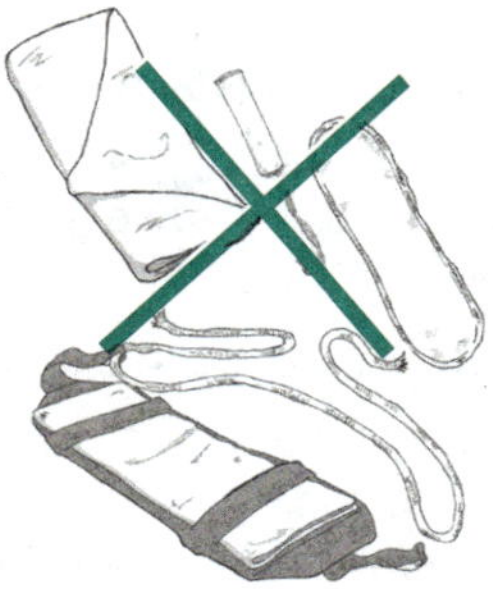

1 Has your monthly bleeding returned?

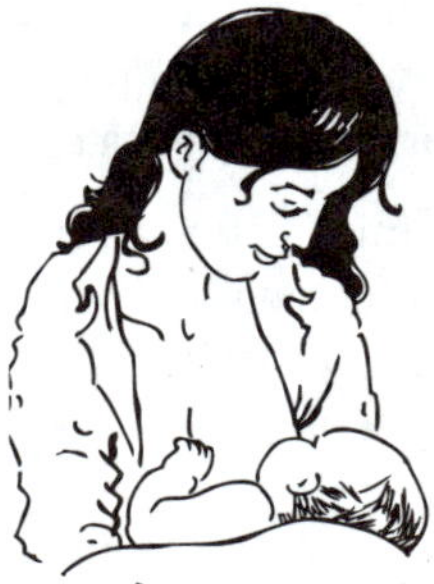

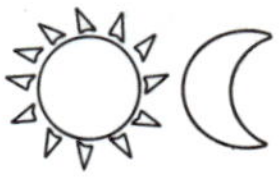

2 Are you regularly giving the baby other food besides breast milk or allowing long periods without breastfeeding, either day or night?

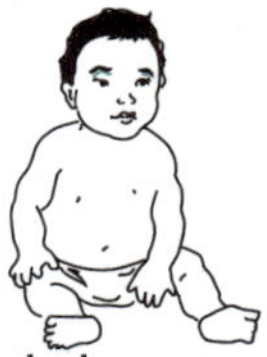

3 Is your baby more than 6 months old?

If the answer to all of these questions is no...

...she can use LAM. There is only a 2% change of pregnancy at this time. A woman may choose another family planning method at any time—but preferably not a method with estrogen while her baby is less than 6 months old. Methods with estrogen include combined oral contraceptives, monthly injectables, the combined patch, and the combined vaginal ring.

But, when the answer to any one of these questions is yes...

...her chances of pregnancy increase. Advise her to begin using another family planning method and to continue breastfeeding for the child's health.

Explaining How to Use

Breastfeed often

- An ideal pattern is feeding on demand (that is, whenever the baby wants to be fed) and at least 10 to 12 times a day in the first few weeks after childbirth and thereafter 8 to 10 times a day, including at least once at night in the first months.
- Daytime feedings should be no more than 4 hours apart, and night-time feedings no more than 6 hours apart.
- Some babies may not want to breastfeed 8 to 10 times a day and may want to sleep through the night. These babies may need gentle encouragement to breastfeed more often.

Start other foods at 6 months

- She should start giving other foods in addition to breast milk when the baby is 6 months old. At this age, breast milk can no longer fully nourish a growing baby.

Plan follow-up visit

- Plan for the next visit while the LAM criteria still apply, so that she can choose another method and continue to be protected from pregnancy.
- If possible, give her condoms or progestin-only pills now. She can start to use them if the baby is no longer fully or nearly fully breastfeeding, if her monthly bleeding returns, or if the baby reaches 6 months of age before she can come back for another method. Plan for a follow-on method. Give her any supplies now.

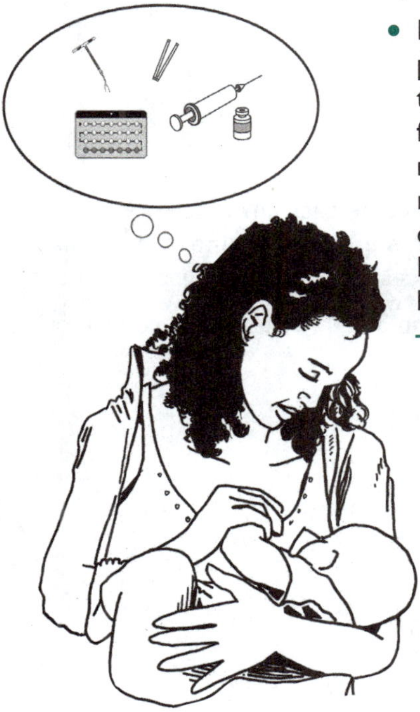

How Can a Partner Help?

The client's partner is welcome to participate in counseling and learn about the method and what support he can give to his partner. A male partner can:

- Support a woman's choice of LAM
- Understand how LAM works and when it will no longer work
- Encourage her to breastfeed often and without giving her baby any supplementary food for the first 6 months
- Make sure that she has extra nutrition and fluids while breastfeeding
- Discuss and plan what method to use when one of the LAM conditions is no longer met – that is, her monthly bleeding returns, she introduces other foods, or the baby reaches 6 months old—or sooner if she prefers
- Start or remind her to start another family planning method as soon as one of the LAM criteria is no longer met
- Help to make sure she has ECPs on hand in case one of the LAM conditions is no longer met and she has not yet started to use another contraceptive
- Use condoms consistently in addition to LAM if he has an STI/HIV or thinks he may be at risk of an STI/HIV

Supporting the User

"Come Back Any Time": Reasons to Return

Assure every client that she is welcome to come back any time—for example, if she has problems, questions, or wants another method; she has a major change in health status; or she thinks she might be pregnant. Also, if:

- She no longer meets one or more of the 3 LAM criteria and so cannot keep relying on LAM.

Helping Continuing Users

Helping Clients Switch to a Continuing Method

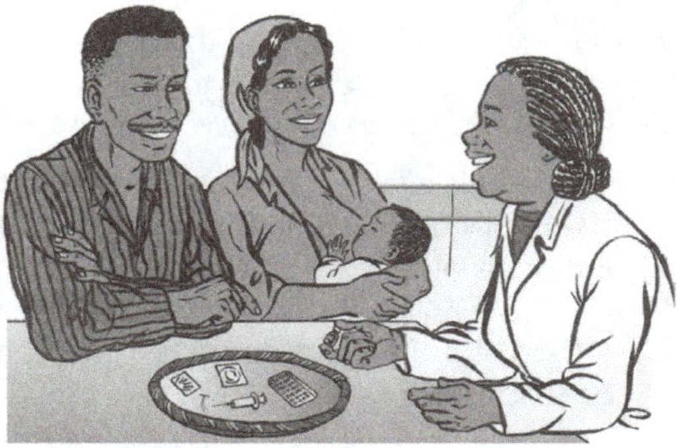

1. A woman can switch to another method any time she wants while using LAM. If she still meets all 3 LAM criteria, it is reasonably certain she is not pregnant. She can start a new method with no need for a pregnancy test, examinations, or evaluation.
2. To continue preventing pregnancy, a woman *must* switch to another method as soon as any one of the 3 LAM criteria no longer applies.
3. Help the woman choose a new method *before* she needs it. If she will continue to breastfeed, she can choose from several hormonal or nonhormonal methods, depending on how much time has passed since childbirth (see Maternal and Newborn Health, Earliest Time That a Woman Can Start a Family Planning Method After Childbirth, p. 351). After 6 months, if a woman wants to continue breastfeeding, she can consider the progesterone-releasing vaginal ring (see p. 127).

Managing Any Problems

Problems With Use

- Problems with breastfeeding or LAM affect women's satisfaction and use of the method. If the client reports any problems, listen to her concerns, give her advice and support, and, if appropriate, treat. Make sure she understands the advice and agrees.
- Offer to help the client choose another method—now, if she wishes, or if problems cannot be overcome.
- For problems with breastfeeding, see Maternal and Newborn Health, Managing Any Breastfeeding Problems, p. 355.

Questions and Answers About the Lactational Amenorrhea Method

1. **Can LAM be an effective method of family planning?**

   Yes. LAM is effective if the woman's monthly bleeding has not returned, she is fully or nearly fully breastfeeding, and her baby is less than 6 months old.

2. **When should a mother start giving her baby other foods besides breast milk?**

   Ideally, when the baby is 6 months old. Along with other foods, breast milk should be a major part of the child's diet through the child's second year or longer.

3. **Can women use LAM if they work away from home?**

   Yes. Women who are able to keep their infants with them at work or nearby and are able to breastfeed frequently can rely on LAM as long as they meet all 3 criteria for LAM. Women who are separated from their infants can use LAM if breastfeeds are less than 4 hours apart. Women can also express their breast milk at least every 4 hours, but pregnancy rates may be slightly higher for women who are separated from their infants. The one study that assessed use of LAM among working women estimated a pregnancy rate of 5 per 100 women during the first 6 months after childbirth, compared with about 2 per 100 women as LAM is commonly used.

4. **What if a woman learns that she has HIV while she is using LAM? Can she continue breastfeeding and using LAM?**

   If a woman is newly infected with HIV, the risk of transmission through breastfeeding may be higher than if she was infected earlier, because there is more HIV in her body. The breastfeeding recommendation is the same as for other HIV-infected women, however. HIV-infected mothers and their infants should receive the appropriate ARV therapy, and mothers should exclusively breastfeed their infants for the first 6 months of life, and then introduce appropriate complementary foods and continue breastfeeding for the first 12 months of life. At 6 months—or earlier if her monthly bleeding has returned or she stops exclusive breastfeeding—she should begin to use another contraceptive method in place of LAM and continue to use condoms. (See also Maternal and Newborn Health, Preventing Mother-to-Child Transmission of HIV, p. 352.)

CHAPTER 21

Serving Diverse Groups

Key Points for Providers and Clients

Adolescents

- **All contraceptives are safe for young people.** Unmarried and married youth may have different sexual and reproductive health needs.

Men

- **Correct information can help men make better decisions about their own health and their partner's health, too.** When couples discuss contraception, they are more likely to make plans that they can carry out.

Women Near Menopause

- **To be sure to avoid pregnancy, a woman should use contraception until she has had no monthly bleeding for 12 months in a row.**

Clients With Disabilities

- **People with disabilities deserve full and sometimes adapted information and the same respectful and conscientious care as other clients.**

Adolescents

Young people may come to a family planning provider not only for contraception but also for advice about physical changes, sex, relationships, family, and problems of growing up. Their needs depend on their particular situations. Some are unmarried and sexually active, others are not sexually active, while still others are already married. Some already have children. Age itself makes a great difference, since young people mature quickly during the adolescent years. These differences make it important to learn about each client first, to understand why that client has come, and to tailor counseling and the offer of services accordingly.

Provide Services with Care and Respect

Young people deserve reproductive health services that meet their needs and are nonjudgmental and respectful, no matter how young the person is. Criticism or unwelcoming attitudes will keep young people away from the care they need. Counseling and services do not encourage young people to have sex. Instead, they help young people protect their health.

Appropriate sexual and reproductive health services, including contraception, should be available and accessible to all adolescents without requiring authorization from a parent or guardian by law, policy, or practice. As much as possible, programs should avoid discouraging adolescents from seeking services and avoid limiting their choice of contraceptives because of cost.

To make services friendly to youth, you can:

- Show young people that you enjoy working with them.
- Offer services that are free or as low cost as possible.
- Offer a wide range of contraceptive methods, including long-acting reversible methods.
- Counsel in private areas where you and the client cannot be seen or overheard. Ensure confidentiality and assure the client of confidentiality.
- Listen carefully and ask open-ended questions such as "How can I help you?" and "What questions do you have?"
- Use simple language and avoid medical terms.
- Use terms that suit young people. Avoid such terms as "family planning," which may seem irrelevant to those who are not married.
- Welcome partners and include them in counseling, if the client desires.
- Try to make sure that a young woman's choices are her own and are not pressured by her partner or her family. In particular, if she is being pressured to have sex, help a young woman think about what she can say and do to resist and reduce that pressure. Practice with her the skills to negotiate condom use.
- Speak without expressing judgment (for example, say "You can" rather than "You should"). Do not criticize even if you do not approve of what the young person is saying or doing. Help young clients make decisions that are in their best interest.
- Take time to fully address questions, fears, and misinformation about sex, sexually transmitted infections (STIs), and contraceptives. Many young people want reassurance that the changes in their bodies and their feelings are normal. Be prepared to answer common questions about puberty, monthly bleeding, masturbation, night-time ejaculation, and genital hygiene.

- Be aware of young people's norms about gender and gently encourage positive, healthful norms. In particular you can help young women feel that they have the right and the power to make their own decisions about sex and contraception. You can help young men to understand the consequences of their sexual behavior for themselves and for their partners.

All Contraceptives Are Safe for Young People

Young people can safely use any contraceptive method. Age is not a medical reason for denying any method to adolescents.

- Young women are often less tolerant of side effects than older women. With counseling, however, they will know what to expect and may be less likely to stop using their methods.
- Unmarried young people may have more sex partners than older people and so may face a greater risk of STIs. It is important when counseling young people to consider STI risk and how to reduce it.

For some contraceptive methods there are specific considerations for young people (see contraceptive method chapters for complete guidance):

Long-acting reversible contraceptives—implants and IUDs

- Implants, copper-bearing IUDs, and LNG-IUDs may be good choices for many young women because:
  - These methods are very effective—fewer than 1 pregnancy per 100 women in the first year of use.
  - Once in place, these methods do not require any action by the user. She does not have to plan in advance for sex.
  - They work for a number of years.
  - They are quickly reversible. Once the implant or IUD is removed, a woman can again become pregnant.
  - It is not obvious that the woman is using a contraceptive method.
- IUDs are more likely to come out among women who have not given birth because their uteruses are small.

Injectable contraceptives

- Injectables can be used without others knowing.

Oral contraceptives

- Some young women find taking a pill every day particularly difficult.

Emergency contraceptive pills (ECPs)

- Young women may have less control than older women over having sex and using contraception. They may need ECPs more often. It is safe to use ECPs multiple times between monthly bleedings. Using combined oral contraceptives or a long-acting reversible method would be more effective in the long run.
- Provide young women with ECPs in advance, for use when needed. ECPs can be used whenever she has any unprotected sex, including sex against her will, or a mistake has occurred when using contraception.

Female sterilization and vasectomy

- Provide with great caution. Young people and people with few or no children are among those most likely to regret sterilization.

Male and female condoms

- Protect against STIs as well as pregnancy. Many young people need protection against both.
- Readily available, and they are affordable and convenient for occasional sex.
- Young men may be less successful than older men at using condoms correctly. They may need practice putting condoms on.

Diaphragms, spermicides, and cervical caps

- Although among the least effective methods, young women can control use of these methods, and they can be used as needed.

Fertility awareness methods

- Until a young woman has regular menstrual cycles, fertility awareness methods should be used with caution.
- Need a backup method or ECPs on hand in case abstinence fails.

Withdrawal

- Requires the man to know when he is about to ejaculate so he can withdraw in time. This may be difficult for some young men.
- One of the least effective methods of pregnancy prevention, but it may be the only method available—and always available—for some young people.

Men

Important Supporters, Important Clients

To health care providers, men are important for 2 reasons. First, they influence women. Many men care about their partner's reproductive health and support them. Others stand in their way or make decisions for them. Thus, men's attitudes can determine whether women can practice healthy behaviors. In some circumstances, such as avoiding HIV infection or getting help quickly in an obstetric emergency, a man's actions can determine whether a woman lives or dies.

Men are also important as clients. Important family planning methods—male condoms and vasectomy—are used by men. Men also have their own sexual and reproductive health needs and concerns—in particular regarding sexually transmitted infections (STIs)—which deserve the attention of the health care system and providers.

Many Ways to Help Men

Providers can give support and services to men both as supporters of women and as clients.

Encourage Couples to Talk

Couples who discuss family planning—with or without a provider's help—are more likely to make plans that they can carry out. Providers can:

- Coach men and women on how to talk with their partners about sex, family planning, and STIs.
- Encourage joint decision-making about sexual and reproductive health matters.

In this handbook most chapters include a box, How Can a Partner Help?. The points in this box can be useful when counseling couples or helping a client get her partner's support with her method.

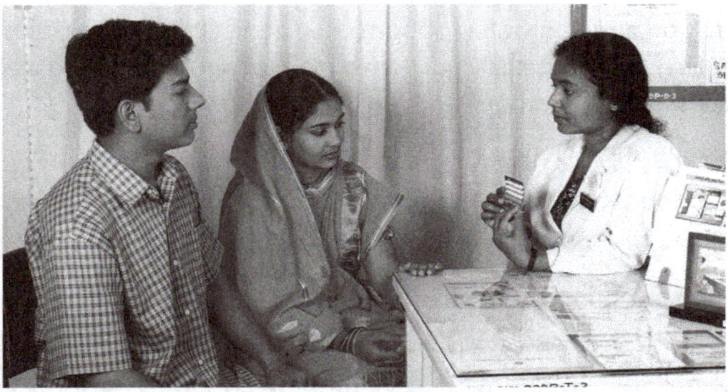

- Invite and encourage women to bring their partners to the clinic for joint counseling, decision-making, and care.
- Encourage the man to understand and support his partner to choose the contraceptive method she prefers.
- Encourage the man to consider taking more responsibility for family planning—for example, by using condoms or vasectomy.
- Suggest to female clients that they tell their partners about health services for men. Give informational materials to take home, if available.

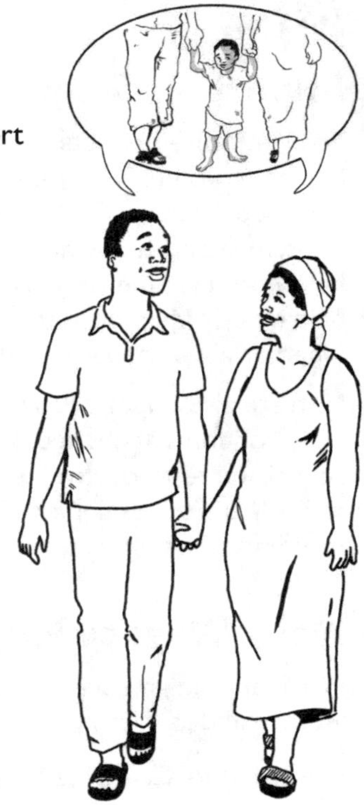

Provide Accurate Information

To inform men's decisions and opinions, they need correct information and correction of misperceptions. Topics important to men include:

- Family planning methods, both for men and for women, including safety and effectiveness
- STIs including HIV—how they are and are not transmitted, signs and symptoms, testing, and treatment
- The benefits of waiting until the youngest child is 2 years old before a woman becomes pregnant again
- Male and female sexual and reproductive anatomy and function
- Safe pregnancy and delivery

Offer Services or Refer

Important services that many men want include:

- Male condoms and vasectomy services
- Information and counseling about other contraceptive methods, particularly methods that must have male cooperation, such as fertility awareness-based methods and female condoms
- Counseling and help for sexual problems
- STI/HIV counseling, testing, and treatment
- Infertility counseling (see Infertility, p. 364)
- Screening for penile, testicular, and prostate cancer

Like women, men of all ages, married or unmarried, have their own sexual and reproductive health needs. They deserve good-quality services and respectful, supportive, and nonjudgmental counseling.

Women Near Menopause

A woman has reached menopause when her ovaries stop releasing eggs (ovulating). Because bleeding does not come every month as menopause approaches, a woman is considered no longer fertile once she has gone 12 months in a row without having any bleeding.

Menopause usually occurs between the ages of 45 and 55. About half of women reach menopause by age 50. By age 55 some 96% of women have reached menopause.

To prevent pregnancy until it is clear that she is no longer fertile, an older woman can use any method, if she has no medical condition that limits its use. By itself, age does not restrict a woman from using any contraceptive method.

Special Considerations About Method Choice

When helping women near menopause choose a method, consider:

Combined hormonal methods (combined oral contraceptives [COCs], monthly injectables, combined patch, combined vaginal ring)

- Women age 35 and older who smoke—regardless of how much—should not use COCs, the patch, or the combined vaginal ring.
- Women age 35 and older who smoke 15 or more cigarettes a day should not use monthly injectables.
- Women age 35 or older should not use COCs, monthly injectables, the patch, or the combined vaginal ring if they have migraine headaches (whether with migraine aura or not).

Progestin-only methods (progestin-only pills, progestin-only injectables, implants)

- A good choice for women who cannot use methods with estrogen.
- During use, DMPA decreases bone mineral density slightly. This may increase the risk of developing osteoporosis and possibly having bone fractures later, after menopause. WHO has concluded that this decrease in bone mineral density does not place age or time limits on use of DMPA.

Emergency contraceptive pills

- Can be used by women of any age, including those who cannot use hormonal methods on a continuing basis.

Female sterilization and vasectomy

- May be a good choice for older women and their partners who know they will not want more children.
- Older women are more likely to have conditions that require delay, referral, or caution for female sterilization.

Male and female condoms, diaphragms, spermicides, cervical caps, and withdrawal

- Protect older women well because of women's reduced fertility in the years before menopause.
- Affordable and convenient for women who may not have sex often.

Intrauterine device (copper-bearing IUDs and LNG-IUDs)

- Expulsion rates fall as women grow older and are lowest in women over 40 years of age.
- Insertion may be more difficult due to tightening of the cervical canal.

Fertility awareness methods

- Lack of regular cycles before menopause makes it more difficult to use these methods reliably.

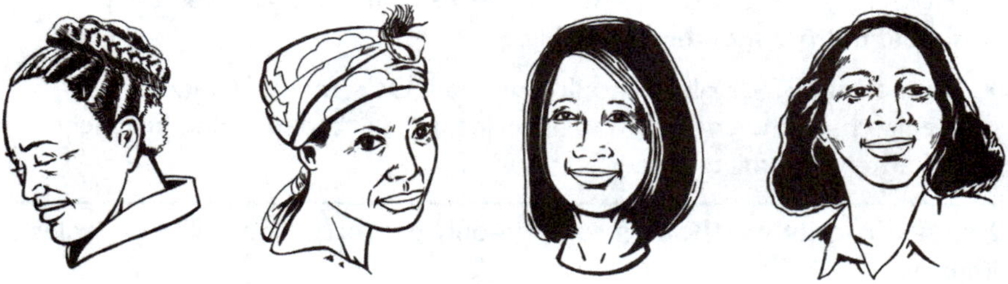

When a Woman Can Stop Using Family Planning

Because bleeding does not come every month in the time before menopause, it is difficult for a woman whose bleeding seems to have stopped to know when to stop using contraception. Thus, it is recommended to continue using a family planning method until 12 months with no bleeding have passed.

Hormonal methods affect bleeding, and so it may be difficult to know if a woman using them has reached menopause. She can switch to a nonhormonal method. She no longer needs contraception once she has had no bleeding for 12 months in a row.

Copper-bearing IUDs can be left in place until after menopause. The IUD should be removed 12 months after a woman's last monthly bleeding.

Relieving Symptoms of Menopause

Women experience physical effects before, during, and after menopause: hot flashes, excess sweating, difficulty holding urine, vaginal dryness that can make sex painful, and difficulty sleeping.

Providers can suggest ways to reduce some of these symptoms:

- Deep breathing from the diaphragm may make a hot flash go away faster. A woman can also try eating foods containing soy or taking 800 international units per day of vitamin E.
- Eat foods rich in calcium (such as dairy products, beans, fish) and engage in moderate physical activity to help slow the loss of bone density that comes with menopause.
- Vaginal lubricants or moisturizers can be used if vaginal dryness persists and causes irritation. During sex, use a commercially available vaginal lubricant, water, or saliva as a lubricant if vaginal dryness is a problem.

Clients with Disabilities

Health care providers should treat people with disabilities in the same way that they should treat people without disabilities: with respect. People with disabilities have the same sexual and reproductive health needs and rights as people without disabilities, but often they are not given information about reproductive and sexual health or adequate care. People with disabilities are more vulnerable to abuse than non-disabled people. They are at increased risk of being infected with HIV and other STIs. Many have been sterilized against their will, forced to have abortions, or forced into unwanted marriages, and many have experienced gender-based violence. Health care programs, including family planning programs, need to follow the relevant articles of the UN Convention on the Rights of Persons with Disabilities, especially the articles that address health, family life, and legal rights.

To counsel clients with disabilities, health care providers need to consider their preferences and the nature of their disability. For example, barrier methods may be difficult for some people with a physical disability, and women with an intellectual disability may have trouble remembering to take a pill each day or dealing with changes in monthly bleeding.

Like all clients, people with disabilities need sexual and reproductive health education to make informed choices. People with intellectual disabilities have the same rights as other people to make their own decisions about contraception, including sterilization. They may need special support to do so. For a client with an intellectual disability who is unable to communicate her or his preferences clearly, someone whom the client trusts should participate and help to make an informed choice that is as consistent as possible with the client's preference. Especially for the choice of sterilization, health care systems should ensure that a process of supported decision-making is available.

> **What is supported decision-making?**
>
> In supported decision-making, supporters, advocates, or others help people with disabilities to make their own decisions, free of conflict of interest or undue influence, and without giving decision-making power to someone else. This process may include documenting informed consent. (See Ensuring Informed Choice, p. 219.)

To care for people with disabilities, programs should make it known in the community that they serve people with disabilities without discrimination. Facilities should be made physically accessible—for example, with ramps for wheelchairs and large bathrooms with grab bars. Outreach programs should make a special effort to identify and reach people in the community who have limited mobility. Print materials should have simple graphics, large print, and Braille, if possible, and information should be available in audio formats, such as CD or cassette tape, as well as in print. Providers may need especially to demonstrate actions as well as describing them, to speak slowly, and to pause often and check comprehension.

Learning to respect the rights of people with disabilities and to care for them should be part of pre-service training for health care providers, and it should be reinforced with in-service training periodically. Moreover, meeting and talking with people with disabilities can give providers valuable information about how to make services more respectful and accessible. Often, the changes needed are easy.

Sexually Transmitted Infections, Including HIV

Key Points for Providers and Clients

- **People with sexually transmitted infections (STIs), including HIV, can use most family planning methods safely and effectively.**
- **Male and female condoms can prevent STIs** when used consistently and correctly.
- **STI risk can be reduced in other ways, too**—limiting number of partners, abstaining from sex, and having a mutually faithful relationship with an uninfected partner.
- **STIs often have no signs or symptoms, particularly in women.** People should seek care if they think that they or their partners might have an STI.
- **Some STIs can be treated.** The sooner treated, the less likely to cause long-term health problems, such as infertility or chronic pain, or to infect a sexual partner or a fetus.
- **In most cases vaginal discharge comes from infections that are not sexually transmitted.**

Family planning providers can help their clients in various ways to prevent STIs, including infection with the human immunodeficiency virus (HIV). Program managers and providers can choose approaches that fit their clients' needs, their training, and resources, and the availability of services for referral.

What Are Sexually Transmitted Infections?

STIs are caused by bacteria, viruses, and parasites spread through sexual contact. Infections can be found in body fluids such as semen, on the skin of the genitals and areas around them, and some also in the mouth, throat, and rectum. Some STIs cause no symptoms. Others can cause discomfort or pain. If not treated, some can cause pelvic inflammatory disease, infertility, chronic pelvic pain, and cervical cancer. Some STIs can also greatly increase the chance of becoming infected with HIV.

STIs spread in a community because an infected person has sex with an uninfected person. The more sexual partners a person has, the greater his or her risk of either becoming infected with STIs or transmitting STIs.

Who Is at Risk?

Many people seeking family planning services are in stable, mutually faithful, long-term relationships and so face little risk of getting an STI. Some clients may be at high risk for STIs, however, or have an STI now. Clients who might benefit most from discussion of STI risk include those who do not have steady partners, unmarried clients, and anyone, married or unmarried, who asks or expresses concern about STIs or HIV or that her or his partner may have other partners.

The risk of acquiring an STI, including HIV, depends on a person's behavior, the behavior of that person's sexual partner or partners, and how common those diseases are in the community. By knowing what STIs are common locally, a health care provider can better help a client assess her or his own risk.

Understanding their own risk for HIV and other STIs helps people decide how to protect themselves and others. People are often the best judges of their own STI risk, especially when they are told what behaviors and situations can increase risk.

Sexual behavior that can increase exposure to STIs includes:

- Sex with a partner who has STI symptoms
- Sex with a partner who has recently been diagnosed with or treated for an STI
- Sex with more than one partner—the more partners, the more risk
- Sex with a partner who has sex with others and does not always use condoms
- Sex without a condom with almost any new partner in a community where many people have STIs

In certain situations people tend to change sexual partners often, to have many partners, or to have a partner who has other partners. All of these behaviors increase the risk of STI transmission. This includes people who:

- Have sex in exchange for money, food, gifts, shelter, or favors
- Move to another area for work, or travel often for work, such as truck drivers
- Have no established long-term sexual relationship, as is common among sexually active adolescents and young adults
- Are the sexual partners of these people

What Causes STIs?

Several types of organisms cause STIs. Those caused by organisms such as bacteria generally can be cured. STIs caused by viruses generally cannot be cured, although they can be treated to relieve symptoms.

STI	Type	Sexual transmission	Nonsexual transmission	Curable?
Chancroid	Bacterial	Vaginal, anal, and oral sex	None	Yes
Chlamydia	Bacterial	Vaginal and anal sex Rarely, from genitals to mouth	From mother to child during pregnancy	Yes
Gonorrhea	Bacterial	Vaginal and anal sex, or contact between mouth and genitals	From mother to child during delivery	Yes
Hepatitis B	Viral	Vaginal and anal sex, or from penis to mouth	In blood, from mother to child during delivery or in breast milk	No
Herpes	Viral	Genital or oral contact with an ulcer, including vaginal and anal sex; also genital contact in area without ulcer	From mother to child during pregnancy or delivery	No
HIV	Viral	Vaginal and anal sex Very rarely, oral sex	In blood, from mother to child during pregnancy or delivery or in breast milk	No
Human papilloma-virus	Viral	Skin-to-skin and genital contact or contact between mouth and genitals	From mother to child during delivery	No
Syphilis	Bacterial	Genital or oral contact with an ulcer, including vaginal and anal sex	From mother to child during pregnancy or delivery	Yes
Tricho-moniasis	Parasite	Vaginal, anal, and oral sex	From mother to child during delivery	Yes

More About HIV

- HIV is the virus that causes acquired immunodeficiency syndrome (AIDS). HIV slowly damages the body's immune system, reducing its ability to fight other diseases.
- People can live with HIV for many years without any signs or symptoms of infection. If not treated, however, eventually the body's immune system breaks down and is unable to fight certain infections, known as opportunistic infections.
- There is no cure for HIV infection, but antiretroviral (ARV) therapy can slow the progress of HIV disease, improve health, prolong life, and reduce the risk of transmission to others. ARVs also can reduce mother-to-child transmission at the time of delivery and during breastfeeding. Opportunistic infections can be treated.
- People at high risk of exposure to HIV can take PrEP—pre-exposure prophylaxis—to prevent HIV infection. PrEP consists of some of the same ARV drugs also used to treat infection. Hormonal contraceptives and PrEP can be taken at the same time. The effectiveness of the contraception and of PrEP are not affected. Condom use while taking PrEP will help prevent both HIV and other STIs.
- Family planning providers can help with prevention and treatment efforts for HIV, particularly in countries where many people are living with HIV, by:
  - Counseling about ways to reduce risk of infection (see Choosing a Dual Protection Strategy, p. 336).
  - Counseling a couple that wants to have a child, and one partner has HIV, about how to conceive while trying to prevent HIV transmission to the uninfected partner (see box, next page).
  - Referring clients for HIV counseling and testing and for HIV care and treatment if the clinic does not offer such services.

For information on family planning methods for people living with HIV, see Contraceptives for Clients with STIs, including HIV, p. 338.

Safer Conception for HIV Serodiscordant Couples

When a couple wants to have a child and one partner has HIV while the other does not (a serodiscordant couple), counseling and care can make these points:

- The partner with HIV should take antiretroviral (ARV) therapy consistently and correctly until the HIV is suppressed to the point that it cannot be detected.
- If the partner with HIV is not virally suppressed on ARV therapy, the partner who does not have HIV (HIV-negative) can consider taking pre-exposure prophylaxis (PrEP) with ARVs during the period when they are trying to conceive (see Fertility Awareness Methods, page 291).
- In some settings where available, if the woman has HIV but the man does not, a safe option for conception is artificial insemination with the uninfected partner's semen.

Both partners should be screened and treated for any other STIs before trying for conception.

Early Identification

Early identification of STIs is not always possible. For example, chlamydia and gonorrhea often have no noticeable signs or symptoms in women. However, early identification, if possible, is important both to avoid passing on the infection and to avoid serious long-term health consequences, such as stillbirth, cervical cancer, and congenital syphilis. To help detect STIs early, a provider can:

- Ask the client's sexual history and assess the risk of having an STI
- Ask whether the client or the client's partner has genital sores or unusual discharge
- Look for signs of STIs when doing a pelvic or genital examination for another reason
- Know how to advise a client who may have an STI
- Promptly diagnose and treat, or else refer for appropriate care, the client who has signs or symptoms
- Advise clients to notice genital sores, warts, or unusual discharge in themselves or in their sexual partners
- For clients without STI signs or symptoms but who are at high risk for STIs, encourage syphilis screening and, when feasible, screening for gonorrhea and chlamydial infection

Common signs and symptoms that may suggest an STI include:

Symptoms	Possible cause
Discharge from the penis—pus, clear or yellow-green drip	Commonly: Chlamydia, gonorrhea Sometimes: Trichomoniasis
Abnormal vaginal discharge or pain during sex	Chlamydia, gonorrhea, pelvic inflammatory disease
Burning or pain during urination	Chlamydia, gonorrhea, herpes
Lower abdominal pain or pain during sex	Chlamydia, gonorrhea, pelvic inflammatory disease
Swollen and/or painful testicles	Chlamydia, gonorrhea
Itching or tingling in the genital area	Commonly: Trichomoniasis Sometimes: Herpes
Blisters or sores on the genitals, anus, surrounding areas, or mouth	Herpes, syphilis, chancroid
Warts on the genitals, anus, or surrounding areas	Human papillomavirus
Unusual cervical discharge—changes from normal vaginal discharge in color, consistency, amount, and/or odor	Most commonly: Bacterial vaginosis, candidiasis (see Common Vaginal Infections That May Not Be Sexually Transmitted, next page) Commonly: Trichomoniasis Sometimes: Chlamydia, gonorrhea

Common Vaginal Infections That May Not Be Sexually Transmitted

The most common vaginal infections usually are due to an overgrowth of organisms normally present in the vagina. They may or may not be sexually transmitted. These infections include candidiasis (also called yeast infection or thrush) and bacterial vaginosis. Candidiasis is not usually sexually transmitted. Recent research links bacterial vaginosis with sexual behavior, but even women who have never had sex can, rarely, develop bacterial vaginosis.

- In most areas these infections are much more common than STIs. Researchers estimate that between 5% and 25% of women have bacterial vaginosis and between 5% and 15% have candidiasis at any given time.
- Vaginal discharge due to these infections may be similar to discharge caused by some STIs such as trichomoniasis. It is important to reassure clients with such symptoms that they may not have an STI—particularly if they have no other symptoms and are at low risk for STIs.
- Bacterial vaginosis can be cured with antibiotics; candidiasis can be cured with anti-fungal medications such as fluconazole. Without treatment, bacterial vaginosis can lead to pregnancy complications, and candidiasis can be transmitted to a newborn during delivery.

Washing the external genital area with unscented soap and clean water, and not using douches, detergents, disinfectants, or vaginal cleaning or drying agents are good hygiene practices. They may also help some women avoid vaginal infections.

Avoiding Sexually Transmitted Infections

Family planning providers can talk to clients about how they can protect themselves both from STIs, including HIV, and pregnancy (dual protection).

Choosing a Dual Protection Strategy

Every family planning client needs to think about preventing STIs, including HIV—even people who assume they face no risk. A provider can discuss what situations place a person at increased risk of STIs, including HIV (see Who Is at Risk?, p. 330), and clients can think about whether these risky situations come up in their own lives. If so, they can consider 5 dual protection strategies.

One person might use different strategies in different situations; one couple might use different strategies at different times. The best strategy is the one that a person is able to practice effectively in the situation that she or he is facing. (Dual protection does not necessarily mean just using condoms along with another family planning method.)

Strategy 1: ***Use a male or female condom correctly with every act of sex.***

- One method helps protect against pregnancy and STIs, including HIV.

Strategy 2: ***Use condoms consistently and correctly plus another family planning method.***

- Adds extra protection from pregnancy in case a condom is not used or is used incorrectly.
- May be a good choice for women who want to be sure to avoid pregnancy but cannot always count on their partners to use condoms.

Strategy 3: ***If both partners know they are not infected, use any family planning method to prevent pregnancy and stay in a mutually faithful relationship.***

- Many family planning clients are in this group and thus are protected from STIs, including HIV.
- Depends on communication and trust between partners.

Other strategies, which do not involve using contraceptives, include:

Strategy 4: ***Engage only in safer sexual intimacy that avoids intercourse or otherwise prevents semen and vaginal fluids from coming in contact with each other's genitals.***

- This strategy will not prevent syphilis, genital herpes, or infection with human papillomavirus. These spread through skin-to-skin contact.
- Depends on communication, trust, and self-control.
- If this is a person's first-choice strategy, it is best to have condoms on hand in case the couple does have sex.

Strategy 5: ***Delay or avoid sexual activity (either avoiding sex any time that it might be risky or abstaining for a longer time).***

- If this is a person's first-choice strategy, it is best to have condoms on hand in case the couple does have sex.
- This strategy is always available in case a condom is not at hand.

People at high risk of HIV infection can take PrEP—pre-exposure prophylaxis. This daily treatment with oral antiretroviral drugs greatly reduces the chances of infection if exposed to HIV. PrEP can be a part of any dual protection strategy. PrEP can be used along with condoms and any other family planning method. Taking PrEP and a hormonal contraceptive at the same time does not reduce the effectiveness of either one.

Many clients will need help, support, and guidance to make their dual protection strategy succeed. For example, they may need help preparing to talk with their partners about STI protection, learning how to use condoms and other methods, and handling practical matters such as where to get supplies and where to keep them. If you can help with such matters, offer to help. If not, refer the client to someone who can provide more counseling or skills-building, such as role-playing to practice negotiating condom use.

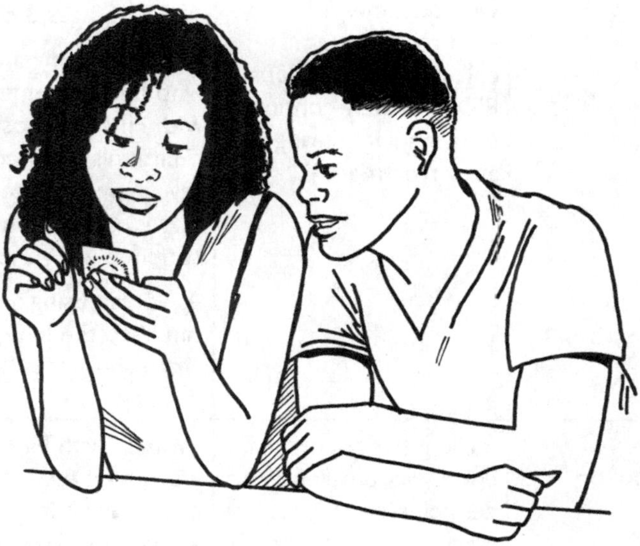

Contraceptives for Clients with STIs, Including HIV

People with STIs and people with HIV, whether or not they are taking antiretroviral (ARV) therapy, can start and continue to use most contraceptive methods safely. There are a few limitations, however. See the table below. (Also, every chapter on a contraceptive method provides more information and considerations for clients with HIV, including those taking ARV medications.)

Special Family Planning Considerations for Clients with STIs, including HIV

Method	Has STIs	Has HIV
Intrauterine device (copper-bearing IUD or LNG-IUD)	Do not insert an IUD in a woman who is at very high individual risk for gonorrhea and chlamydia, or who currently has gonorrhea, chlamydia, purulent cervicitis, or PID. (A current IUD user who becomes infected with gonorrhea or chlamydia or develops PID can safely continue using an IUD during and after treatment.)	A woman with HIV clinical disease that is mild or with no symptoms, including a woman on ARV therapy, can have an IUD inserted. Generally, a woman should not have an IUD inserted if she has HIV clinical disease that is severe or advanced (WHO Stages 3 or 4). A woman using an IUD who becomes infected with HIV or whose HIV clinical disease becomes severe or advanced (WHO Stages 3 or 4) can safely continue using the IUD. A woman using an IUD can keep the IUD in place when she starts ARV therapy.
Female sterilization	If client has gonorrhea, chlamydia, purulent cervicitis, or PID, delay sterilization until the condition is treated and cured.	Women with HIV, including women on ARV therapy, can safely undergo female sterilization. The procedure may need to be delayed if she currently has an HIV-related illness.

Method	Has STIs	Has HIV
Vasectomy	If client has scrotal skin infection, active STI, or swollen, tender tip of penis, sperm ducts, or testicles, delay sterilization until the condition is treated and cured.	Men who are living with HIV, including men on ARV therapy, can safely undergo vasectomy. The procedure may need to be delayed if he currently has an HIV-related illness.
Spermicides (including when used with diaphragm or cervical cap)	Can safely use spermicides.	Should not use spermicides if at high risk of HIV. Generally, should not use spermicides if she has HIV infection.
Combined oral contraceptives, monthly injectables, combined patch, combined ring	Can safely use combined hormonal methods.	Can safely use combined hormonal methods.
Progestin-only pills, injectables, and implants	Can safely use progestin-only methods.	Can safely use progestin-only methods. There is some concern that using a progestin-only injectable could make a woman more likely to develop HIV infection if exposed to the virus (see Progestin-Only Injectables, Question 2, p. 92). However, a woman who already has HIV can safely use a progestin-only injectable.

Cervical Cancer

What Is Cervical Cancer?

Cervical cancer results from uncontrolled, untreated growth of abnormal cells in the cervix. Infection with a sexually transmitted virus, the human papillomavirus (HPV), causes such cells to develop and grow.

HPV is found on skin in the genital area and also in the tissues of the vagina, cervix, and mouth. It is primarily transmitted through skin-to-skin contact. Vaginal, anal, and oral sex also can spread HPV. Over 50 types of HPV can infect the cervix; 7 of them account for nearly all cervical cancers, with 2 types accounting for about 70% of cancers. Two other types of HPV cause most cases of genital warts.

An estimated 50% to 80% of sexually active women are infected with HPV at least once in their lives. In most cases the HPV infection clears on its own. In some women, however, HPV persists and causes precancerous growths, which can develop into cancer. Overall, less than 5% of women with persistent HPV infection get cervical cancer.

Cancer of the cervix usually takes 10 to 20 years or more to develop, and so there is a long period of opportunity to detect and treat changes and precancerous growths before they become cancer. This is the goal of cervical cancer screening.

Who Is at Greatest Risk?

Some factors make women more likely to be infected by HPV. Other factors make infection with the most risky types of HPV progress to cervical cancer more quickly. A woman with any of these characteristics would benefit especially from screening:

- Has many sexual partners now or over the years
- Has a sexual partner who has or has had many other sexual partners
- Has a weak immune system (includes women living with HIV)
- Has other sexually transmitted infections, such as herpes simplex, chlamydia, and gonorrhea
- Has had many births (the more births, the greater the risk)
- Was young when she first gave birth
- Smokes tobacco
- Has used combined oral contraceptives for more than 5 years. (This factor is weak. WHO notes that it is not in a woman's interest to discourage or prevent her from using COCs. See Facts About Combined Oral Contraceptives and Cancer, p. 4.)

Screening and Treatment

Screening for cervical cancer is simple, quick, and generally not painful. Women age 30 years and older and women of any age living with HIV should be screened for cervical cancer. The screening should be repeated every 3 to 5 years. Any precancerous cervical changes that are detected can be treated successfully.

Three screening methods are recommended, depending on the capacity and conditions in a region. These methods are HPV testing, cytology (Papanicolaou, or Pap) screening, and/or visual inspection with acetic acid (VIA). The first 2 methods involve scraping a small sample of cells from the cervix. VIA involves looking at the cervix after it is coated with a weak vinegar solution. All three methods generally require a woman to go to a facility for testing (although HPV testing can use self-collected vaginal samples). Then she may have to return for the test results. VIA and some HPV tests can provide results at the first visit, and any preventive treatment needed can be offered at the same visit.

If a test finds precancerous changes, they must be treated to prevent progression to cancer. These changes can be removed by freezing with a probe (cryotherapy) or cut away using a hot wire loop (loop electrosurgical excision procedure [LEEP]). Freezing is less effective for larger growths, but LEEP requires electricity and more extensive training. No hospital stay is needed for either type of treatment. Both treatments are generally well-tolerated and effective.

Treatment for cervical cancer includes surgery or radiation therapy, sometimes together with chemotherapy. Treatment can be effective if the cancer is detected early. Women with advanced cervical cancer, however, have a high mortality rate.

Vaccine Available for Prevention

In the mid 2000s the European Union and the United States Food and Drug Administration approved 2 vaccines against cervical cancer, precancer, and genital warts. One vaccine, called Gardasil, protects against infection by 4 types of HPV that account for about 70% of all cervical cancers and an estimated 90% of all genital warts. The other vaccine, Cervarix, protects against the 2 main cancer-causing HPV types. Both vaccines are most effective when administered to girls before they become sexually active. They are available through GAVI—the Global Alliance for Vaccines and Immunization—and they are offered by programs around the world. A new vaccine protecting against 9 HPV types, which will protect against the great majority of cervical cancers, has recently been approved and will likely become available globally in 2018.

Questions and Answers About Sexually Transmitted Infections, Including HIV

1. **Does having another STI place a person at greater risk of infection if they are exposed to HIV?**

   Yes. In particular, infections that cause sores on the genitals such as chancroid and syphilis increase a person's risk of becoming infected if exposed to HIV. Other STIs, too, can increase the risk of HIV infection.

2. **Does using a condom only some of the time offer any protection from STIs, including HIV?**

   For best protection, a condom should be used with every act of sex. In some cases, however, occasional use can be protective. For example, if a person has a regular, faithful partner and has one act of sex outside of the relationship, using a condom for that one act can be very protective. For people who are frequently exposed to STIs, including HIV, however, using a condom only some of the time will offer only limited protection.

3. **Who is more at risk of becoming infected with an STI, men or women?**

   If exposed to STIs, women are more likely to become infected than men due to biological factors. Women have a greater area of exposure than men (the cervix and the vagina), and small tears may occur in the vaginal tissue during sex, making an easy pathway for infection.

4. **Can STIs be transmitted through oral sex (mouth on penis or vagina)?**

   Yes. Herpes, syphilis, hepatitis B, chlamydia, and gonorrhea can be transmitted through oral sex.

5. **Can STIs be transmitted through anal sex (penis in anus)?**

   Yes. STIs, including HIV, are commonly transmitted through anal sex. Unprotected anal sex carries the highest sexual risk of HIV transmission.

6. **Can HIV be transmitted through hugging? Shaking hands? Mosquito bites?**

   HIV cannot be transmitted through casual contact. This includes closed mouth kissing, hugging, shaking hands, and sharing food, clothing, or toilet seats. The virus cannot survive long outside of the human body. Mosquitoes cannot transmit HIV, either.

7. **Is there any truth to rumors that condoms are coated with HIV?**

   No, these rumors are false. Some condoms are covered with a wet or a powder-like material such as spermicide or cornstarch, but these are materials used for lubrication, to make sex smoother.

8. **Will having sex with a virgin cure someone with an STI, including HIV?**

   No. Instead, this practice only risks infecting the person who has not yet had sex.

9. **Will washing the penis or vagina after sex lower the risk of becoming infected with an STI?**

   Genital hygiene is important and a good practice. There is no evidence, however, that washing the genitals prevents STI infection. In fact, vaginal douching increases a woman's risk of acquiring STIs, including HIV, and pelvic inflammatory disease. If exposure to HIV is certain, treatment with antiretroviral medications (post-exposure prophylaxis), where available, can help reduce HIV transmission. If exposure to other STIs is certain, a provider can treat presumptively for those STIs—that is, treat the client as if he or she were infected.

10. **Why is it especially important to prevent HIV infection during pregnancy?**

    If a woman becomes infected with HIV during pregnancy, the chances that HIV will be transmitted to her baby during pregnancy, delivery, and childbirth may be at their highest because she will have a high level of virus in her blood. If a pregnant woman thinks that she may have HIV, she should seek HIV testing. Resources may be available to help her prevent transmitting HIV to her baby during pregnancy, delivery, and childbirth. It is not clear whether a woman who is exposed to HIV is more likely to become infected if she is pregnant.

11. **Is pregnancy especially risky for women with HIV and their infants?**

    Pregnancy will not make the woman's condition worse. HIV infection may increase some health risks of pregnancy, however, and may also affect the health of the infant. Women living with HIV are at greater risk of developing anemia and infection after vaginal delivery or caesarean section. The level of risk depends on such factors as a woman's health during pregnancy, her nutrition, and the medical care she receives. Also, the risk of these health problems increases if HIV infection progresses. Further, women living with HIV are at greater risk of having preterm births, stillbirths, and low birthweight babies.

12. How well do condoms help protect against HIV infection?

On average, condoms are 80% to 95% effective in protecting people from HIV infection when used correctly with every act of sex. This means that condom use prevents 80% to 95% of HIV transmissions that would have occurred without condoms. (It does *not* mean that 5% to 20% of condom users will become infected with HIV.) For example, among 10,000 uninfected women whose partners have HIV, if each couple has vaginal sex just once and has no additional risk factors for infection, on average:

- If all 10,000 did not use condoms, about 10 women would likely become infected with HIV.
- If all 10,000 used condoms correctly, 1 or 2 women would likely become infected with HIV.

The chances that a person who is exposed to HIV will become infected can vary greatly. These chances depend on the partner's stage of HIV infection (early and late stages are more infectious), whether the person exposed has other STIs (increases susceptibility), and male circumcision status (uncircumcised men are more likely to become infected with HIV), among other factors. On average, women face twice the risk of infection, if exposed, that men do.

CHAPTER 23

Maternal and Newborn Health

Key Points for Providers and Clients

- **Wait until the youngest child is at least 2 years old before trying to become pregnant again.** Spacing births is good for the mother's and the baby's health.
- **Make the first antenatal care contact within the first 12 weeks of pregnancy and schedule at least 8 contacts during the pregnancy.**
- **Plan ahead for family planning after delivery.**
- **Prepare for childbirth.** Have a plan for normal delivery and an emergency plan, too.
- **Breastfeed for a healthier baby.**

Health care providers see many women who want to become pregnant, who are pregnant, or who have recently given birth. They also see adolescent girls who are pregnant. Providers can help women plan pregnancies, plan for contraception after delivery, prepare for childbirth, and care for their babies. Attentive care can help women see pregnancy as a positive experience.

Planning Pregnancy

A woman who wants to have a child can use advice about preparing for safe pregnancy and delivery and having a healthy child:

- It is best to wait at least 2 years after giving birth before stopping contraception to become pregnant again.
- At least 3 months before stopping contraception to get pregnant, a woman should begin to eat a healthy, balanced diet, and she should continue doing so throughout pregnancy. A healthy diet includes adequate energy, protein, vitamins, and minerals from green and orange vegetables, meat, fish, beans, nuts, whole grains, and fruit.

Folic acid and iron are particularly important.

- Folic acid is found in such foods as legumes (beans, bean curd, lentils, and peas), citrus fruits, whole grains, and green leafy vegetables. Folic acid tablets are recommended.
- Iron is found in such foods as meat and poultry, fish, green leafy vegetables, and legumes. Iron tablets are recommended.

- If a woman has a sexually transmitted infection (STI) or may have been exposed to an STI, including HIV, treatment can reduce the chances that her child will be born with the infection. If a woman thinks she has been exposed or might be infected, she should seek testing, if available (see also Safer Conception for HIV Serodiscordant Couples, p. 333).

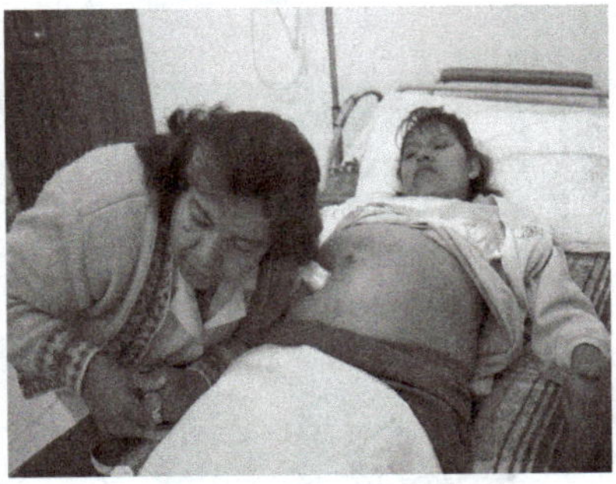

During Pregnancy

The first antenatal care contact should come early in pregnancy, ideally before week 12. For most women, 8 contacts with a health care provider during pregnancy are appropriate. Women with certain health conditions or complications of pregnancy may need more contacts.

Health Promotion and Disease Prevention

- Counsel women about good nutrition. Pregnant women should eat foods that contain iron, folate, vitamin A, calcium, and iodine. They should avoid using tobacco and breathing second-hand smoke, drinking alcohol, and taking drugs (except medications recommended by a health care provider). Pregnant women should take daily oral iron and folic acid supplements if available.
- Encourage women to stay active. Physical activity is healthy for a pregnant woman and helps her avoid gaining too much weight.
- If a woman has had hyperglycemia (high blood sugar) first diagnosed during a pregnancy, it should be classified as either gestational diabetes mellitus, which will resolve for most women after pregnancy, or diabetes mellitus in pregnancy, which will require continuing treatment after pregnancy. High blood sugar increases the chances of adverse outcomes of pregnancy.
- Assess gestational age with an ultrasound scan, if available, before 24 weeks' gestation.

- Help pregnant women protect themselves from infections and to get treatment if infected.
  - If she is at risk for STIs, discuss condom use or abstinence during pregnancy (see Sexually Transmitted Infections, Including HIV, p. 329).
  - Ensure that pregnant women are immunized against tetanus.
  - To prevent or treat anemia where hookworm infection is common, provide treatment (antihelminthic therapy) after the first trimester.
  - Screen pregnant women for bacteriuria (bacteria in the urine) according to program guidelines. Cases with symptoms and cases without symptoms should be treated with antibiotics. Bacteriuria without symptoms increases the chances of preterm birth and low birth weight.
- Help pregnant women protect their babies from infections.
  - Test for syphilis as early in pregnancy as possible, and treat as needed.
  - Offer HIV testing and counseling.
  - Pregnant women are particularly likely to get malaria. Provide insecticide-treated bed nets for malaria prevention and effective malaria treatment to every pregnant woman in areas where malaria is widespread, whether or not malaria is diagnosed (presumptive treatment). Monitor pregnant women for malaria and provide immediate treatment if diagnosed.
- For common symptoms during pregnancy, these treatments may help:
  - Nausea in early pregnancy: ginger, chamomile, vitamin B6, acupuncture
  - Heartburn: avoid large, fatty meals and alcohol; stop smoking; take antacids (at least 2 hours before or after taking iron and folic acid supplements)
  - Leg cramps: magnesium, calcium
  - Low back pain and pelvic pain: regular exercise, physiotherapy, support belts, acupuncture
  - Constipation: wheat bran or other fiber supplements
  - Varicose veins and edema: compression stockings, leg elevation, soaking in water
- To improve continuity and quality of care, each pregnant woman should be given her clinic case notes or records about her pregnancy and asked to take them to any health facility that she visits.

Planning for Family Planning After Delivery

Help pregnant women and new mothers decide how they will avoid pregnancy after childbirth. Ideally, family planning counseling should start during antenatal care.

- Waiting until her baby is at least 2 years old before a woman tries to become pregnant again is best for the baby and good for the mother, too.
- A woman who is not fully or nearly fully breastfeeding is able to become pregnant as soon as 4 to 6 weeks after childbirth.
- A woman who is fully or nearly fully breastfeeding is able to become pregnant as soon as 6 months postpartum (see Lactational Amenorrhea Method, p. 309).
- For maximum protection, a woman should not wait until the return of monthly bleeding to start a contraceptive method. Instead, she should start as soon as guidance allows (see Earliest Time That a Woman Can Start a Family Planning Method After Childbirth, p. 351).

Preparing for Childbirth and Complications

Potentially life-threatening complications develop in about 15% of pregnancies, and all of these women need immediate care. Over 70% of maternal deaths are due to complications of pregnancy and childbirth, such as hemorrhage, hypertension, infection, and abortion. Most complications cannot be predicted, but providers can help women and their families be prepared for them in case they happen.

- Help women arrange for skilled attendance at birth, and ensure that they know how to contact the skilled birth attendant at the first signs of labor.
- Explain danger signs during pregnancy and childbirth to women and their families (see next page).

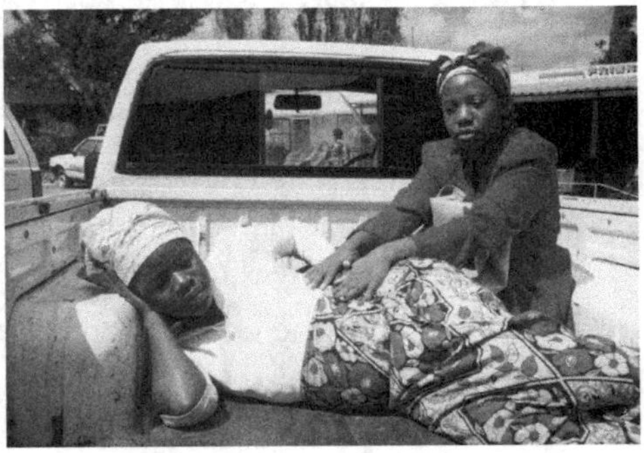

- Help the woman and her family plan how she will reach emergency care if complications arise: Where will she go? Who will take her there? What transport will they use? How will she pay for medical help? Are there people ready to donate blood?

Health facilities caring for pregnant women should have providers who are trained to:

- Monitor labor
- Care for the newborn at birth and during the first week

- Manage pre-eclampsia and eclampsia and their complications
- Manage difficult labor
- Manage postpartum hemorrhage, the leading cause of preventable maternal mortality
- Perform newborn resuscitation
- Manage preterm labor and care for preterm and small babies
- Manage maternal and newborn infections
- Communicate effectively. Providers need to be supportive, respectful, and sensitive to the needs of the pregnant woman and her family. Women should feel involved and informed so that they can make informed choices about their care.

Facilities must have a referral system in place for complications that need to be handled at a higher-level facility.

Danger Signs During Pregnancy and Childbirth

If any of these signs appears, the family should follow their emergency plan and get the woman to emergency care immediately.

- Fever (38°C/101°F or higher)
- Foul-smelling discharge from vagina
- Severe headache/blurred vision
- Decreased or no fetal movements
- Green or brown fluid leaking from vagina
- High blood pressure
- Vaginal bleeding
- Difficulty breathing
- Convulsions, fainting
- Severe abdominal pain

After Childbirth

- Mothers and newborns should receive routine postnatal care. Four routine postpartum contacts are recommended:
    1. In the facility for the first 24 hours or at home within the first 24 hours
    2. On day 3
    3. In days 7 through 14
    4. At 6 weeks
- Coordinate family planning visits with an infant's immunization schedule.
- Optimal breastfeeding offers triple value: important improvements in child survival and health, better health for mothers, and temporary contraception (see Lactational Amenorrhea Method, p. 309). Still, any breastfeeding is better than none (except if a woman has HIV; see Preventing Mother-to-Child Transmission of HIV, p. 352).

Guidelines for Best Breastfeeding

1. Begin breastfeeding the newborn as soon as possible—within 1 hour after delivery

- This stimulates uterine contractions that may help prevent heavy bleeding.
- It helps the infant to establish suckling early, which stimulates milk production.
- Colostrum, the yellowish milk produced in the first days after childbirth, provides important nutrients for the child and transfers immunities from mother to child.

2. Fully or nearly fully breastfeed for 6 months

- Mother's milk alone can fully nourish a baby for the first 6 months of life.
- Avoids the risks of feeding the baby contaminated liquids or foods.
- Full breastfeeding provides contraceptive benefits for the first 6 months as long as monthly bleeding has not returned (see Lactational Amenorrhea Method, p. 309).

3. At 6 months, add other foods to breastfeeding

- After 6 months babies need a variety of foods in addition to breast milk.
- At each feeding breastfeed before giving other foods.
- Breastfeeding can and should continue through the child's second year or longer.

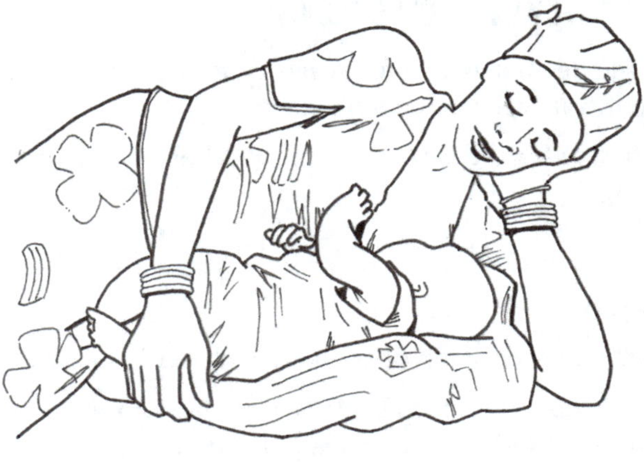

Earliest Time That a Woman Can Start a Family Planning Method After Childbirth

Family Planning Method	Fully or Nearly Fully Breastfeeding	Partially Breastfeeding or Not Breastfeeding
Lactational Amenorrhea Method	Immediately	(Not applicable)
Vasectomy	Immediately or during partner's pregnancy‡	
Male or female condoms **Spermicides**	Immediately	
Progestin-only pills **Implants**	Immediately	
Copper-bearing IUD **Levonorgestrel IUD**	Within 48 hours. Otherwise wait 4 weeks.	
Female sterilization	Within 7 days. Otherwise wait 6 weeks.	
Progesterone-releasing vaginal ring	4–9 weeks postpartum	If breastfeeding at least 4 times a day, start at 4–9 weeks postpartum Not breastfeeding: Does not apply
Diaphragm	Can be fitted 6 weeks after childbirth	
Fertility awareness methods	Start when normal secretions have returned (for symptoms-based methods) or she has had 3 regular menstrual cycles (for calendar-based methods). This will be later for breastfeeding women than for women who are not breastfeeding.	

‡ *If a man has a vasectomy during the first 6 months of his partner's pregnancy, it will be effective by the time she delivers her baby.*

(Continued on next page)

Family Planning Method	Fully or Nearly Fully Breastfeeding	Partially Breastfeeding or Not Breastfeeding
Progestin-only injectables	6 weeks after childbirth§	Immediately if not breastfeeding§ 6 weeks after childbirth if partially breastfeeding§
Combined oral contraceptives **Monthly injectables** **Combined patch** **Combined vaginal ring**	6 months after childbirth§	21 days after childbirth if not breastfeeding§ 6 weeks after childbirth if partially breastfeeding§

§ *Earlier use is not usually recommended unless other, more appropriate methods are not available or not acceptable.*

Preventing Mother-to-Child Transmission of HIV

A woman living with HIV can pass HIV to her child during pregnancy, delivery, or breastfeeding. Treatment can greatly reduce the chances of this.

Lifelong antiretroviral therapy (ART) is recommended for all adults and children from the time their HIV-positive status is known. A woman who started ART before pregnancy or when tested during pregnancy greatly reduces the chances that her baby will be infected in the uterus or during delivery. ART for the mother also greatly reduces the chances of passing HIV to her infant through breast milk.

Also, the newborns of mothers living with HIV should receive 2 anti-retroviral drugs (ARVs) for the first 6 weeks of life. This further reduces the chances of HIV passing from mother to child in the period around birth.

How can family planning providers help prevent mother-to-child transmission of HIV?

- *Help women—and men—avoid HIV infection* (see Sexually Transmitted Infections, Including HIV, Avoiding Sexually Transmitted Infections, p. 336). Women and men at high risk of HIV infection can take PrEP, pre-exposure prophylaxis, a daily oral treatment with ARVs.
- *Prevent unintended pregnancies:* Help women who do not want a child to choose a contraceptive method that they can use effectively.

- *Offer HIV counseling and testing:* In all settings offer counseling and testing in family planning facilities to all pregnant women and to the partners of women with HIV. Where HIV is common, offer testing to all women. Testing in family planning facilities can be helpful because a woman's HIV status might affect her choice of a family planning method. If testing in family planning facilities is not possible, refer clients to an HIV testing service or offer self-testing so that they can learn their HIV status.
- *Refer for prevention of HIV transmission:* Refer women with HIV who are pregnant, or who want to become pregnant, to services for prevention of mother-to-child transmission, if available. If a couple wants to have a child, and one partner has HIV while the other does not, they can take steps to reduce the chances of passing HIV while trying for conception (see Sexually Transmitted Infections, Including HIV, Safer Conception for HIV Serodiscordant Couples, p. 333).
- *Promote and support appropriate infant feeding:* In each country national authorities decide which of 2 infant feeding practices should be promoted to pregnant women and mothers living with HIV and that all health facilities should support. The 2 practices are either (1) breastfeeding while mothers receive ART or (2) avoiding all breastfeeding (while mothers still receive ART). Countries decide which practice will lead to more children surviving free of HIV, depending on conditions in the country.

  Where national authorities have decided to promote and support breastfeeding and ART for mothers with HIV:

  - Counsel all women, including women with HIV, that breastfeeding, and especially early and exclusive breastfeeding, is the best way to promote the child's survival.
  - Mothers living with HIV and their infants should receive appropriate ART, and mothers should exclusively breastfeed their infants for the first 6 months of life, then introduce appropriate complementary foods and continue breastfeeding. All children need complementary foods from 6 months of age.
  - Mothers living with HIV should breastfeed for at least 12 months and may continue breastfeeding for up to 24 months or more (like other women) while being fully supported to keep taking ART.
  - Breastfeeding should stop only when a nutritionally adequate and safe diet without breast milk can be provided.

(Continued on next page)

- When mothers decide to stop breastfeeding, they should stop gradually within one month, and infants should be given safe and adequate replacement feeds to enable normal growth and development. Stopping breastfeeding abruptly is not advised.
- Even when ART is not available, breastfeeding (exclusive breastfeeding in the first 6 months of life and continued breastfeeding for the first 12 months of life) may still give infants born to mothers living with HIV a greater chance of survival while avoiding HIV infection than not breastfeeding at all.
- If a woman is temporarily unable to breastfeed—for example, she or the infant is sick, she is weaning, or her supply of ARVs has run out—she may express and heat-treat breast milk to destroy the HIV before feeding it to the infant. Milk should be heated to the boiling point in a small pot and then cooled by letting the milk stand or by placing the pot in a container of cool water. This approach should be used only short-term, not throughout breastfeeding.
- Women with HIV who are breastfeeding need support to maintain their own nutritional status and keep their breasts healthy. Infection of the milk ducts in the breast (mastitis), a pocket of pus under the skin (breast abscess), and cracked nipples increase the risk of HIV transmission. If a problem does occur, prompt and appropriate care is important (see Sore or cracked nipples, p. 356).

Where national authorities have decided to recommend that mothers living with HIV should avoid all breastfeeding even where ART is provided:

- Mothers living with HIV should receive skilled counseling to ensure that they provide a replacement food that is safe and adequate and is safely prepared, stored, and given to their infant.
  - *For infants less than 6 months of age,* the recommended alternative to breastfeeding is commercial infant formula, as long as home conditions outlined below are met. Home-modified animal milk is not recommended as a replacement food in the first 6 months of life.
- *For infants more than 6 months of age*, alternatives to breastfeeding include:
  - Commercial infant formula milk, as long as home conditions outlined on the next page are met

- Animal milk (boiled for infants under 12 months), as part of a diet providing adequate micronutrients. Children should be fed meals, including milk-only feeds, other foods, and combination of milk feeds and other foods, 4 or 5 times per day.

- All children need complementary foods from 6 months of age.
- Mothers living with HIV should consider replacement feeding only if all the following conditions are met:
  - safe water and sanitation are ensured in the household and community; and
  - the mother or caregiver can reliably provide sufficient infant formula to support the infant's normal growth and development; and
  - the mother or caregiver can prepare it cleanly and frequently enough so that it is safe enough and carries a low risk of diarrhea and malnutrition; and
  - the mother or caregiver can give the replacement feeding exclusively in the first 6 months; and
  - the family supports this practice; and
  - the mother or caregiver can obtain comprehensive child health services.
- If infants and young children are known to be living with HIV, mothers should be strongly encouraged to exclusively breastfeed for the first 6 months of life and continue breastfeeding up to 2 years or beyond.

Managing Any Breastfeeding Problems

If a client reports any of these common problems, listen to her concerns and give advice and support. Make sure she understands the advice and agrees.

Baby is not getting enough milk

- Reassure the woman that most women can produce enough breast milk to feed their babies.
- If the newborn is gaining more than 500 grams a month, weighs more than birth weight at 2 weeks, or urinates at least 6 times a day, reassure her that her baby is getting enough breast milk.

- Tell her to breastfeed her newborn about every 2 hours to increase milk supply.
- Recommend that she reduce any supplemental foods and/or liquids if the baby is less than 6 months of age.

Sore breasts

- If her breasts are full, tight, and painful, then she may have engorged breasts. If one breast has tender lumps, then she may have blocked ducts. Engorged breasts or blocked ducts may progress to red and tender infected breasts. Treat breast infection with antibiotics according to clinic guidelines. To aid healing, advise her to:
  - Continue to breastfeed often
  - Massage her breasts before and during breastfeeding
  - Apply heat or a warm compress to breasts
  - Try different breastfeeding positions
  - Ensure that the infant attaches properly to the breast
  - Express some milk before breastfeeding

Sore or cracked nipples

- If her nipples are cracked, she can continue breastfeeding. Assure her that they will heal with time.
- To aid healing, advise her to:
  - Apply drops of breast milk to the nipples after breastfeeding and allow to air-dry.
  - After feeding, use a finger to break suction first before removing the baby from the breast.
  - Do not wait until the breast is full to breastfeed. If full, express some milk first.
- Teach her about proper attachment and how to check for signs that the baby is not attaching properly.
- Tell her to clean her nipples with only water only once a day and to avoid soaps and alcohol-based solutions.
- Examine her nipples and the baby's mouth and buttocks for signs of fungal infection (thrush).

CHAPTER 24

Reproductive Health Issues

Key Points for Providers and Clients

Postabortion Care

- **Fertility returns quickly, within a few weeks, after abortion or miscarriage.** Women need to start using a family planning method almost immediately to avoid unwanted pregnancy.

Violence Against Women

- **Violence is not the woman's fault.** It is very common. All health care providers can do something to help.

Infertility

- **Infertility often can be prevented.** Avoiding sexually transmitted infections and receiving prompt treatment for these and other reproductive tract infections can reduce a client's risk of infertility.

Family Planning in Postabortion Care

Women who have just been treated for postabortion complications need easy and immediate access to family planning services. Many different health care providers can offer these women family planning services, including those who provide postabortion care. When such services are integrated with postabortion care, are offered immediately postabortion, or are nearby, women are more likely to use contraception when they face the risk of unintended pregnancy.

Help Women Obtain Family Planning

Counsel with Compassion

A woman who has had postabortion complications needs support. A woman who has faced the double risk of pregnancy and unsafe induced abortion especially needs help and support. Good counseling gives support to the woman who has just been treated for postabortion complications. In particular:

- Try to understand what she has been through
- Treat her with respect and avoid judgment and criticism
- Ensure privacy and confidentiality
- Ask if she wants someone she trusts to be present during counseling

Provide Important Information

A woman has important choices to make after receiving postabortion care. To make decisions about her health and fertility, she needs to know:

- Fertility returns quickly—within 2 weeks after a first-trimester abortion or miscarriage and within 4 weeks after a second-trimester abortion or miscarriage. Therefore, she needs protection from pregnancy almost immediately.
- She can choose among many different family planning methods that she can start at once (see next page). Methods that women should not use immediately after giving birth pose no special risks after treatment for abortion complications.
- She can wait before choosing a contraceptive for ongoing use, but she should consider using a backup method* in the meantime if she has sex. If a woman decides not to use contraceptives at this time, providers can offer information on available methods and where to obtain them. Also, providers can offer condoms, oral contraceptives, and also emergency contraceptive pills for women to take home and use later.
- To avoid infection, she should not have sex until bleeding stops—about 5 to 7 days. If being treated for infection or vaginal or cervical injury, she should wait to have sex again until she has fully healed.
- If she wants to become pregnant again soon, encourage her to wait. Waiting at least 6 months may reduce the chances of low birth weight, premature birth, and maternal anemia.

A woman receiving postabortion care may need other reproductive health services. In particular, a provider can help her consider if she might have been exposed to sexually transmitted infections.

* *Backup methods include abstinence, male or female condoms, spermicides, and withdrawal. She can use spermicides if she has no vaginal or cervical injury. Tell her that spermicides and withdrawal are the least effective contraceptive methods. If possible, give her condoms.*

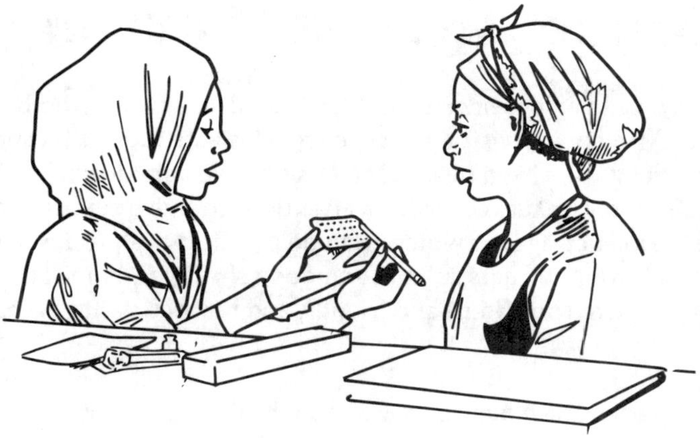

When to Start Contraceptive Methods

- Combined oral contraceptives, progestin-only pills, progestin-only injectables, monthly injectables, combined patch, implants, male condoms, female condoms, and withdrawal can be started immediately in every case, even if the woman has injury to the genital tract or has a possible or confirmed infection.
- IUDs, female sterilization, and fertility awareness methods can be started once infection is ruled out or resolved.
- IUDs, combined vaginal ring, spermicides, diaphragms, cervical caps, female sterilization, and fertility awareness methods can be started once any injury to the genital tract has healed.

Special considerations:

- *IUD* insertion immediately after a second-trimester abortion requires a specifically trained provider.
- *Female sterilization* must be decided upon in advance, and not while a woman is sedated, under stress, or in pain. Counsel carefully and be sure to mention available reversible methods (see Female Sterilization, Because Sterilization Is Permanent, p. 220).
- The *combined vaginal ring, spermicides, diaphragms,* and *cervical caps* can be used immediately, even in cases of uncomplicated uterine perforation.
- The *diaphragm* must be refitted after uncomplicated first-trimester miscarriage or abortion. After uncomplicated second-trimester miscarriage or abortion, use should be delayed 6 weeks for the uterus to return to normal size, and then the diaphragm should be refitted.
- *Fertility awareness methods:* A woman can start symptoms-based methods once she has no infection-related secretions or bleeding due to injury to the genital tract. She can start calendar-based methods with her next monthly bleeding, if she is not having bleeding due to injury to the genital tract.

Violence Against Women

Every family planning provider probably sees many women who have experienced violence. Physical violence includes acts such as hitting, slapping, kicking, punching, beating, and using a weapon. Sexual violence includes unwanted sexual contact or attention, coercive sex, and forced sex (rape). Violence against women can be psychological, too, such as insults, intimidation, threats to hurt someone she loves, humiliation, isolating a woman from family and friends, and restricting her access to resources.

Women experiencing violence have special health needs, many of them sexual and reproductive health needs. Providers of reproductive health care are in a good position to identify women who experience violence and to attend to their physical health needs as well as provide psychosocial support.

Women who experience violence often seek health services, although many will not mention the violence. Violence can lead to a range of health problems, including injuries, unwanted pregnancy, sexually transmitted infections (STIs) including HIV, decreased sexual desire, pain during sex, and chronic pelvic pain. Violence may start or become worse during a pregnancy, placing the fetus at risk as well. A man's violence or the threat of violence can deprive a woman of her right to make her own choice about whether to use family planning or what method to use.

What Can Family Planning Providers Do?

1. **Help women feel welcome, safe, and free to talk.** Help women feel comfortable speaking freely about any personal issue, including violence. Assure every woman that her visit will be confidential.

   Give a woman opportunities to discuss issues that concern her—for example, her partner's attitudes toward her use of family planning or any possible problems with using family planning—or you can ask simply if there is anything she would like to discuss. Most women will not bring up that they are being abused, but some may disclose it if asked. Be alert to symptoms, injuries, or signs that suggest violence. Violence at home may lead a woman to refuse or to insist on a specific family planning method, to resist family planning counseling, or to insist on reversal of female sterilization. Many pregnancies close together or requests for pregnancy termination also may reflect violence at home. (Of course, there could be many other reasons for these preferences and behaviors.)

2. If you suspect violence, ask about it.
Some tips for bringing up the topic of violence:

- To increase trust, explain why you are asking—because you want to help.
- Use language that is comfortable for you and best fits your own style.
- Do not ask such questions when a woman's partner or anyone else is present or when privacy cannot be ensured.

"Should I ask all my clients about violence?"

Health care providers should routinely ask all clients about violence only if they are trained in asking about violence and offering first-line support, if privacy and confidentiality can be ensured, and if referral linkages to other support services are in place.

To explore whether a client is experiencing partner violence and to support her disclosure of violence, you can first approach the topic indirectly. You can say, for example:

– "Many women experience problems with their husband or partner or someone else they live with."

– "I have seen women with problems like yours who have been having trouble at home."

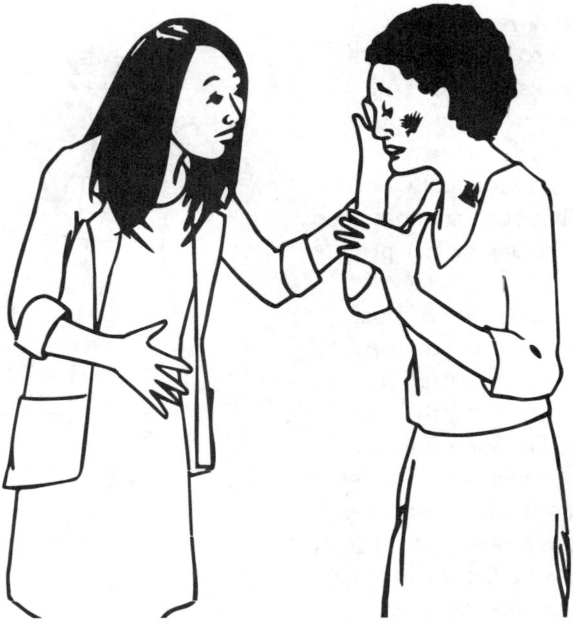

24 Reproductive Health Issues

You can follow it up with more direct questions, such as these:

- "Are you afraid of your husband (or partner)?"
- "Has your husband (or partner) or someone else at home ever threatened to hurt you or physically harm you in some way? If so, when has this happened?"
- "Does your husband (or partner) or someone at home bully you or insult you or try to control you?"
- "Has your husband (or partner) forced you into sex or forced you to have any sexual contact you did not want?"

To explore further how violence affects a woman's reproductive and sexual life, you can ask these 4 questions:

1. Has your partner ever told you not to use contraception, blocked you from getting a method, or hidden or taken away your contraception?
2. Has your partner ever tried to force you or pressure you to become pregnant?
3. Has your partner ever refused to use a condom?
4. Has your partner ever made you have sex without using contraception so that you would become pregnant?

3. Offer first-line support.

In response to a disclosure of violence, you should offer first-line support. First-line support provides practical care and responds to a woman's emotional, physical, safety, and support needs, without intruding on her privacy.

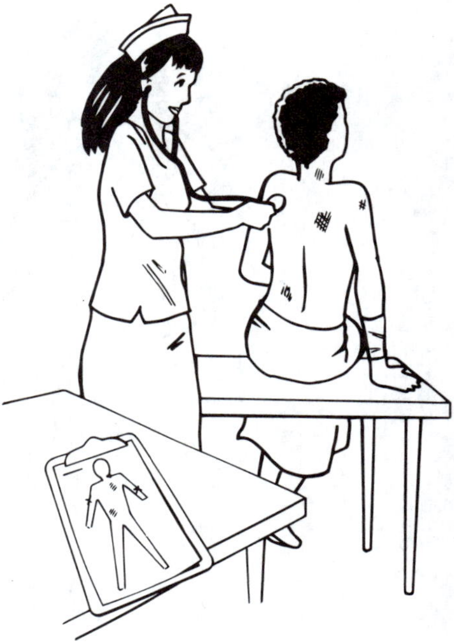

First-line support is the most important care that you can provide. Even if this is all you can do, you will have greatly helped your client. First-line support involves 5 simple tasks. The letters in the word "LIVES" can remind you of these 5 tasks that protect women's lives—**L**isten, **I**nquire about needs and concerns, **V**alidate, **E**nhance safety, **S**upport.

LISTEN	Listen to the woman closely, with empathy, and without judging. Give her a chance to say what she wants to say in a safe, confidential, and private place to a caring person who wants to help. **Listening is the most important part of good communication and the basis of first-line support.** If she does not want to talk about violence, assure her that you are available whenever she needs you.
INQUIRE ABOUT NEEDS AND CONCERNS	Assess and respond to her various needs and concerns. As you listen to the woman's story, pay particular attention to what she says about her needs and concerns—and what she does not say but implies with words or body language. She may let you know about physical needs, emotional needs, or economic needs, her safety concerns, or social support that she needs. **Respect her ability and her right to make her own choices about her life.**
VALIDATE	**Show her that you understand and believe her.** Validating another person's experience means letting the person know that you are listening closely, that you understand what she is saying, and that you believe what she says without judgment or conditions. Some important things that you can say: – "It's not your fault. You are not to blame." – "This happens to many women." – "You are not alone, and help is available."
ENHANCE SAFETY	Discuss a plan to protect herself from further harm if violence occurs again. Explain that partner violence is not likely to stop on its own. It tends to continue and may become worse and happen more often. You can ask: – "Are you or your children in danger now?" – "Do you feel safe to go home?" – "Is there a friend or relative who can help you with the situation at home?" **If the woman faces immediate danger, help her consider various courses of action. If not in immediate danger, help her make a longer-term plan.**
SUPPORT	**Support her by helping her connect to information, services, and social support.** Women's needs generally go beyond what you can provide in the clinic. You can help by discussing the woman's needs with her, telling her about other sources of help, such as shelter, social services, child protection, police, legal aid, financial aid, peer support, and assisting her to get help if she wants it.

4. **Provide appropriate care. Tailor your care and counseling to a woman's circumstances.**
   - **Treat any injuries** or see that she gets treatment.
   - **Discuss** with her how she can make the best choices for family planning in her circumstances.
     - If your client wants a method that would be hard for her partner to detect or to interfere with, an injectable may be her best choice. You might also discuss IUDs and implants. Be sure to point out that even these methods can sometimes be detected.
     - Make clear that these methods do not protect her against sexually transmitted infections (STIs), including HIV. Condoms are the only family planning method that protects against STIs as well as pregnancy. Give information and offer referral to support services, if available, for women's empowerment and skills building on condom use negotiation and safer sexual practices.
     - Provide emergency contraceptive pills if appropriate and wanted.
5. **Document the abuse experienced by the woman.** Carefully and confidentially document the woman's history of abuse along with symptoms or injuries and the cause of the injuries if relevant. Record the relationship of the perpetrator to the woman.

Infertility

What Is Infertility?

Involuntary infertility is a disease of the reproductive system: the inability to become pregnant when desired. Involuntary childlessness is the inability to give birth to desired children, whether due to inability to achieve pregnancy or due to stillbirth or miscarriage. These conditions occur in couples who have never had children (primary infertility) and, more often, in couples who have had children previously (secondary infertility). Infertility is "defined by the failure to establish a clinical pregnancy after 12 months of regular unprotected sexual intercourse" between a man and a woman. (On average, 85% of women would be pregnant by then.)

Worldwide, infertility affects about 12% of couples who are seeking to have a child—about 2% who have never had children and about 10% who have had children previously. There are differences among regions.

In some countries or communities, infertility or childlessness can have drastic consequences, especially for women but also with significant impact on men. These consequences can include economic deprivation, divorce, stigma and discrimination, isolation, intimate partner violence, murder, mental health disorders, and suicide.

What Causes Infertility?

Globally, infertility has many causes, which vary depending on the setting. Although often the woman is blamed, the cause of infertility can be in either the man or the woman or in both.

Medically, causes of infertility range from the effects of sexually transmitted infections (STIs) in one or both partners to hormonal imbalances and defects of the uterus in women and low sperm count, low sperm motility, and malformed sperm in men. Lifestyle factors include smoking, alcohol, and drug abuse as well as obesity and nutritional deficiencies. Exposures to chemicals in the environment that disrupt the endocrine system as well as other environmental and stress-related factors are suspected as well.

A large WHO study in the late 1970s found that STIs were a major cause of infertility in developing countries. It is not known how much STIs contribute to infertility now.

However, the evidence is clear that, if left untreated, gonorrhea and chlamydia can infect the fallopian tubes, the uterus, and the ovaries in women. This is known as pelvic inflammatory disease (PID). Clinical PID is painful, but sometimes PID has no symptoms and goes unnoticed (silent PID). Gonorrhea and chlamydia can scar women's fallopian tubes, blocking eggs from traveling down the tubes to meet sperm. Similarly, untreated gonorrhea and chlamydia in men can cause scarring and blockage in the sperm duct (epididymis) and urethra (see Female Anatomy, p. 432, and Male Anatomy, p. 435).

Other factors or conditions that can reduce fertility or cause infertility include:

- Other reproductive tract infections, including genital tuberculosis (TB) in both men and women
- HIV
- Medical procedures that introduce infection into a woman's upper reproductive tract or uterus, including postpartum and postabortion infections
- Mumps that develop after puberty in men
- Certain disorders of the reproductive tract, such as endometriosis, polycystic ovaries, and fibroids (myomas)
- Anatomical, endocrine, genetic, or immune system problems in both men and women
- Surgical interventions that adversely affect reproductive tissues or organs
- Cancer treatments that affect reproductive health and the capacity to reproduce
- Aging in both women and men

Preventing Involuntary Infertility

Involuntary infertility often can be prevented. Providers can:

- Counsel clients about STI prevention (see Sexually Transmitted Infections, Including HIV, Avoiding Sexually Transmitted Infections, p. 336). Encourage clients to seek treatment as soon as they think they might have an STI or might have been exposed.
- Treat or refer clients with signs and symptoms of STIs and clinical PID (see Sexually Transmitted Infections, including HIV, Symptoms of Sexually Transmitted Infections, p. 334). Treating these infections can help to prevent infertility.
- Avoid causing infection by following proper infection-prevention practices when performing medical procedures that pass instruments from the vagina into the uterus, such as IUD insertion (see Infection Prevention in the Clinic, p. 376).
- Treat or refer clients with signs or symptoms of infection postpartum or postabortion.
- Help clients with fertility problems become aware of risks to fertility—not only infections but also lifestyle and environmental factors.
- Counsel clients about available options for their future childbearing—that is, fertility preservation techniques such as sperm freezing for men and in vitro fertilization or freezing eggs—if they are being treated or are having surgery for cancer or other diseases that may affect reproductive tissues or organs.

Contraceptives Do Not Cause Infertility

- With most modern contraceptive methods, there is no significant delay in the time to desired pregnancy after contraception is stopped. On average, pregnancy occurs after 3 to 6 months of unprotected sex. There is great variation around this average, however, related to the age and the health status of the individuals in the couple. When counseling couples who stop contraception and want to have a child, aging and other factors affecting the fertility of the woman and the man need to be considered.
- The return of fertility after injectable contraceptives are stopped usually takes longer than with most other methods (see Progestin-Only Injectables, Questions 7 and 8, pp. 93–94, and Monthly Injectables, Questions 10 and 11, p. 118). In time, however, a woman is as fertile as before using the method, taking aging into account.
- Among women with current gonorrhea or chlamydia, IUD insertion slightly increases the risk of pelvic inflammatory disease in the first 20 days after insertion. However, research has not found that former IUD users are more likely to be infertile than other women (see Copper-Bearing IUD, Question 4, p. 179).

Counseling Clients With Fertility Problems

- Counsel both partners together, if possible. A man may blame his partner for infertility when he himself may be responsible for the inability of the woman to become pregnant or to maintain a pregnancy.
- Explain that a man is just as likely to have fertility problems as a woman. In more than 40% of couples with fertility problems, it is because of semen or sperm abnormalities, or other health problems of the male partner. In 20% of couples with fertility problems, both male and female factors reduce fertility. Sometimes it is not possible to find the cause of the problem,
- Recommend that the couple attempt pregnancy with unprotected sex for at least 12 months before they suspect infertility. Provide educational materials and guidance on risks to fertility.
- The most fertile time of a woman's cycle is several days before and at the time of ovulation (when an ovary releases an egg) (see The Menstrual Cycle, p. 434). Fertility awareness methods can help couples identify the most fertile time of each cycle (see Fertility Awareness Methods, p. 291). Provide educational material about these methods and/or refer the couple to a fertility care provider or specialist.
- If, after one year, following the suggestions above has not resulted in a pregnancy or live birth, refer both partners to a qualified fertility care provider for evaluation and assessment, if available. Referral to a fertility care provider or specialist may be particularly helpful in the following situations: the couple is affected by HIV or suspected genital TB; the woman is age 35 or older; she has polycystic ovary syndrome or has been diagnosed with endometriosis; the woman or the man suspects they had an STI and it was not treated; either had been treated for a cancer or had surgery that may have affected the reproductive tissues or organs.
- The couple also may want to consider adoption or other alternatives to having children or more children of their own, such as taking in nieces and nephews.

CHAPTER 25

Family Planning Provision

Importance of Selected Procedures for Providing Family Planning Methods

The table on the next page shows how important various examinations and tests are when providing specific family planning methods.

Most methods do not require any of these exams or tests (Class C). However, these exams and tests may be useful as part of a general health check-up or for the diagnosis or monitoring of other health conditions.

Key to the chart:

Class A: Essential and mandatory in all circumstances for safe and effective use of the contraceptive method. A pelvic or genital examination is essential for IUD insertion, most diaphragms, female sterilization, and vasectomy. STI risk assessment also is essential before IUD insertion. Blood pressure screening is essential before female sterilization.

Class B: Contributes substantially to safe and effective use. If the test or examination cannot be done, however, the risk of not performing it should be weighed against the benefits of making the contraceptive method available. Laboratory screening for STIs and a hemoglobin test would contribute to the safety of IUD insertion. A hemoglobin test also would contribute to the safety of female sterilization.

Class C: Does not contribute substantially to safe and effective use of the contraceptive method. These tests and exams are not required or helpful for hormonal contraceptive methods, male or female condoms, or spermicides.

These classifications apply to people who are presumed to be healthy. For a person with a known medical condition or other special condition, refer to the Medical Eligibility Criteria for Contraceptive Use, p. 388.

For information on ruling out pregnancy, see p. 439. Ruling out pregnancy is essential for IUD insertion and helpful for deciding when to start hormonal methods.

Specific situation	Combined oral contraceptives*	Monthly injectables	Progestin-only pills	Progestin-only injectables	Implants	Cu- and LNG-IUDs	Male and female condoms	Diaphragms and cervical caps	Spermicides	Female sterilization	Vasectomy
Breast examination by provider	C	C	C	C	C	C	C	C	C	C	NA
Pelvic/genital examination	C	C	C	C	C	A	C	A	C	A	A
Cervical cancer screening	C	C	C	C	C	C	C	C	C	C	NA
Routine laboratory tests	C	C	C	C	C	C	C	C	C	C	C
Hemoglobin test	C	C	C	C	C	B	C	C	C	B	C
STI risk assessment: medical history and physical examination	C	C	C	C	C	A**	C	C†	C†	C	C
STI/HIV screening: laboratory tests	C	C	C	C	C	B**	C	C†	C†	C	C
Blood pressure screening	‡	‡	‡	‡	‡	C	C	C	C	A	C§

Note: No tests or examinations are needed before using fertility awareness-based methods, lactational amenorrhea method, or emergency contraceptive pills.

NA=Not applicable

* *Includes patch and combined vaginal ring.*

** *If a woman has a very high individual likelihood of exposure to STIs, she generally should not have an IUD inserted unless other methods are not available or not acceptable. If she has current purulent cervicitis, gonorrhea, or chlamydia, she should not have an IUD inserted until these conditions are resolved and she is otherwise medically eligible.*

† *Women at high risk of HIV infection should not use spermicides. Using spermicides alone or diaphragms or cervical caps with spermicides is not usually recommended for women with HIV infection unless other, more appropriate methods are not available or acceptable.*

‡ *Desirable, but in settings where the risks of pregnancy are high, and hormonal methods are among the few methods widely available, women should not be denied use of hormonal methods solely because their blood pressure cannot be measured.*

§ *For procedures performed using only local anesthesia.*

Successful Counseling

Good counseling helps clients choose and use family planning methods that suit them. Clients differ, their situations differ, and they need different kinds of help. The best counseling is tailored to the individual client.

Client Type	Usual Counseling Tasks
Returning clients with no problems	• Provide more supplies or routine follow-up • Ask a friendly question about how the client is doing with the method
Returning clients with problems	• Understand the problem and help resolve it—whether the problem is side effects, trouble using the method, an uncooperative partner, or another problem
New clients with a method in mind	• Check that the client's understanding is accurate • Support the client's choice, if client is medically eligible • Discuss how to use method and how to cope with any side effects
New clients with no method in mind	• Discuss the client's situation, plans, and what is important to her or him about a method • Help the client consider methods that might suit her or him. If needed, help her or him reach a decision • Support the client's choice, give instructions on use, and discuss how to cope with any side effects

Give time to clients who need it. Many clients are returning with no problems and need little counseling. Returning clients with problems and new clients with no method in mind need the most time, but usually they are few.

Tips for Successful Counseling

- Show every client respect, and help each client feel at ease.
- Encourage the client to explain needs, express concerns, ask questions.
- Let the client's wishes and needs guide the discussion.
- Be alert to related needs such as protection from sexually transmitted infections including HIV, and support for condom use.
- Talk with the client in a private place, where no one else can hear.
- Assure the client of confidentiality—that you will not tell others about your conversation or the client's decisions.
- Listen carefully. Listening is as important as giving correct information.

- Give just *key* information and instructions. Use words the client knows.
- Respect and support the client's informed decisions.
- Bring up side effects, if any, and take the client's concerns seriously.
- Check the client's understanding.
- Invite the client to come back any time for any reason.

Counseling has succeeded when:

- Clients feel they got the help they wanted
- Clients know what to do and feel confident that they can do it
- Clients feel respected and appreciated
- Clients come back when they need to
- And, most important, clients use their methods effectively and with satisfaction.

Counseling About Effectiveness

The effectiveness of a family planning method is very important to most clients. The effectiveness of family planning methods varies greatly (see Appendix A, Contraceptive Effectiveness, p. 383). Describing and discussing effectiveness is an important part of counseling.

Describing effectiveness to clients takes thought and care. Instead of talking about pregnancy rates, which can be hard to understand, it may be more useful to compare the effectiveness of methods and to discuss whether the client feels able to use the method effectively.

The chart on the back cover can help. The chart groups contraceptive methods according to their effectiveness as commonly used. Also, it points out how the user can obtain the greatest possible effectiveness.

- In general, **methods that require *little or no* action by clients are the most effective.** The 4 most effective methods—implants, IUDs, female sterilization, and vasectomy—are shown in the top row of the chart. All 4 methods need a health care provider's help to get started, but then they need little or no action by the user. These methods are very effective for everyone who uses them—less than one pregnancy in 100 women in 1 year of use. Moreover, implants and IUDs are highly effective for 4 to 5 years or more, and female sterilization and vasectomy are permanent.
- Methods in the second row can be highly effective when used correctly and consistently. They require some repeated action by the user, however—some seldom, such as getting 4 injections a year, and some

often, such as taking a pill every day, 365 days a year. As a result, they are less effective, on average, than methods in the top row, but still effective. Pregnancy rates for these methods range from 2 to 7 pregnancies in 100 women in a year.

- The methods in the lower rows of the chart usually have much higher pregnancy rates—as high as 20 or more pregnancies in 100 women in 1 year of use for the least effective methods. The effectiveness of these methods depends greatly on the user taking correct action repeatedly, such as using a condom with every act of sexual intercourse. Particularly for these methods, some highly motivated couples are much more successful than average. Others make more mistakes and are more likely than average to get pregnant.

Women tend to underestimate the effectiveness of the methods on the upper rows of the chart and overestimate the effectiveness of the methods on the lower rows. This may lead them to make misinformed decisions and to choose a contraceptive method that does not meet their needs. Counseling may need to gently correct these common misperceptions.

In counseling it is not possible or necessary to provide complete information about every method. Clients do, however, benefit from key information, especially about the method that they want. The goal of counseling about method choice is to help the client find a method that she or he can use successfully and with satisfaction. Well-informed clients are more likely to be satisfied with their method and to use it longer. Clients need to understand how that method works, how effective it is, how to make the method most effective, what are the most likely side effects, and what to do if such side effects occur. With this knowledge and understanding, clients are better able to exercise their right to make a truly informed choice.

Who Provides Family Planning?

Many different people can learn to inform and advise people about family planning and to provide family planning methods. When more types of health workers are authorized and trained to provide family planning methods, more people have access to them.

The types of health care providers who can and do provide family planning include the following:

Type of Health Worker	Examples
Specialist doctor	• Gynecologist, obstetrician
Non-specialist doctor	• Family doctor, general practitioner
Advanced associate and associate clinician	• Assistant medical officer, clinical officer, medical licentiate practitioner, health officer, physician assistant, surgical technician, non-physician clinician, medical assistant, nurse practitioner
Midwife	• Registered midwife, midwife, community midwife, nurse-midwife
Nurse	• Registered nurse, clinical nurse specialist, licensed nurse, BSc nurse
Auxiliary nurse-midwife	• Auxiliary midwife
Auxiliary nurse	• Auxiliary nurse, nurse assistant, enrolled nurse
Pharmacist	• Pharmacist, chemist, clinical pharmacist, community pharmacist
Pharmacy worker	• Pharmacy assistant, pharmacy technician dispenser, pharmacist aide
Lay health worker	• Community health worker (CHW), village health worker, community health volunteer
User/self	• Woman, man, client

In addition, some methods can be offered by health workers but do not *require* health workers. For example, condoms are sold in shops and by vendors and in vending machines. Also, lay health workers in the community and experienced and successful users can teach others how to use their method—for example, fertility awareness methods, male and female condoms, LAM, and withdrawal—and they can support and advise new users of many other methods. Users of injectables can learn to give themselves injections with a special formulation of DMPA in the Uniject delivery device (see Progestin-Only Injectables, Self-injection Can Be an Option, p. 83). Programs can support self-injection with information and training, strong referral links to health care providers, and monitoring and follow-up.

Task-Sharing: WHO Recommendations

Many countries and programs are changing their policies or regulations to allow more types of providers to offer contraceptive methods—a change known as task-sharing. Task-sharing refers to expanding the levels of health care providers who can appropriately deliver health services. Task-sharing helps to:

- address shortages and uneven distribution of providers, particularly in rural and remote areas
- give higher-level clinicians more time to use their specialized skills
- provide more family planning methods at the primary care level, and
- overall, increase access to safe and timely care

To encourage and guide task-sharing, WHO has developed recommendations on which types of health workers can safely and effectively provide specific family planning methods. WHO based these recommendations on evidence that a wide variety of providers can safely and effectively provide contraception. The table on the next page summarizes the WHO recommendations.

Specific competency-based training and continued educational support help all types of health care providers do a better job at providing family planning. They are particularly important when providers take on new tasks. Some tasks and some providers require more training and support than others. Training needs to cover skills in informing and counseling clients about choosing and using specific methods, including their side effects, as well as any specific technical skills such as how to give injections or insert and remove an IUD or an implant. Even specialist doctors need training in specific techniques—for example, no-scalpel vasectomy and laparoscopic tubal sterilization. Checklists and other job aids can help a wide range of providers and managers in various ways, such as screening clients for medical eligibility criteria, making sure all steps in a process are carried out (such as infection prevention), and ensuring good quality of services.

As programs plan for task-sharing and carrying it out, maintaining quality and safety are the top concerns. Successful task-sharing requires that a program pay attention to:

- training and support
- supplying the new providers with the method
- supervision
- referral for managing any complications
- changes to protocols, regulations, and training programs
- salaries or payment that reflect the providers' scope of practice.

Family Planning Methods and Services Typically Offered by Various Types of Service Providers

National policies and service delivery guidelines specify which cadres of providers can offer specific family planning services. The chart below shows the family planning methods that are typically offered by these cadres of providers based on recommendations from WHO.

CONTRACEPTIVE SERVICE	Lay Health Workers (Such as CHWs)	Pharmacy Workers	Pharmacists	Auxiliary Nurses	Auxiliary Nurse-Midwives	Nurses	Midwives	Associate/ Advanced Associate Clinicians	Non-specialist Doctor	Specialist Doctor
• Informed choice counselling • Combined oral contraceptives (COCs) • Progestin-only oral contraceptives POPs) • Emergency contraceptive pills (ECPs) • Standard Days Method and TwoDay Method • Lactational amenorrhea method (LAM) • Condoms (male & female), diaphragms, caps, spermicides	✔*	✔*	✔*	✔*	✔*	✔*	✔*	✔*	✔*	✔*
• Injectable contraceptives (DMPA, NET-EN, combined monthly injectables)	(✔)	(✔)	✔	✔	✔	✔*	✔*	✔*	✔*	✔*
• Implant insertion and removal	(R✔)	✖	✖	(✔)	(✔)	✔	✔	✔*	✔*	✔*
• Intrauterine devices (IUD)	✖	✖	✖	(R✔)	✔	✔	✔	✔*	✔*	✔*
• Vasectomy (male sterilization)	⊗*	⊗*	⊗*	(R✔)	(R✔)	(R✔)	(R✔)	✔*	✔*	✔*
• Tubal ligation (female sterilization)	⊗*	⊗*	⊗*	⊗*	⊗*	(R✔)	(R✔)	✔*	✔*	✔*

LEGEND

- ✔ Recommended
- ✔* Considered within typical scope of practice; evidence not assessed.
- (✔) Recommended in specific circumstances
- (R✔) Recommended in the context of rigorous research
- ✖ Recommended against
- ⊗* Considered outside the typical scope of practice; evidence not assessed.

All of the recommendations assume that the assigned health workers will receive task-specific training prior to offering services. Adopting task-sharing also requires functioning mechanisms for monitoring, supervision, and referral.

The recommendations are applicable in both high- and low-resource settings. They provide for a range of types of health workers who can perform the task safely and effectively. The options are intended to be inclusive and do not imply either a preference for or an exclusion of any particular type of provider. The choice of the type of health worker for a specific task will depend upon local needs and conditions.

Infection Prevention in the Clinic

Infection-prevention procedures are simple, effective, and inexpensive. Germs (infectious organisms) of concern in the clinic include bacteria (such as staphylococcus), viruses (particularly HIV and hepatitis B), fungi, and parasites. In the clinic infectious organisms can be found in blood, body fluids with visible blood, and tissue. (Feces, nasal secretions, saliva, sputum, sweat, tears, urine, and vomit are not considered potentially infectious unless they contain blood.) The organisms can be passed through mucous membranes or broken skin, such as cuts and scratches, and by needle sticks with used needles and other puncture wounds. Infectious organisms can pass from clinics to communities when waste disposal is not proper or staff members do not wash their hands properly before leaving the clinic.

Basic Rules of Infection Prevention

These rules apply the universal precautions for infection prevention to the family planning clinic.

Wash hands

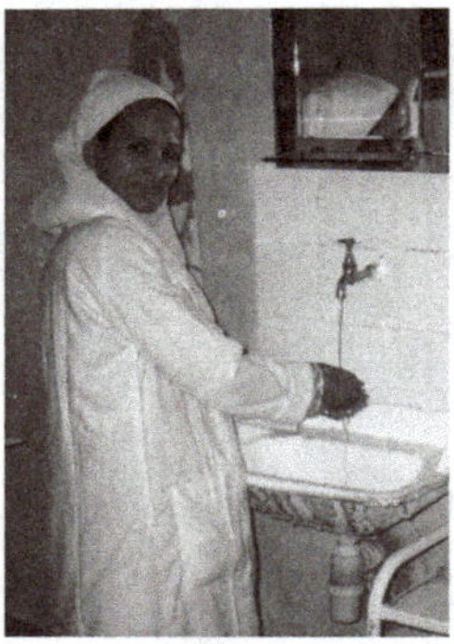

- *Hand washing may be the single most important infection-prevention procedure.*
- Wash hands before and after examining or treating each client. (Hand washing is not necessary if clients do not require an examination or treatment.)
- Use clean water and plain soap, and rub hands for at least 10 to 15 seconds. Be sure to clean between the fingers and under fingernails. Wash hands after handling soiled instruments and other items or touching mucous membranes, blood, or other body fluids. Wash hands before putting on gloves, after taking off gloves, and whenever hands get dirty. Wash hands when you arrive at work, after you use the toilet or latrine, and when you leave work. Dry hands with a paper towel or a clean, dry cloth towel that no one else uses, or air-dry.
- If clean water and soap are not available, a hand sanitizer containing at least 60% alcohol can reduce the number of germs on the hands. Sanitizers do not eliminate all types of germs and might not remove harmful chemicals.

Process instruments that will be reused

- High-level disinfect or sterilize instruments that touch intact mucous membranes or broken skin.
- Sterilize instruments that touch tissue beneath the skin (see The 4 Steps of Processing Equipment, p. 379).

Wear gloves	• Wear gloves for any procedure that risks touching blood, other body fluids, mucous membranes, broken skin, soiled items, dirty surfaces, or waste. Wear surgical gloves for surgical procedures such as insertion of implants. Wear single-use examination gloves for procedures that touch intact mucous membranes or generally to avoid exposure to body fluids. Gloves are not necessary for giving injections. • Change gloves between procedures on the same client and between clients. • Do not touch clean equipment or surfaces with dirty gloves or bare hands. • Wash hands before putting on gloves. Do not wash gloved hands instead of changing gloves. Gloves are not a substitute for hand washing. • Wear clean utility gloves when cleaning soiled instruments and equipment, handling waste, and cleaning blood or body fluid spills.
Do pelvic examinations only when needed	• Pelvic examinations are not needed for most family planning methods—only for female sterilization, the IUD, diaphragm, and cervical cap (see Importance of Selected Procedures for Providing Family Planning Methods, p. 368). Pelvic examinations should be done only when there is a reason—such as suspicion of sexually transmitted infections, when the examination could help with diagnosis or treatment.
For injections, use new auto-disable syringes and needles	• Auto-disable syringes and needles are safer and more reliable than standard single-use disposable syringes and needles, and any disposable syringes and needles are safer than sterilizing reusable syringes and needles. Sterilizing and reusing syringes and needles should be avoided. It might be considered only when single-use injection equipment is not available and the program can document the quality of sterilization. • Cleaning the client's skin before the injection is not needed unless the skin is dirty. If it is, wash with soap and water and dry with a clean towel. Wiping with an antiseptic has no added benefit.
Wipe surfaces with chlorine solution	• Wipe examination tables, bench tops, and other surfaces that come in contact with unbroken skin with 0.5% chlorine solution after each client.

Dispose of single-use equipment and supplies properly and safely 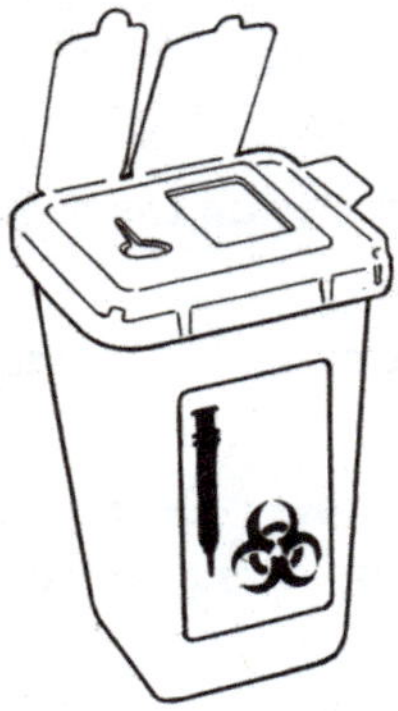	• Use personal protective equipment—goggles, mask, apron, and closed protective shoes—when handling wastes. • Needles and syringes meant for single use must not be reused. Do not take apart the needle and syringe. Used needles should not be broken, bent, or recapped. Put used needles and syringes immediately into a puncture-proof container for disposal. (If needles and syringes will not be incinerated, they should be decontaminated by flushing with 0.5% chlorine solution before they are put into the puncture-proof container.) The puncture-proof sharps container should be sealed and either burned, incinerated, or deeply buried when three-fourths full. • Dressings and other soiled solid waste should be collected in plastic bags and, within 2 days, burned and buried in a deep pit. Liquid wastes should be poured down a utility sink drain or a flushable toilet, or poured into a deep pit and buried. • Clean waste containers with detergent and rinse with water. • Remove utility gloves and clean them whenever they are dirty and at least once every day. • Wash hands before and after disposing of soiled equipment and waste.
Wash linens	• Wash linens (for example, bedding, caps, gowns, and surgical drapes) by hand or machine and line-dry or machine-dry. When handling soiled linens, wear gloves, hold linens away from your body, and do not shake them.

Little Risk of HIV Infection in the Clinic

Health care providers may be exposed to HIV through needle sticks, mucous membranes, or broken skin, but the risk of infection is low:

- Needle sticks or cuts cause most infections in health care settings. The average risk of HIV infection after a needle-stick exposure to HIV-infected blood is 3 infections per 1,000 needle sticks.
- The risk after exposure of the eye, nose, or mouth to HIV-infected blood is estimated to be about 1 infection per 1,000 exposures.

Following universal precautions is the best way that providers can avoid workplace exposure to HIV and other fluid-borne infections. Post-exposure prophylaxis (PEP) with antiretroviral medicines will help to prevent HIV infection if a needle stick might have exposed a provider to HIV.

Make Infection Prevention a Habit

With each and every client, a health care provider should think, "What infection prevention is needed?" Any client or provider may have an infection without knowing it and without obvious symptoms. Infection prevention is a sign of good health care that can attract clients. For some clients cleanliness is one of the most important signs of quality.

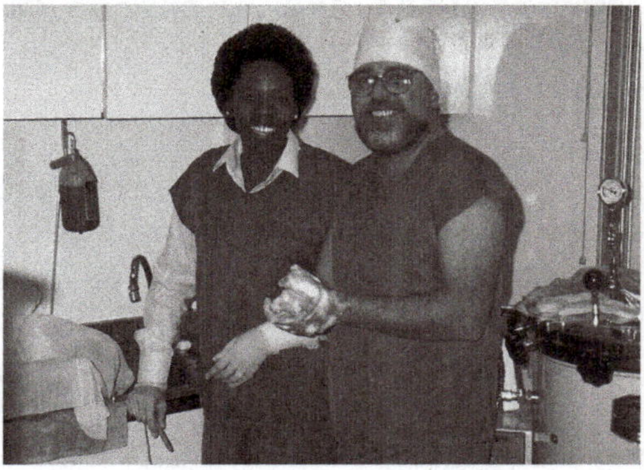

The 4 Steps of Processing Equipment

1. *Decontaminate to kill infectious organisms such as HIV and hepatitis B* and to make instruments, gloves, and other objects safer for people who clean them. Soak in 0.5% chlorine solution for 10 minutes. Rinse with clean cool water or clean immediately.
2. *Clean to remove body fluids, tissue, and dirt.* Wash or scrub with a brush with liquid soap or detergent and water. Avoid bar soap or powdered soap, which can stay on the equipment. Rinse and dry. While cleaning, wear utility gloves and personal protective equipment—goggles, mask, apron, and enclosed shoes.
3. *High-level disinfect or sterilize.*
   - High-level disinfect to kill all infectious organisms except some bacterial endospores (a dormant, resistant form of bacteria) by boiling, by steaming, or with chemicals. High-level disinfect instruments or supplies that touch intact mucous membranes or broken skin, such as vaginal specula, uterine sounds, and gloves for pelvic examinations.
   - Sterilize to kill all infectious organisms, including bacterial endospores, with a high-pressure steam autoclave, a dry-heat oven, chemicals, or radiation. Sterilize instruments such as scalpels and needles that touch tissue beneath the skin. If sterilization is not possible or practical (for example, for laparoscopes), instruments must be high-level disinfected.
4. *Store instruments and supplies to protect them from contamination.* They should be stored in a high-level disinfected or sterilized container in a clean area away from clinic traffic. The equipment used to sterilize and high-level disinfect instruments and supplies also must be guarded against contamination.

Managing Contraceptive Supplies

Good-quality reproductive health care requires a continuous supply of contraceptives and other commodities. Family planning providers are the most important link in the contraceptive supply chain that moves commodities from the manufacturer to the client.

Accurate and timely reports and orders from providers help supply chain managers determine what products are needed, how much to buy, and where to distribute them. Clinic staff members do their part when they properly manage contraceptive inventory, accurately record and report what is provided to clients, and promptly order new supplies. In some facilities one staff member is assigned all the logistics duties. In other facilities different staff members may help with logistics as needed. Clinic staff members need to be familiar with, and work within, whatever systems are in place to make certain that they have the supplies they need.

Logistics Responsibilities in the Clinic

Each supply chain operates according to specific procedures that work in a specific setting, but typical contraceptive logistics responsibilities of clinic staff include these common activities:

Daily

- Track the number and types of contraceptives dispensed to clients using the appropriate recording form (typically called a "daily activity register").
- Maintain proper storage conditions for all supplies: clean, dry storage, away from direct sun and protected from extreme heat.
- Provide contraceptives to clients by "First Expiry, First Out" management of the stock of supplies. "First Expiry, First Out," or FEFO, sees to it that products with the earliest labeled expiry dates are the first products issued or dispensed. FEFO clears out older stock first to prevent waste due to expiry.

Regularly (monthly or quarterly, depending on the logistics system)

- Count the amount of each method on hand in the clinic and determine the quantity of contraceptives to order (often done with a clinic pharmacist). This is a good time to inspect the supplies, looking for such problems as products past their expiry date, damaged containers and packages, IUD or implant packaging that has come open, or discoloration of condoms.

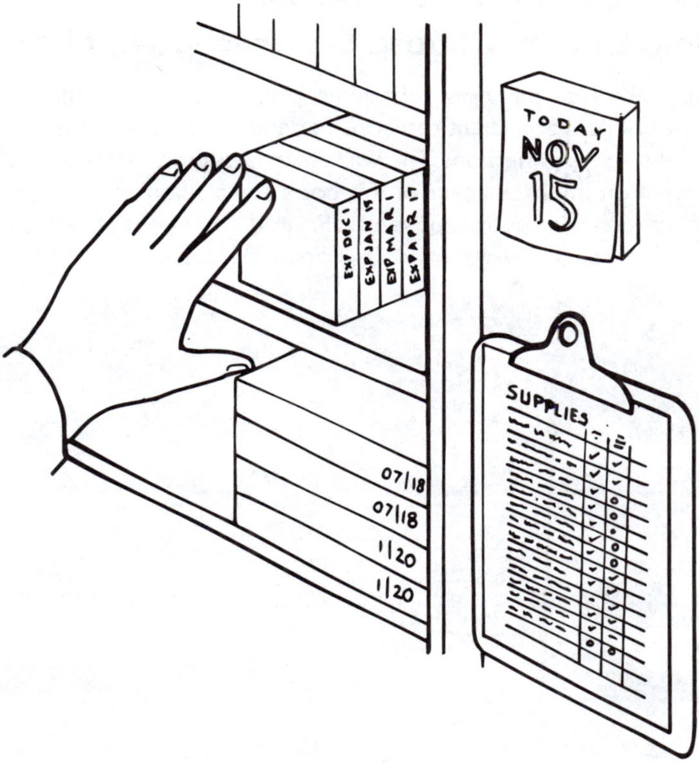

- Work with any community-based distribution agents supervised by clinic staff, reviewing their consumption records and helping them complete their order forms. Issue contraceptive supplies to community-based agents based on their orders. A record of the date of expiry of these supplies can help with retrieving supplies that have not been distributed and are out of date.
- Report to and make requests of the family planning program coordinator or health supplies officer (typically at the district level), using the appropriate reporting and ordering form or forms. The quantity that is ordered is the amount that will bring the stock up to the level that will meet expected need until the next order is received. (A plan should be made in advance to place emergency orders or borrow supplies from neighboring facilities if there are sudden increases in demand, potential for running out of inventory, or large losses, for example, if a warehouse is flooded.)
- Receive the ordered contraceptive supplies from the clinic pharmacist or other appropriate person in the supply chain. Receipts should be checked against what was ordered.

Wall Chart Available

To Help Clients Choose Contraceptive Methods

The wall chart "Do you know your family planning choices?" offers important points that a client can consider, and a provider can discuss, about many family planning methods. The wall chart includes the effectiveness chart shown on the back cover of this book and a summary of medical eligibility criteria for contraceptive use. Printed copies of the wall chart can be ordered online at: www.fphandbook.org/order-form.

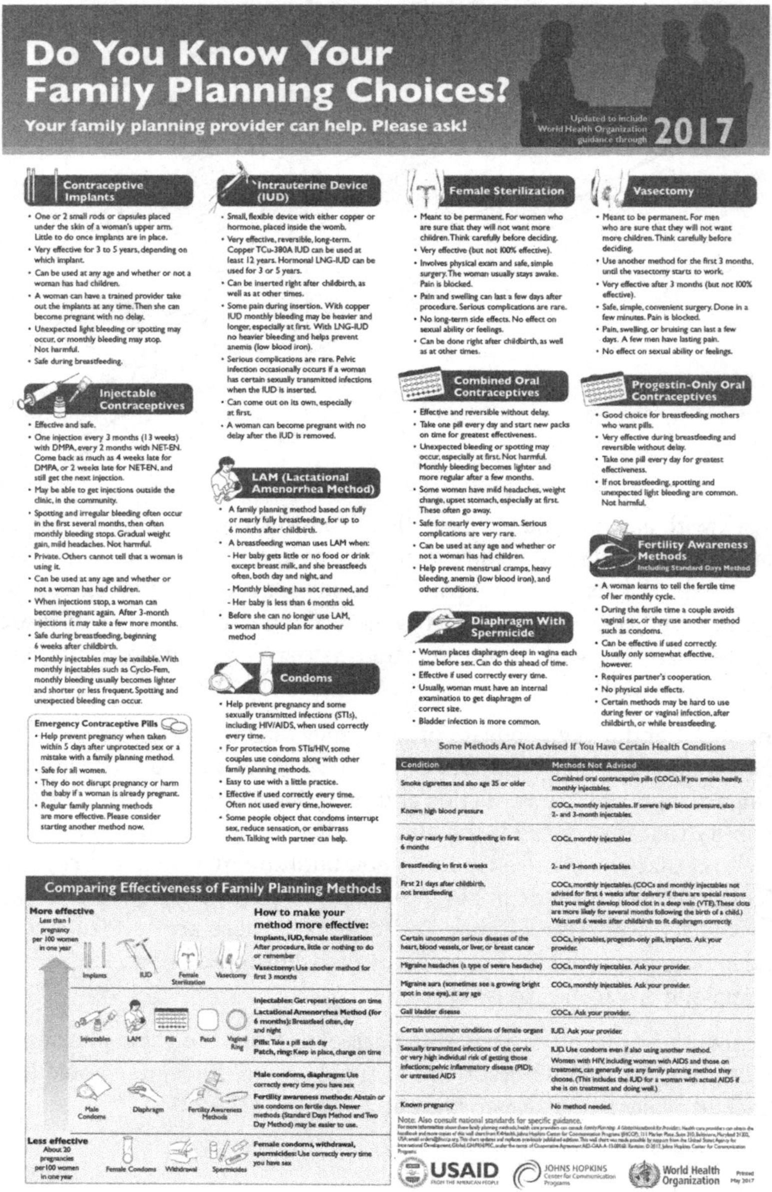

Do You Know Your Family Planning Choices?

Your family planning provider can help. Please ask!

Updated to include World Health Organization guidance through 2017

Contraceptive Implants

- One or 2 small rods or capsules placed under the skin of a woman's upper arm. Little to do once implants are in place.
- Very effective for 3 to 5 years, depending on which implant.
- Can be used at any age and whether or not a woman has had children.
- A woman can have a trained provider take out the implants at any time. Then she can become pregnant with no delay.
- Unexpected light bleeding or spotting may occur, or monthly bleeding may stop. Not harmful.
- Safe during breastfeeding.

Injectable Contraceptives

- Effective and safe.
- One injection every 3 months (13 weeks) with DMPA, every 2 months with NET-EN. Come back as much as 4 weeks late for DMPA, or 2 weeks late for NET-EN, and still get the next injection.
- May be able to get injections outside the clinic, in the community.
- Spotting and irregular bleeding often occur in the first several months, then often monthly bleeding stops. Gradual weight gain, mild headaches. Not harmful.
- Private. Others cannot tell that a woman is using it.
- Can be used at any age and whether or not a woman has had children.
- When injections stop, a woman can become pregnant again. After 3-month injections it may take a few more months.
- Safe during breastfeeding, beginning 6 weeks after childbirth.
- Monthly injectables may be available. With monthly injectables such as Cyclo-Fem, monthly bleeding usually becomes lighter and shorter or less frequent. Spotting and unexpected bleeding can occur.

Emergency Contraceptive Pills

- Help prevent pregnancy when taken within 5 days after unprotected sex or a mistake with a family planning method.
- Safe for all women.
- They do not disrupt pregnancy or harm the baby if a woman is already pregnant.
- Regular family planning methods are more effective. Please consider starting another method now.

Intrauterine Device (IUD)

- Small, flexible device with either copper or hormone, placed inside the womb.
- Very effective, reversible, long-term. Copper TCu-380A IUD can be used at least 12 years. Hormonal LNG-IUD can be used for 3 or 5 years.
- Can be inserted right after childbirth, as well as at other times.
- Some pain during insertion. With copper IUD monthly bleeding may be heavier and longer, especially at first. With LNG-IUD no heavier bleeding and helps prevent anemia (low blood iron).
- Serious complications are rare. Pelvic infection occasionally occurs if a woman has certain sexually transmitted infections when the IUD is inserted.
- Can come out on its own, especially at first.
- A woman can become pregnant with no delay after the IUD is removed.

LAM (Lactational Amenorrhea Method)

- A family planning method based on fully or nearly fully breastfeeding, for up to 6 months after childbirth.
- A breastfeeding woman uses LAM when:
  - Her baby gets little or no food or drink except breast milk, and she breastfeeds often, both day and night, and
  - Monthly bleeding has not returned, and
  - Her baby is less than 6 months old.
- Before she can no longer use LAM, a woman should plan for another method

Condoms

- Help prevent pregnancy and some sexually transmitted infections (STIs), including HIV/AIDS, when used correctly every time.
- For protection from STIs/HIV, some couples use condoms along with other family planning methods.
- Easy to use with a little practice.
- Effective if used correctly every time. Often not used every time, however.
- Some people object that condoms interrupt sex, reduce sensation, or embarrass them. Talking with partner can help.

Female Sterilization

- Meant to be permanent. For women who are sure that they will not want more children. Think carefully before deciding.
- Very effective (but not 100% effective).
- Involves physical exam and safe, simple surgery. The woman usually stays awake. Pain is blocked.
- Pain and swelling can last a few days after procedure. Serious complications are rare.
- No long-term side effects. No effect on sexual ability or feelings.
- Can be done right after childbirth, as well as at other times.

Combined Oral Contraceptives

- Effective and reversible without delay.
- Take one pill every day and start new packs on time for greatest effectiveness.
- Unexpected bleeding or spotting may occur, especially at first. Not harmful. Monthly bleeding becomes lighter and more regular after a few months.
- Some women have mild headaches, weight change, upset stomach, especially at first. These often go away.
- Safe for nearly every woman. Serious complications are very rare.
- Can be used at any age and whether or not a woman has had children.
- Help prevent menstrual cramps, heavy bleeding, anemia (low blood iron), and other conditions.

Diaphragm With Spermicide

- Woman places diaphragm deep in vagina each time before sex. Can do this ahead of time.
- Effective if used correctly every time.
- Usually, woman must have an internal examination to get diaphragm of correct size.
- Bladder infection is more common.

Vasectomy

- Meant to be permanent. For men who are sure that they will not want more children. Think carefully before deciding.
- Use another method for the first 3 months, until the vasectomy starts to work.
- Very effective after 3 months (but not 100% effective).
- Safe, simple, convenient surgery. Done in a few minutes. Pain is blocked.
- Pain, swelling, or bruising can last a few days. A few men have lasting pain.
- No effect on sexual ability or feelings.

Progestin-Only Oral Contraceptives

- Good choice for breastfeeding mothers who want pills.
- Very effective during breastfeeding and reversible without delay.
- Take one pill every day for greatest effectiveness.
- If not breastfeeding, spotting and unexpected light bleeding are common. Not harmful.

Fertility Awareness Methods
Including Standard Days Method

- A woman learns to tell the fertile time of her monthly cycle.
- During the fertile time a couple avoids vaginal sex, or they use another method such as condoms.
- Can be effective if used correctly. Usually only somewhat effective, however.
- Requires partner's cooperation.
- No physical side effects.
- Certain methods may be hard to use during fever or vaginal infection, after childbirth, or while breastfeeding.

Comparing Effectiveness of Family Planning Methods

More effective Less than 1 pregnancy per 100 women in one year

Implants, IUD, Female Sterilization, Vasectomy

Injectables, LAM, Pills, Patch, Vaginal Ring

Male Condoms, Diaphragm, Fertility Awareness Methods

Female Condoms, Withdrawal, Spermicides

Less effective About 20 pregnancies per 100 women in one year

How to make your method more effective:

Implants, IUD, female sterilization: After procedure, little or nothing to do or remember

Vasectomy: Use another method for first 3 months

Injectables: Get repeat injections on time

Lactational Amenorrhea Method (for 6 months): Breastfeed often, day and night

Pills: Take a pill each day

Patch, ring: Keep in place, change on time

Male condoms, diaphragm: Use correctly every time you have sex

Fertility awareness methods: Abstain or use condoms on fertile days. Newer methods (Standard Days Method and Two Day Method) may be easier to use.

Female condoms, withdrawal, spermicides: Use correctly every time you have sex

Some Methods Are Not Advised If You Have Certain Health Conditions

Condition	Methods Not Advised
Smoke cigarettes and also age 35 or older	Combined oral contraceptive pills (COCs). If you smoke heavily, monthly injectables.
Known high blood pressure	COCs, monthly injectables. If severe high blood pressure, also 2- and 3-month injectables.
Fully or nearly fully breastfeeding in first 6 months	COCs, monthly injectables
Breastfeeding in first 6 weeks	2- and 3-month injectables
First 21 days after childbirth, not breastfeeding	COCs, monthly injectables. (COCs and monthly injectables not advised for first 6 weeks after delivery if there are special reasons that you might develop blood clot in a deep vein (VTE). These clots are more likely for several months following the birth of a child.) Wait until 6 weeks after childbirth to fit diaphragm correctly.
Certain uncommon serious diseases of the heart, blood vessels, or liver, or breast cancer	COCs, injectables, progestin-only pills, implants. Ask your provider.
Migraine headaches (a type of severe headache)	COCs, monthly injectables. Ask your provider.
Migraine aura (sometimes see a growing bright spot in one eye), at any age	COCs, monthly injectables. Ask your provider.
Gall bladder disease	COCs. Ask your provider.
Certain uncommon conditions of female organs	IUD. Ask your provider.
Sexually transmitted infections of the cervix or very high individual risk of getting those infections; pelvic inflammatory disease (PID); or untreated AIDS	IUD. Use condoms even if also using another method. Women with HIV, including women with AIDS and those on treatment, can generally use any family planning method they choose. (This includes the IUD for a woman with actual AIDS if she is on treatment and doing well.)
Known pregnancy	No method needed.

Note: Also consult national standards for specific guidance.

USAID FROM THE AMERICAN PEOPLE · JOHNS HOPKINS Center for Communication Programs · World Health Organization · Printed May 2017

APPENDIX A

Contraceptive Effectiveness

Rates of Unintended Pregnancies per 100 Women

	First-Year Pregnancy Rate[a] (Trussell & Aiken[b])		12-Month Pregnancy Rate[c] (Polis et al.[d])
Family planning method	Consistent and correct use	As commonly used	As commonly used
Implants	0.1	0.1	0.6
Vasectomy	0.1	0.15	
Female sterilization	0.5	0.5	
Levonorgestrel IUD	0.5	0.7	
Copper-bearing IUD	0.6	0.8	1.4
LAM (for 6 months)	0.9[e]	2[e]	
Monthly injectable	0.05[e]	3[e]	
Progestin-only injectable	0.2	4	1.7
Combined oral contraceptives	0.3	7	5.5
Progestin-only pills	0.3	7	
Combined patch	0.3	7	
Combined vaginal ring	0.3	7	
Male condoms	2	13	5.4
Standard Days Method	5	12	
TwoDay Method	4	14	
Ovulation method	3	23	
Other fertility awareness methods		15	
Diaphragms with spermicide	16	17	
Withdrawal	4	20	13.4
Female condoms	5	21	
Spermicide	16	21	
Cervical cap[f]	26[g], 9[h]	32[g], 16[h]	
No method	85	85	

Key

Key	
0–0.9	Very effective
1–9	Effective
10–19	Moderately effective
20+	Less effective

[a] Rates largely from the United States. Data from best available source as determined by authors.
[b] Trussell J and Aiken ARA, Contraceptive efficacy. In: Hatcher RA et al. Contraceptive Technology, 21st revised edition. New York, Ardent Media, 2018.
[c] Rates from developing countries. Data from self-reports in population-based surveys.
[d] Polis CB et al. Contraceptive failure rates in the developing world: an analysis of Demographic and Health Survey data in 43 countries. New York: Guttmacher Institute, 2016.
[e] Source: Hatcher R et al. Contraceptive technology. 20th ed. New York, Ardent Media, 2011.
[f] Source: Trussell J. Contraceptive failure in the United States. Contraception. 2004:70(2): 89–96.
[g] Pregnancy rate for women who have given birth
[h] Pregnancy rate for women who have never given birth

APPENDIX B

Signs and Symptoms of Serious Health Conditions

The table below lists signs and symptoms of some serious health conditions. These conditions are mentioned under Health Risks or Managing Any Problems in the chapters on contraceptive methods. These conditions occur rarely to extremely rarely among users of the method. They also occur rarely among people of reproductive age generally. Still, it is important to recognize possible signs of these conditions and to take action or refer for care if a client reports them. In some cases clients who develop one of these conditions may need to choose another contraceptive method.

Condition	Description	Signs and Symptoms
Deep vein thrombosis	A blood clot that develops in the deep veins of the body, generally in the legs	Persistent, severe pain in one leg, sometimes with swelling or red skin.
Ectopic pregnancy	Pregnancy in which the fertilized egg implants in tissue outside the uterus, most commonly in a fallopian tube but sometimes in the cervix or abdominal cavity	In the early stages of ectopic pregnancy, symptoms may be absent or mild, but eventually they become severe. A combination of these signs and symptoms should increase suspicion of ectopic pregnancy: • Unusual abdominal pain or tenderness • Abnormal vaginal bleeding or no monthly bleeding—especially if a change from her usual bleeding pattern • Light-headedness or dizziness • Fainting
Heart attack	Occurs when the blood supply to the heart is blocked, usually due to a build-up of cholesterol and other substances in the coronary arteries	Chest discomfort or uncomfortable pressure; fullness, squeezing, or pain in the center of the chest that lasts longer than a few minutes or that comes and goes; spreading pain or numbness in one or both arms, back, jaw, or stomach; shortness of breath; cold sweats; nausea.

Condition	Description	Signs and Symptoms
Liver disorders	Infection with hepatitis inflames the liver; cirrhosis scars tissue, which blocks blood flow through the liver	Yellow eyes or skin (jaundice) and abdominal swelling, tenderness, or pain, especially in the upper abdomen.
Pelvic inflammatory disease (PID)	An infection of the upper genital tract, caused by various types of bacteria	Lower abdominal pain; pain during sex, pelvic examination, or urination; abnormal vaginal bleeding or discharge; fever; cervix bleeds when touched. In a pelvic examination, signs of PID include tenderness in the ovaries or fallopian tubes, yellowish cervical discharge containing mucus and pus, bleeding easily when the cervix is touched with a swab, or a positive swab test, and tenderness or pain when moving the cervix and uterus during pelvic examination.
Pulmonary embolism	A blood clot that travels through the bloodstream to the lungs	Sudden shortness of breath, which may worsen with a deep breath, cough that may bring up blood, fast heart rate, and a light-headed feeling.
Ruptured ectopic pregnancy	When a fallopian tube breaks due to an ectopic pregnancy	Sudden sharp or stabbing pain in lower abdomen, sometimes on one side. Possible right shoulder pain. Usually, within hours the abdomen becomes rigid and the woman goes into shock.
Severe allergic reaction to latex	When a person's body has a strong reaction to contact with latex	Rash over much of the body, dizziness brought on by a sudden drop in blood pressure, difficult breathing, loss of consciousness (anaphylactic shock).
Stroke	When arteries to the brain become blocked or burst, preventing normal blood flow and leading to the death of brain tissue	Numbness or weakness of the face, arm or leg, especially on one side of the body; confusion or trouble speaking or understanding; trouble seeing in one or both eyes; trouble walking, dizziness, loss of balance or coordination; severe headache with no other known cause. Signs and symptoms develop suddenly.
Toxic shock syndrome	A severe reaction throughout the body to toxins released by bacteria	High fever, body rash, vomiting, diarrhea, dizziness, muscle aches. Signs and symptoms develop suddenly.

APPENDIX C

Medical Conditions That Make Pregnancy Especially Risky

Some common medical conditions make pregnancy riskier to a woman's health. The effectiveness of her contraceptive method thus has special importance. For a comparison of the effectiveness of family planning methods, see Contraceptive Effectiveness, p. 383.

Some methods depend more on their users for effectiveness than do others. Mostly, the methods that require correct use with every act of sex or abstaining during fertile days are the less effective methods, as commonly used:

- Spermicides
- Withdrawal
- Fertility awareness methods
- Cervical caps
- Diaphragms
- Female condoms
- Male condoms

If a woman says that she has any of the common conditions listed below:

- She should be told that pregnancy could be especially risky to her health and in some cases to the health of her baby.
- During counseling, focus special attention on the effectiveness of methods. Clients who are considering a method that requires correct use with every act of sex should think carefully whether they can use it effectively.

Reproductive Tract Infections and Disorders

- Breast cancer
- Endometrial cancer
- Ovarian cancer
- Some sexually transmitted infections (gonorrhea, chlamydia)
- Some vaginal infections (bacterial vaginosis)
- Malignant gestational trophoblastic disease

Cardiovascular Disease

- High blood pressure (systolic blood pressure higher than 160 mm Hg or diastolic blood pressure higher than 100 mm Hg)
- Complicated valvular heart disease
- Ischemic heart disease (heart disease due to narrowed arteries)
- Stroke
- Thrombogenic mutations

Other Infections

- HIV (see Sexually Transmitted Infections Including HIV, Question 11, p. 343)
- Tuberculosis
- Schistosomiasis with fibrosis of the liver

Endocrine Conditions

- Diabetes if insulin dependent, with damage to arteries, kidneys, eyes, or nervous system (nephropathy, retinopathy, neuropathy), or of more than 20 years' duration

Anemia

- Sickle cell disease

Gastrointestinal Conditions

- Severe (decompensated) cirrhosis of the liver
- Malignant (cancerous) liver tumors (hepatoma) and hepatocellular carcinoma of the liver

Neurologic Conditions

- Epilepsy

Rheumatic Conditions

- Systemic lupus erythematosus

APPENDIX D

Medical Eligibility Criteria for Contraceptive Use

The table on the following pages summarizes the World Health Organization Medical Eligibility Criteria for Contraceptive Use. These criteria are the basis for the Medical Eligibility Criteria checklists in most chapters of this handbook on family planning methods. These checklists are based on the 2-level system for providers with limited clinical judgment (see table below). The checklist questions address conditions in MEC categories 3 or 4 that the woman knows of. The boxes "Using Clinical Judgment in Special Cases" list conditions that are in MEC category 3: The method can be provided if other, more appropriate methods are not available or acceptable to the client, and a qualified provider can carefully assess the specific woman's condition and situation.

Categories for Temporary Methods

Category	With Clinical Judgment	With Limited Clinical Judgment
1	Use method in any circumstances	Yes (Use the method)
2	Generally use method	
3	Use of method not usually recommended unless other more appropriate methods are not available or not acceptable	No (Do not use the method)
4	Method not to be used	

Note: In the table beginning on the next page, category 3 and 4 conditions are shaded to indicate that the method should not be provided where clinical judgment is limited. Categories that are new or changed since the 2011 edition of this handbook are shown in **dark type**.

For vasectomy, male and female condoms, spermicides, diaphragms, cervical caps, and the lactational amenorrhea method, see pp. 397–399. For fertility awareness methods, see p. 399.

Categories for Female Sterilization and Vasectomy

Accept (A)	There is no medical reason to deny the method to a person with this condition or in this circumstance.
Caution (C)	The method is normally provided in a routine setting, but with extra preparation and precautions.
Delay (D)	Use of the method should be delayed until the condition is evaluated and/or corrected. Alternative, temporary methods of contraception should be provided.
Special (S)	The procedure should be undertaken in a setting with an experienced surgeon and staff, equipment needed to provide general anesthesia, and other backup medical support. The capacity to decide on the most appropriate procedure and anesthesia support also is needed. Alternative, temporary methods of contraception should be provided if referral is required or there is otherwise any delay.

	= Use the method
(shaded)	= Do not use the method
I	= Initiation of the method
C	= Continuation of the method
—	= Condition not listed; does not affect eligibility for method
NA	= Not applicable

Condition	Combined oral contraceptives	Monthly injectables	Combined patch and combined vaginal ring	Progestin-only pills	Progestin-only injectables	Implants	Emergency contraceptive pills*	Copper-bearing intrauterine device	Levonorgestrel intrauterine device	Female sterilization*
PERSONAL CHARACTERISTICS AND REPRODUCTIVE HISTORY										
Pregnant	NA	NA	NA	NA	NA	NA	NA	4	4	D
Age	Menarche to < 40 years			Menarche to < 18 years				Menarche to < 20 years		Young age
	1	1	1	1	2	1	—	2	2	C
	≥ 40 years			18 to 45 years				≥ 20 years		
	2	2	2	1	1	1	—	1	1	
				> 45						
				1	2	1	—			
Parity										
Nulliparous (has not given birth)	1	1	1	1	1	1	—	2	2	A
Parous (has given birth)	1	1	1	1	1	1	—	1	1	A
Breastfeeding										
< 6 weeks postpartum	4	4	4	2	3[a]	2	1 UPA=2	b	b	*
≥ 6 weeks to < 6 months postpartum (primarily breastfeeding)	3	3	3	1	1	1	1 UPA=2	b	b	A
≥ 6 months postpartum	2	2	2	1	1	1	1 UPA=2	b	b	A
Postpartum (not breastfeeding)										
< 21 days	3	3	3	1	1	1	—	b	b	
With other added VTE risk factors	4	4	4							*
21–42 days	2	2	2	1	1	1	—	b	b	
With other added VTE risk factors	3	3	3							
> 42 days	1	1	1	1	1	1	—	1	1	A
Postabortion										
First trimester	1	1	1	1	1	1	—	1	1	
Second trimester	1	1	1	1	1	1	—	2	2	*
Immediate post-septic abortion	1	1	1	1	1	1	—	4	4	

(Continued)

* For additional conditions relating to emergency contraceptive pills and female sterilization, see p. 397.

[a] In settings where pregnancy morbidity and mortality risks are high and this method is one of few widely available contraceptives, it may be made accessible to breastfeeding women immediately postpartum.

[b] Postpartum IUD use: For the copper-bearing IUD, insertion at <48 hours is category 1. For the LNG-IUD, insertion at <48 hours is category 2 for breastfeeding women and category 1 for women not breastfeeding. For all women and both IUD types, insertion from 48 hours to <4 weeks is category 3; ≥4 weeks, category 1; and puerperal sepsis, category 4.

Condition	Combined oral contraceptives	Monthly injectables	Combined patch and combined vaginal ring	Progestin-only pills	Progestin-only injectables	Implants	Emergency contraceptive pills*	Copper-bearing intrauterine device	Levonorgestrel intrauterine device	Female sterilization*
Past ectopic pregnancy	1	1	1	2	1	1	1	1	1	A
History of pelvic surgery	1	1	1	1	1	1	—	1	1	C*
Smoking										
Age < 35 years	2	2	2	1	1	1	—	1	1	A
Age ≥ 35 years										
< 15 cigarettes/day	3	2	3	1	1	1	—	1	1	A
≥ 15 cigarettes/day	4	3	4	1	1	1	—	1	1	A
Obesity										
≥ 30 kg/m² body mass index	2	2	2	1	1[†]	1	1	1	1	C
Blood pressure measurement unavailable	NA[c]	NA[c]	NA[c]	NA[c]	NA[c]	NA[c]	—	NA	NA	NA
CARDIOVASCULAR DISEASE										
Multiple risk factors for arterial cardiovascular disease (older age, smoking, diabetes, and hypertension)	3/4[d]	3/4[d]	3/4[d]	2	3	2	—	1	2	S
Hypertension[e]										
History of hypertension, where blood pressure CANNOT be evaluated (including hypertension in pregnancy)	3	3	3	2[c]	2[c]	2[c]	—	1	2	NA
Adequately controlled hypertension, where blood pressure CAN be evaluated	3	3	3	1	2	1	—	1	1	C
Elevated blood pressure (properly measured)										
Systolic 140–159 or diastolic 90–99	3	3	3	1	2	1	—	1	1	C[f]
Systolic ≥ 160 or diastolic ≥ 100[g]	4	4	4	2	3	2	—	1	2	S[f]

Key:
- (white box) = Use the method
- (shaded box) = Do not use the method
- I = Initiation of the method
- C = Continuation of the method
- — = Condition not listed; does not affect eligibility for method
- NA = Not applicable

[†] From menarche to age <18 years, ≥30 kg/m² body mass index is category 2 for DMPA, category 1 for NET-EN.

[c] In settings where pregnancy morbidity and mortality risks are high and this method is one of few widely available contraceptives, women should not be denied access simply because their blood pressure cannot be measured.

[d] When multiple major risk factors exist, any of which alone would substantially increase the risk of cardiovascular disease, use of the method may increase her risk to an unacceptable level. However, a simple addition of categories for multiple risk factors is not intended. For example, a combination of factors assigned a category 2 may not necessarily warrant a higher category.

[e] Assuming no other risk factors for cardiovascular disease exist. A single reading of blood pressure is not sufficient to classify a woman as hypertensive.

[f] Elevated blood pressure should be controlled before the procedure and monitored during the procedure.

☐ = Use the method ▒ = Do not use the method I = Initiation of the method C = Continuation of the method — = Condition not listed; does not affect eligibility for method NA = Not applicable **Condition**	Combined oral contraceptives	Monthly injectables	Combined patch and combined vaginal ring	Progestin-only pills	Progestin-only injectables	Implants	Emergency contraceptive pills*	Copper-bearing intrauterine device	Levonorgestrel intrauterine device	Female sterilization*
Vascular disease	4	4	4	2	3	2	—	1	2	S
History of high blood pressure during pregnancy (where current blood pressure is measurable and normal)	2	2	2	1	1	1	—	1	1	A
Deep venous thrombosis (DVT)/**Pulmonary embolism** (PE)										
History of DVT/PE	4	4	4	2	2	2	*	1	2	A
Acute DVT/PE	4	4	4	3	3	3	*	1	3	D
DVT/PE and on anticoagulant therapy	4	4	4	2	2	2	*	1	2	S
Family history of DVT/PE (first-degree relatives)	2	2	2	1	1	1	*	1	1	A
Major surgery										
With prolonged immobilization	4	4	4	2	2	2	—	1	2	D
Without prolonged immobilization	2	2	2	1	1	1	—	1	1	A
Minor surgery without prolonged immobilization	1	1	1	1	1	1	—	1	1	A
Known thrombogenic mutations (e.g., factor V Leiden, prothrombin mutation; protein S, protein C, and antithrombin deficiencies)[g]	4	4	4	2	2	2	*	1	2	A
Superficial venous disorders										
Varicose veins	1	1	1	1	1	1	—	1	1	A
Superficial venous thrombosis	2	2	2	1	1	1	—	1	1	A
Ischemic heart disease[g]				I / C		I / C			I / C	
Current	4	4	4	2 / 3	3	2 / 3	*	1	2 / 3	D
History of	4	4	4	2 / 3	3	2 / 3	*	1	2 / 3	C
Stroke (history of cerebrovascular accident)[g]	4	4	4	2 / 3	3	2 / 3	*	1	2	C
Known dyslipidemias without other known cardiovascular risk factors[h]	**2**	**2**	**2**	2	2	2	—	1	2	A

(Continued)

[g] This condition may make pregnancy an unacceptable health risk. Women should be advised that because of relatively higher pregnancy rates, as commonly used, spermicides, withdrawal, fertility awareness methods, cervical caps, diaphragms, or female or male condoms may not be the most appropriate choice.

[h] Routine screening is not appropriate because of the rarity of the condition and the high cost of screening.

Legend:
- (white box) = Use the method
- (shaded box) = Do not use the method
- I = Initiation of the method
- C = Continuation of the method
- — = Condition not listed; does not affect eligibility for method
- NA = Not applicable

In cells with two values, "I" gives the category for initiation and "C" the category for continuation of the method.

Condition	Combined oral contraceptives	Monthly injectables	Combined patch and combined vaginal ring	Progestin-only pills	Progestin-only injectables	Implants	Emergency contraceptive pills*	Copper-bearing intrauterine device	Levonorgestrel intrauterine device	Female sterilization*
Valvular heart disease										
Uncomplicated	2	2	2	1	1	1	—	1	1	C[i]
Complicated[‡, g]	4	4	4	1	1	1	—	2[i]	2[i]	S*
Systemic lupus erythematosus					I / C			I / C		
Positive (or unknown) antiphospholipid antibodies	4	4	4	3	I 3 / C 3	3	—	I 1 / C 1	3	S
Severe thrombocytopenia	2	2	2	2	I 3 / C 2	2	—	I 3 / C 2	2	S
Immunosuppresive treatment	2	2	2	2	I 2 / C 2	2	—	I 2 / C 1	2	S
None of the above	2	2	2	2	I 2 / C 2	2	—	I 1 / C 1	2	C
NEUROLOGICAL CONDITIONS										
Headaches[j]	I / C	I / C	I / C	I / C	I / C	I / C			I / C	
Nonmigrainous (mild or severe)	I 1 / C 2	I 1 / C 2	I 1 / C 2	I 1 / C 1	I 1 / C 1	I 1 / C 1	—	1	I 1 / C 1	A
Migraine							2			
Without aura	I / C	I / C	I / C	I / C	I / C	I / C			I / C	
Age < 35	I 2 / C 3	I 2 / C 3	I 2 / C 3	I 1 / C 2	I 2 / C 2	I 2 / C 2	—	1	I 2 / C 2	A
Age ≥ 35	I 3 / C 4	I 3 / C 4	I 3 / C 4	I 1 / C 2	I 2 / C 2	I 2 / C 2	—	1	I 2 / C 2	A
With aura, at any age	I 4 / C 4	I 4 / C 4	I 4 / C 4	I 2 / C 3	I 2 / C 3	I 2 / C 3	—	1	I 2 / C 3	A
Epilepsy	1[k]	1[k]	1[k]	1[k]	1[k]	1[k]	—	1		C
DEPRESSIVE DISORDERS										
Depressive disorders	1[l]	1[l]	1[l]	1[l]	1[l]	1[l]	—	1	1[l]	C
REPRODUCTIVE TRACT INFECTIONS AND DISORDERS										
Vaginal bleeding patterns									I / C	
Irregular pattern without heavy bleeding	1	1	1	2	2	2	—	1	I 1 / C 1	A
Heavy or prolonged bleeding (including regular and irregular patterns)	1	1	1	2	2	2	—	2	I 1 / C 2	A
Unexplained vaginal bleeding (suspicious for serious condition), before evaluation	2	2	2	2	3	3	—	I 4 / C 2	I 4 / C 2	D
Endometriosis	1	1	1	1	1	1	—	2	1	S
Benign ovarian tumors (including cysts)	1	1	1	1	1	1	—	1	1	A
Severe dysmenorrhea	1	1	1	1	1	1	—	2	1	A

‡ Pulmonary hypertension, atrial fibrillation, history of subacute bacterial endocarditis.

i Prophylactic antibiotics are advised before providing the method.

j Category is for women without any other risk factors for stroke.

k If taking anticonvulsants, refer to section on drug interactions, p. 396.

l Certain medications may interact with the method, making it less effective.

[ ] = Use the method
[shaded] = Do not use the method
I = Initiation of the method
C = Continuation of the method
— = Condition not listed; does not affect eligibility for method
NA = Not applicable

Condition	Combined oral contraceptives	Monthly injectables	Combined patch and combined vaginal ring	Progestin-only pills	Progestin-only injectables	Implants	Emergency contraceptive pills*	Copper-bearing intrauterine device	Levonorgestrel intrauterine device	Female sterilization*
Gestational trophoblastic disease										
Decreasing or undetectable ß-hCG levels	1	1	1	1	1	1	—	3	3	A
Persistently elevated ß-hCG levels or malignant disease[g]	1	1	1	1	1	1	—	4	4	D
Cervical ectropion	1	1	1	1	1	1	—	1	1	A
Cervical intraepithelial neoplasia (CIN)	2	2	2	1	2	2	—	1	2	A
Cervical cancer (awaiting treatment)	2	2	2	1	2	2	—	I: 4; C: 2	I: 4; C: 2	D
Breast disease										
Undiagnosed mass	2	2	2	2	2	2	—	1	2	A
Benign breast disease	1	1	1	1	1	1	—	1	1	A
Family history of cancer	1	1	1	1	1	1	—	1	1	A
Breast cancer										
Current[g]	4	4	4	4	4	4	—	1	4	C
Past, no evidence of disease for at least 5 years	3	3	3	3	3	3	—	1	3	A
Endometrial cancer[g]	1	1	1	1	1	1	—	I: 4; C: 2	I: 4; C: 2	D
Ovarian cancer[g]	1	1	1	1	1	1	—	I: 3; C: 2	I: 3; C: 2	D
Uterine fibroids										
Without distortion of the uterine cavity	1	1	1	1	1	1	—	1	1	C
With distortion of the uterine cavity	1	1	1	1	1	1	—	4	4	C
Anatomical abnormalities										
Distorted uterine cavity	—	—	—	—	—	—	—	4	4	—
Other abnormalities not distorting the uterine cavity or interfering with IUD insertion (including cervical stenosis or lacerations)	—	—	—	—	—	—	—	2	2	—
Pelvic inflammatory disease (PID)										
Past PID (assuming no current risk factors for STIs)								I / C	I / C	
With subsequent pregnancy	1	1	1	1	1	1	—	I: 1; C: 1	I: 1; C: 1	A
Without subsequent pregnancy	1	1	1	1	1	1	—	I: 2; C: 2	I: 2; C: 2	C

(Continued)

(blank box)	= Use the method
(shaded box)	= Do not use the method
I	= Initiation of the method
C	= Continuation of the method
—	= Condition not listed; does not affect eligibility for method
NA	= Not applicable

Condition	Combined oral contraceptives	Monthly injectables	Combined patch and combined vaginal ring	Progestin-only pills	Progestin-only injectables	Implants	Emergency contraceptive pills*	Copper-bearing intrauterine device		Levonorgestrel intrauterine device		Female sterilization*
Current PID	1	1	1	1	1	1	—	4	2[m]	4	2[m]	D
Sexually transmitted infections (STIs)[g]								I	C	I	C	
Current purulent cervicitis, chlamydia, or gonorrhea	1	1	1	1	1	1	—	4	2	4	2	D
Other STIs (excluding HIV and hepatitis)	1	1	1	1	1	1	—	2	2	2	2	A
Vaginitis (including trichomonas vaginalis and bacterial vaginosis)	1	1	1	1	1	1	—	2	2	2	2	A
Increased risk of STIs	1	1	1	1	1	1	—	2 / 3[n]	2	2 / 3[n]	2	A
HIV/AIDS[g]												
								I	C	I	C	
High risk of HIV	1	1	1	1	2	1	—	2	2	2	2	A
Asymptomatic or mild HIV clinical disease (WHO stage 1 or 2)	1	1	1	1	1	1	—	2	2	2	2	A
Severe or advanced HIV clinical disease (WHO stage 3 or 4)	1	1	1	1	1	1	—	3	2	3	2	S[o]
Antiretroviral therapy												
Treated with nucleoside reverse transcriptase inhibitors (NRTIs)**	1	1	1	1	1	1	—	2 / 3[p]	2	2 / 3[p]	2	—
Treated with non-nucleoside reverse transcriptase inhibitors (NNRTIs)												
Efavirenz (EFV) or nevirapine (NVP)	2	2	2	2	DMPA 1 NET-EN 2	2	—	2 / 3[p]	2	2 / 3[p]	2	—
Etravirine (ETR) or rilpivirine (RPV)	1	1	1	1	1	1	—	2 / 3[p]	2	2 / 3[p]	2	—
Treated with protease inhibitors (PIs)††	2	2	2	2	DMPA 1 NET-EN 2	2	—	2 / 3[p]	2	2 / 3[p]	2	—

†† PIs include: ritonavir-boosted atazanavir (ATV/r), ritonavir-boosted lopinavir (LPV/r), ritonavir-boosted darunavir (DRV/r), ritonavir (RTV).

** NRTIs include: abacavir (ABC), tenofovir (TDF), zidovudine (AZT), lamivudine (3TC), didanosine (DDI), emtricitabine (FTC), stavudine (D4T).

m Treat PID using appropriate antibiotics. There is usually no need to remove the IUD if the client wishes to continue use.

n The condition is category 3 if a woman has a very high individual likelihood of STIs.

o Presence of an AIDS-related illness may require a delay in the procedure.

p Condition is category 2 for IUD insertion for asymptomatic or mild HIV clinical disease (WHO stage 1 or 2), category 3 for severe or advanced HIV clinical disease (WHO stage 3 or 4).

Condition	Combined oral contraceptives	Monthly injectables	Combined patch and combined vaginal ring	Progestin-only pills	Progestin-only injectables	Implants	Emergency contraceptive pills*	Copper-bearing intrauterine device	Levonorgestrel intrauterine device	Female sterilization*
Treated with integrase inhibitors (raltegravir [RAL])	1	1	1	1	1	1	—	I: 2/3[p]; C: 2	I: 2/3[p]; C: 2	—
OTHER INFECTIONS										
Schistosomiasis										
Uncomplicated	1	1	1	1	1	1	—	1	1	A
Fibrosis of liver (if severe, see cirrhosis, next page)[g]	1	1	1	1	1	1	—	1	1	C
Tuberculosis[g]								I / C	I / C	
Non-pelvic	1	1	1	1	1	1	—	I: 1; C: 1	I: 1; C: 1	A
Known pelvic	1	1	1	1	1	1	—	I: 4; C: 3	I: 4; C: 3	S
Malaria	1	1	1	1	1	1	—	1	1	A
ENDOCRINE CONDITIONS										
Diabetes										
History of gestational diabetes	1	1	1	1	1	1	—	1	1	A[q]
Non-vascular diabetes										
Non-insulin dependent	2	2	2	2	2	2	—	1	2	C[i,q]
Insulin dependent[g]	2	2	2	2	2	2	—	1	2	C[i,q]
With kidney, eye, or nerve damage[g]	3/4[r]	3/4[r]	3/4[r]	2	3	2	—	1	2	S
Other vascular disease or diabetes of > 20 years' duration[g]	3/4[r]	3/4[r]	3/4[r]	2	3	2	—	1	2	S
Thyroid disorders										
Simple goiter	1	1	1	1	1	1	—	1	1	A
Hyperthyroid	1	1	1	1	1	1	—	1	1	S
Hypothyroid	1	1	1	1	1	1	—	1	1	C
GASTROINTESTINAL CONDITIONS										
Gallbladder disease										
Symptomatic										
Treated by cholecystectomy	2	2	2	2	2	2	—	1	2	A
Medically treated	3	2	3	2	2	2	—	1	2	A
Current	3	2	3	2	2	2	—	1	2	D

Key:
- (unshaded box) = Use the method
- (shaded box) = Do not use the method
- I = Initiation of the method
- C = Continuation of the method
- — = Condition not listed; does not affect eligibility for method
- NA = Not applicable

(Continued)

[q] If blood glucose is not well controlled, referral to a higher-level facility is recommended.

[r] Assess according to severity of condition.

- ☐ = Use the method
- (shaded) = Do not use the method
- I = Initiation of the method
- C = Continuation of the method
- — = Condition not listed; does not affect eligibility for method
- NA = Not applicable

Condition	Combined oral contraceptives	Monthly injectables	Combined patch and combined vaginal ring	Progestin-only pills	Progestin-only injectables	Implants	Emergency contraceptive pills*	Copper-bearing intrauterine device	Levonorgestrel intrauterine device	Female sterilization*
Asymptomatic	2	2	2	2	2	2	—	1	2	A
History of cholestasis										
Pregnancy-related	2	2	2	1	1	1	—	1	1	A
Past combined oral contraceptives-related	3	2	3	2	2	2	—	1	2	A
Viral hepatitis	I | C	I | C	I | C							
Acute or flare	3/4[r] | 2	3 | 2	3/4[r,s] | 2	1	1	1	2	1	1	D
Carrier	1	1	1	1	1	1	—	1	1	A
Chronic	1	1	1	1	1	1	—	1	1	A
Cirrhosis										
Mild (compensated)	1	1	1	1	1	1	—	1	1	A
Severe (decompensated)[g]	4	3	4	3	3	3	—	1	3	S[t]
Liver tumors										
Focal nodular hyperplasia	2	2	2	2	2	2	—	1	2	A
Hepatocellular adenoma	4	3	4	3	3	3	—	1	3	C[t]
Malignant (hepatoma)[g]	4	3/4	4	3	3	3	—	1	3	C[t]
ANEMIAS										
Thalassemia	1	1	1	1	1	1	—	2	1	C
Sickle cell disease[g]	2	2	2	1	1	1	—	2	1	C
Iron-deficiency anemia	1	1	1	1	1	1	—	2	1	D/C[u]
DRUG INTERACTIONS (for antiretroviral drugs, see HIV/AIDS)										
Anticonvulsant therapy										
Certain anticonvulsants (barbiturates, carbamazepine, oxcarbazepine, phenytoin, primidone, topiramate)	3[l]	2	3[l]	3[l]	DMPA 1, NET-EN 2	2[l]	—	1	1	—
Lamotrigine	3[§]	3[§]	3[§]	1	1	1	—	1	1	—
Antimicrobial therapy										
Broad-spectrum antibiotics	1	1	1	1	1	1	—	1	1	—

[s] In women with symptomatic viral hepatitis, withhold these methods until liver function returns to normal or 3 months after she becomes asymptomatic, whichever is earlier.

[t] Liver function should be evaluated.

[u] For hemoglobin < 7 g/dl, delay. For hemoglobin ≥ 7 to < 10 g/dl, caution.

[§] Combined hormonal contraceptives may reduce the effectiveness of lamotrigine.

☐ = Use the method
▨ = Do not use the method
I = Initiation of the method
C = Continuation of the method
— = Condition not listed; does not affect eligibility for method
NA = Not applicable

Condition	Combined oral contraceptives	Monthly injectables	Combined patch and combined vaginal ring	Progestin-only pills	Progestin-only injectables	Implants	Emergency contraceptive pills*	Copper-bearing intrauterine device	Levonorgestrel intrauterine device	Female sterilization*
Antifungals and antiparasitics	1	1	1	1	1	1	—	1	1	—
Rifampicin or rifabutin therapy	3[1]	2	3[1]	3[1]	DMPA 1 NET-EN 2	2	—	1	1	—

*Additional conditions relating to emergency contraceptive pills:

Category 1: Repeated use; rape; **CYP3A4 inducers** (e.g., rifampicin, phenytoin, phenobarbital, carbamazepine, efavirenz, fosphenytoin, nevirapine, oxcarbazepine, primidone, rifabutin, St. John's wort/Hypericum perforatum).

Category 2: History of severe cardiovascular complications (ischemic heart disease, cerebrovascular attack, or other thromboembolic conditions, and angina pectoralis).

*Additional conditions relating to female sterilization:

Caution: Diaphragmatic hernia; kidney disease; severe nutritional deficiencies; previous abdominal or pelvic surgery; concurrent with elective surgery.

Delay: Abdominal skin infection; acute respiratory disease (bronchitis, pneumonia); systemic infection or gastroenteritis; emergency surgery (without previous counseling); surgery for an infectious condition; certain postpartum conditions (7 to 41 days after childbirth); severe pre-eclampsia/eclampsia; prolonged rupture of membranes (24 hours or more); fever during or immediately after delivery; sepsis after delivery; severe hemorrhage; severe trauma to the genital tract; cervical or vaginal tear at time of delivery); certain postabortion conditions (sepsis, fever, or severe hemorrhage; severe trauma to the genital tract; cervical or vaginal tear at time of abortion; acute hematometra); subacute bacterial endocarditis; unmanaged atrial fibrillation.

Special arrangements: Coagulation disorders; chronic asthma, bronchitis, emphysema, or lung infection; fixed uterus due to previous surgery or infection; abdominal wall or umbilical hernia; postpartum uterine rupture or perforation; postabortion uterine perforation.

Conditions relating to vasectomy:

No special considerations: High risk of HIV, asymptomatic or mild HIV clinical disease, sickle cell disease.

Caution: Young age; depressive disorders; diabetes; previous scrotal injury; large varicocele or hydrocele; cryptorchidism (may require referral); lupus with positive (or unknown) antiphospholipid antibodies; lupus and on immunosuppressive treatment.

Delay: Active STIs (excluding HIV and hepatitis); scrotal skin infection; balanitis; epididymitis or orchitis; systemic infection or gastroenteritis; filariasis; elephantiasis; intrascrotal mass.

Special arrangements: Severe or advanced HIV clinical disease may require delay; coagulation disorders; inguinal hernia; lupus with severe thrombocytopenia.

Conditions relating to male and female condoms, spermicides, diaphragms, cervical caps, and the lactational amenorrhea method:

All other conditions listed on the previous pages that do not appear here are a category 1 or NA for male and female condoms, spermicides, diaphragms, and cervical caps, and not listed in the Medical Eligibility Criteria for the lactational amenorrhea method.

[ ] = Use the method

[shaded] = Do not use the method

[—] = Condition not listed; does not affect eligibility for method

NA = Not applicable

Condition	Male and female condoms	Spermicides	Diaphragms	Cervical caps	Lactational amenorrhea method[##]
REPRODUCTIVE HISTORY					
Parity					
Nulliparous (has not given birth)	1	1	1	1	—
Parous (has given birth)	1	1	2	2	—
< 6 weeks postpartum	1	1	NA[v]	NA[v]	—
CARDIOVASCULAR DISEASE					
Complicated valvular heart disease (pulmonary hypertension, risk of atrial fibrillation, history of subacute bacterial endocarditis)[g]	1	1	2	2	—
REPRODUCTIVE TRACT INFECTIONS AND DISORDERS					
Cervical intraepithelial neoplasia	1	1	1	4	—
Cervical cancer	1	2	1	4	—
Anatomical abnormalities	1	1	NA[w]	NA[x]	—
HIV/AIDS[g]					
High risk of HIV	1	4	4	4	—
Asymptomatic or mild HIV clinical disease (WHO stage 1 or 2)	1	3	3	3	C[y]
Severe or advanced HIV clinical disease (WHO stage 3 or 4)	1	3	3	3	C[y]
OTHERS					
History of toxic shock syndrome	1	1	3	3	—
Urinary tract infection	1	1	2	2	—
Allergy to latex[z]	3	1	3	3	—

[v] Wait to fit/use until uterine involution is complete.

[w] Diaphragm cannot be used in certain cases of uterine prolapse.

[x] Cap use is not appropriate for a client with severely distorted cervical anatomy.

[y] Caution: Women living with HIV should receive appropriate ARV therapy and exclusively breastfeed for the first 6 months of a baby's life, introduce appropriate complementary foods at 6 months, and continue breastfeeding through 12 months. (See Maternal and Newborn Health, Preventing Mother-to-Child Transmission of HIV, p. 352.)

[z] Does not apply to plastic condoms, diaphragms, and cervical caps.

[##]For additional conditions relating to the lactational amenorrhea method, see next page.

‡Additional conditions relating to the lactational amenorrhea method:

Conditions affecting the newborn that may make breastfeeding difficult: Congenital deformities of the mouth, jaw, or palate; newborns who are small-for-date or premature and needing intensive neonatal care; and certain metabolic disorders.

Medication used during breastfeeding: To protect infant health, breastfeeding is not recommended for women using such drugs as anti-metabolites, bromocriptine, certain anticoagulants, corticosteroids (high doses), cyclosporine, ergotamine, lithium, mood-altering drugs, radioactive drugs, and reserpine.

Conditions relating to fertility awareness methods:

A = Accept C = Caution D = Delay **Condition**	Symptoms-based methods	Calendar-based methods
Age: post menarche or perimenopause	C	C
Breastfeeding < 6 weeks postpartum	D	D[aa]
Breastfeeding ≥ 6 weeks postpartum	C[bb]	D[bb]
Postpartum, not breastfeeding	D[cc]	D[aa]
Postabortion	C	D[dd]
Irregular vaginal bleeding	D	D
Vaginal discharge	D	A
Taking drugs that affect cycle regularity, hormones, and/or fertility signs	D/C[ee]	D/C[ee]
Diseases that elevate body temperature		
Acute	D	A
Chronic	C	A

[aa] Delay until she has had 3 regular menstrual cycles.
[bb] Use caution after monthly bleeding or normal secretions return (usually at least 6 weeks after childbirth).
[cc] Delay until monthly bleeding or normal secretions return (usually < 4 weeks postpartum).
[dd] Delay until she has had one regular menstrual cycle.
[ee] Delay until the drug's effect has been determined, then use caution.

Conditions relating to the progesterone-releasing vaginal ring:

Pregnancy	**N/A**
Breastfeeding ≥ 4 weeks postpartum	**1**

Glossary

abscess A pocket of **pus** surrounded by inflammation, caused by a bacterial infection and marked by persistent pain.

acquired immunodeficiency syndrome (AIDS) The condition, due to infection with **human immunodeficiency virus** (HIV), when the body's immune system breaks down and is unable to fight certain infections.

AIDS See **acquired immunodeficiency syndrome.**

amenorrhea See **vaginal bleeding.**

anaphylactic shock See Severe allergic reaction to latex, Appendix B, p. 385.

anemia A condition in which the body lacks adequate **hemoglobin**, commonly due to iron deficiency or excessive blood loss. As a result, tissues do not receive adequate oxygen.

antiretroviral (ARV) therapy A group of drugs used to treat HIV infection. There are several ARV classes, which work against HIV in different ways. Patients take a combination of several drugs at once.

atrial fibrillation A heart rhythm disorder in which the upper heart chambers contract in an abnormal or disorganized manner.

aura See **migraine aura.**

backup method A contraceptive method used when mistakes are made with using an ongoing method of contraception, or to help ensure that a woman does not become pregnant when she first starts to use a contraceptive method. Include abstinence, male or female condoms, spermicides, and withdrawal.

bacterial endocarditis Infection that occurs when bacteria from the bloodstream colonize damaged heart tissue or valves.

bacterial vaginosis A common condition caused by overgrowth of bacteria normally found in the **vagina.**

balanitis Inflammation of the tip of the **penis.**

benign breast disease Growth of abnormal but noncancerous breast tissue.

benign ovarian tumor Noncancerous growth that develops on or in the ovary.

blood pressure The force of the blood against the walls of blood vessels. Generally, normal systolic (pumping) blood pressure is less than 140 mm Hg, and normal diastolic (resting) blood pressure is less than 90 mm Hg (see **hypertension**).

bone density A measure of how dense and strong a bone is. When old bone breaks down faster than new bone tissue is formed, bones become less dense, increasing risk of fractures.

breakthrough bleeding See **vaginal bleeding.**

breast cancer Malignant (cancerous) growth that develops in breast tissue.

breastfeeding Feeding an infant with milk produced by the breasts (see also Lactational Amenorrhea Method, p. 309). Breastfeeding patterns include:

- **exclusive breastfeeding** Giving the infant only breast milk with no supplementation of any type—not even water—except for perhaps vitamins, minerals, or medication.
- **fully breastfeeding** Giving the infant breast milk almost exclusively but also water, juice, vitamins, or other nutrients infrequently.
- **nearly fully breastfeeding** Giving the infant some liquid or food in addition to breast milk, but more than three-fourths of feedings are breastfeeds.
- **partially breastfeeding** Any breastfeeding less than nearly fully breastfeeding, giving the infant more supplementation with other liquids or food. Less than three-fourths of feedings are breastfeeds.

candidiasis A common vaginal infection caused by a yeast-like fungus. Also known as yeast infection or thrush. Not usually sexually transmitted.

cardiovascular disease Any disease of the heart, blood vessels, or blood circulation.

cerebrovascular disease Any disease of the blood vessels of the brain.

cervical cancer Malignant (cancerous) growth that occurs in the **cervix**, usually due to persistent infection with certain types of **human papillomavirus**.

cervical ectropion A nonserious condition in which the mucus-producing cells found in the cervical canal begin to grow on the area around the opening of the **cervix**.

cervical intraepithelial neoplasia (CIN) Abnormal, precancerous cells in the cervix. Mild forms may go away on their own, but more severe abnormalities may progress to **cervical cancer** if not treated. Also called cervical dysplasia or precancer.

cervical laceration See **laceration**.

cervical mucus A thick fluid plugging the opening of the **cervix**. Most of the time it is thick enough to prevent **sperm** from entering the **uterus**. At the midpoint of the **menstrual cycle**, however, the mucus becomes thin and watery, and sperm can more easily pass through.

cervical stenosis When the cervical opening is narrower than normal.

cervicitis See **purulent cervicitis**.

cervix The lower portion of the **uterus** extending into the upper **vagina** (see Female Anatomy, p. 432).

chancroid A **sexually transmitted infection** caused by a bacterium, which causes an ulcer to grow on the genitals.

chlamydia A **sexually transmitted infection** caused by a bacterium. If left untreated, it can cause infertility.

cholecystectomy Surgical removal of the gallbladder.

cholestasis Reduced flow of bile secreted by the liver.

cirrhosis (of the liver) See Liver disorders, Appendix B, p. 385.

cryptorchidism Failure of one or both **testes** to descend into the **scrotum** after birth.

decontaminate (medical equipment) To remove infectious organisms in order to make instruments, gloves, and other objects safer for people who clean them.

deep vein thrombosis See Deep vein thrombosis, Appendix B, p. 384.

depression A mental condition typically marked by dejection, despair, lack of hope, and sometimes either extreme tiredness or agitation.

diabetes (diabetes mellitus) A chronic disorder that occurs when blood glucose levels become too high because the body does not produce enough insulin or cannot use the insulin properly.

disinfection See **high-level disinfection**.

dual protection Avoiding both pregnancy and **sexually transmitted infection**.

dysmenorrhea Pain during **vaginal bleeding**, commonly known as menstrual cramps.

eclampsia A condition of late pregnancy, labor, and the period immediately after delivery characterized by convulsions. In serious cases, sometimes followed by coma and death.

ectopic pregnancy See Ectopic pregnancy, Appendix B, p. 384.

ejaculation The release of **semen** from the **penis** at orgasm.

elephantiasis A chronic and often extreme swelling and hardening of skin and tissue just beneath the skin, especially of the legs and **scrotum**, due to an obstruction in the lymphatic system (see **filariasis**).

embryo The product of fertilization of an egg (**ovum**) by a **sperm** during the first 8 weeks of development.

endometrial cancer Malignant (cancerous) growth in the lining of the **uterus**.

endometriosis A condition in which tissue of the **endometrium** grows outside the **uterus**. Tissue may attach itself to the reproductive organs or to other organs in the abdominal cavity. Can cause pelvic pain and impair fertility.

endometrium The membrane that lines the inner surface of the **uterus**. It thickens and is then shed once a month, causing **monthly bleeding**. During pregnancy, this lining is not shed but instead changes and produces hormones, helping to support the pregnancy (see Female Anatomy, p. 432).

engorgement (breast engorgement) A condition during breastfeeding that occurs when more milk accumulates in the breasts than the infant consumes. May make breasts feel full, hard, tender, and warm. Can be prevented (or relieved) by breastfeeding often and on demand.

epididymis A coiled tube (duct) attached to and lying on the **testes**. Developing **sperm** reach maturity and develop their swimming capabilities within this duct. The matured sperm leave the epididymis through the **vas deferens** (see Male Anatomy, p. 435).

epididymitis Inflammation of the **epididymis**.

epilepsy A chronic disorder caused by disturbed brain function. May involve convulsions.

estrogen Hormone responsible for female sexual development. Natural estrogens, especially the **hormone** estradiol, are secreted by a mature ovarian **follicle**, which surrounds the egg (**ovum**). Also, a group of synthetic drugs that have effects similar to those of natural estrogen; some are used in some hormonal contraceptives.

expulsion When a contraceptive implant or intrauterine device fully or partially comes out of place.

fallopian tube Either of a pair of slender ducts that connect the **uterus** to the region of each **ovary**. **Fertilization** of an egg (**ovum**) by **sperm** usually takes place in one of the fallopian tubes (see Female Anatomy, p. 432).

fertilization Union of an **ovum** with a **sperm**.

fetus The product of **fertilization** from the end of the 8th week of pregnancy until birth (see **embryo**).

fibroid See **uterine fibroid.**

fibrosis The excess formation of fibrous tissue, as in reaction to organ damage.

filariasis A chronic parasitic disease caused by filarial worms. May lead to inflammation and permanent clogging of channels in the lymphatic system and **elephantiasis**.

fixed uterus A **uterus** that cannot be moved out of place, often as a result of **endometriosis**, past surgery, or infection.

follicle A small round structure in the **ovary**, each of which contains an egg (**ovum**). During **ovulation** a follicle on the surface of the ovary opens and releases a mature egg.

foreskin Hood of skin covering the end of the **penis** (see Male Anatomy, p. 435).

fully breastfeeding See **breastfeeding**.

gallbladder diseases Conditions that affect the gallbladder, a sac located under the liver that stores bile used in fat digestion. May include inflammation, infection, or obstruction, gallbladder cancer, or gall stones (when the components of bile solidify within the organ).

gastroenteritis Inflammation of the stomach and intestine.

genital herpes A disease caused by a virus, spread by sexual contact.

genital warts Growths on the **vulva**, the vaginal wall, and the **cervix** in women, and on the **penis** in men. Caused by certain types of **human papillomavirus**.

gestational trophoblast disease Disease during pregnancy involving abnormal cell growth of the trophoblast, the outermost layer of cells of the developing **embryo**, which develops into the **placenta**.

goiter A noncancerous enlargement of the thyroid.

gonorrhea A **sexually transmitted infection** caused by a bacterium. If not treated, can cause **infertility**.

heart attack See Heart attack, Appendix B, p. 384. See also **ischemic heart disease**.

heavy bleeding See **vaginal bleeding**.

hematocrit The percentage of whole blood that is made up of red blood cells. Used as a measurement of **anemia**.

hematoma A bruise or area of skin discoloration caused by broken blood vessels beneath the skin.

hematometra An accumulation of blood in the **uterus**, which may occur following spontaneous or induced abortion.

hemoglobin The iron-containing material in red blood cells that carries oxygen from the lungs to the tissues of the body.

hepatitis See Liver disorders, Appendix B, p. 385.

hernia The projection of an organ, part of an organ, or any bodily structure through the wall that normally contains it.

herpes See **genital herpes**.

high-level disinfection (medical instruments) To destroy all living microorganisms except some forms of bacteria. Compare with **sterilize**.

HIV See **human immunodeficiency virus**.

hormone A chemical substance formed in one organ or part of the body and carried in the blood to another organ or part, where it works through chemical action. Also, manufactured chemical substances that function as hormones.

human immunodeficiency virus (HIV) The virus that causes **acquired immunodeficiency syndrome** (AIDS).

human papillomavirus (HPV) A common, highly contagious virus spread by sexual activity and skin-to-skin contact in the genital area. Certain subtypes of HPV are responsible for most cases of **cervical cancer**; others cause **genital warts**.

hydrocele The collection of fluid in a body cavity, especially in the **testes** or along the **spermatic cord**.

hyperlipidemia High level of fats in the blood that increases the risk of heart disease.

hypertension Higher **blood pressure** than normal; 140 mm Hg or higher (systolic) or 90 mm Hg or higher (diastolic).

hyperthyroidism Too much production of thyroid **hormones**.

hypothyroidism Not enough production of thyroid **hormones**.

implantation The embedding of the **embryo** in the **endometrium** of the **uterus**, where it establishes contact with the woman's blood supply for nourishment.

infertility The inability of a couple to produce living children.

informed choice A freely made decision based on clear, accurate, and relevant information. A goal of family planning counseling.

infrequent bleeding See **vaginal bleeding**.

inguinal hernia A **hernia** in the groin.

intercourse See **sex**.

irregular bleeding See **vaginal bleeding**.

ischemic heart disease, ischemia Ischemia is reduced blood flow to tissues of the body. When this reduced flow is in the arteries of the heart, it is called ischemic heart disease.

jaundice Abnormal yellowing of the skin and eyes. Usually a symptom of **liver disease**.

labia The inner and outer lips of the **vagina**, which protect the internal female organs (see Female Anatomy, p. 432).

laceration A wound or irregular tear of the flesh anywhere on the body, including the **cervix** and **vagina**.

laparoscope A device consisting of a tube with lenses for viewing the inside of an organ or body cavity. Used in diagnosis and in some female sterilization procedures.

laparoscopy A procedure performed with a laparoscope.

latex allergy When a person's body has a reaction to contact with latex, including persistent or recurring severe redness, itching, or swelling. In extreme cases, may lead to anaphylactic shock (see Severe allergic reaction to latex, Appendix B, p. 385).

lesion A disturbed or diseased area of skin or other body tissue.

liver disease Includes tumors, **hepatitis**, and **cirrhosis**.

mastitis An inflammation of breast tissue due to infection that may cause fever, redness, and pain.

menarche The beginning of cycles of **monthly bleeding**. Occurs during puberty after girls start producing **estrogen** and **progesterone**.

menopause The time in a woman's life when monthly bleeding stops permanently. Occurs when a woman's **ovaries** stop releasing eggs (ova). A woman is considered menopausal after she has had no bleeding for 12 months.

menorrhagia See **vaginal bleeding**.

menses, menstrual period, menstruation See **monthly bleeding**.

menstrual cycle A repeating series of changes in the **ovaries** and **endometrium** that includes **ovulation** and **monthly bleeding.** Most women have cycles that each last between 24 and 35 days (see The Menstrual Cycle, p. 434).

migraine aura A nervous system disturbance that affects sight and sometimes touch and speech (see Identifying Migraine Headaches and Auras, p. 436).

migraine headache A type of severe, recurrent headache (see Identifying Migraine Headaches and Auras, p. 436).

minilaparotomy A female sterilization technique performed by bringing the **fallopian tubes** to a small incision in the abdomen and then usually tying and cutting them.

miscarriage Natural loss of pregnancy during the first 20 weeks.

monthly bleeding Monthly flow of bloody fluid from the **uterus** through the **vagina** in adult women, which takes place between **menarche** and **menopause**. Also, the monthly vaginal flow of bloody fluid that women have while using combined hormonal contraceptives (a withdrawal bleed).

mucous membrane Membrane lining passages and cavities of the body that come in contact with air.

nearly fully breastfeeding See **breastfeeding**.

nephropathy Kidney disease, including damage to the small blood vessels in the kidneys from long-standing diabetes.

neuropathy Nervous system or nerve disease, including nerve degeneration due to damage to the small blood vessels in the nervous system from long-standing diabetes.

nonsteroidal anti-inflammatory drug (NSAID) A class of drugs used to reduce pain, fever, and swelling.

orchitis Inflammation of a **testis** (see Male Anatomy, p. 435).

ovarian cyst Fluid-filled sac that develops in the **ovary** or on its surface. Usually disappears on its own but may rupture and cause pain and complications.

ovaries A pair of female sex glands that store and release ova (see **ovum**) and produce the sex **hormones estrogen** and **progesterone** (see Female Anatomy, p. 432).

ovulation The release of an **ovum** from an **ovary**.

ovum Reproductive egg cell produced by the **ovaries**.

partially breastfeeding See **breastfeeding**.

pelvic inflammatory disease See Pelvic inflammatory disease, Appendix B, p. 385.

pelvic tuberculosis Infection of the pelvic organs by **tuberculosis** bacteria from the lungs.

pelvis The skeletal structure located in the lower part of the human torso, resting on the legs and supporting the spine. In females, also refers to the hollow portion of the pelvic bone structure through which the **fetus** passes during birth.

penis The male organ for urination and sexual intercourse (see Male Anatomy, p. 435).

perforation A hole in the wall of an organ or the process of making the hole, as with a medical instrument.

placenta The organ that nourishes a growing **fetus**. The placenta (afterbirth) is formed during pregnancy and comes out of the **uterus** within a few minutes after the birth of a baby.

postpartum After childbirth; the first 6 weeks after childbirth.

pre-eclampsia **Hypertension** with either excess protein in the urine, or local or generalized swelling, or both (but without convulsions) after 20 weeks of pregnancy. May progress to **eclampsia**.

premature birth A birth that occurs before 37 weeks of pregnancy.

preventive measures Actions taken to prevent disease, such as washing hands or providing drugs or other therapy.

progesterone A steroid **hormone** that is produced by the **ovary** after **ovulation**. Prepares the **endometrium** for **implantation** of a fertilized egg (**ovum**), protects the **embryo,** enhances development of the **placenta**, and helps prepare the breasts for **breastfeeding**.

progestin (progestogen) Any of a large group of synthetic drugs that have effects similar to those of **progesterone.** Some are used in hormonal contraceptives.

prolonged bleeding See **vaginal bleeding**.

prolonged rupture of membranes Occurs when the fluid-filled sac surrounding a pregnant woman's fetus breaks 24 hours or more before delivery of the infant.

prophylaxis See **preventive measures**.

prostate Male reproductive organ where some of the **semen** is produced (see Male Anatomy, p. 435).

puerperal sepsis Infection of the reproductive organs during the first 42 days **postpartum** (puerperium).

pulmonary embolism See Pulmonary embolism, Appendix B, p. 385.

pulmonary hypertension Continuous **hypertension** in the pulmonary artery, impeding blood flow from the heart to the lungs.

purulent cervicitis Inflammation of the **cervix** accompanied by a **pus**-like discharge. Often indicates infection with gonorrhea or chlamydia.

pus A yellowish-white fluid formed in infected tissue.

retinopathy Disease of the retina (nerve tissue lining the back of the eye), including damage to the small blood vessels to the retina from long-standing diabetes.

ruptured ectopic pregnancy See Ruptured ectopic pregnancy, Appendix B, p. 385.

schistosomiasis A parasitic disease caused by a flatworm living in a snail host. People become infected while wading or bathing in water containing larvae of the infected snails.

scrotum The pouch of skin behind the **penis** that contains the **testes** (see Male Anatomy, p. 435).

semen The thick, white fluid produced by a man's reproductive organs and released through the **penis** during **ejaculation**. Contains **sperm** unless the man has had a vasectomy.

seminal vesicles Male organs where **sperm** mixes with **semen** (see Male Anatomy, p. 435).

sepsis The presence of various **pus**-forming and disease-causing organisms, or poisonous substances that they produce, in the blood or body tissues.

septic abortion Induced or **spontaneous abortion** involving infection.

sex, sexual intercourse Sexual activity in which the penis is inserted into a body cavity.

- **anal** Sex involving the anus.
- **oral** Sex involving the mouth.
- **vaginal** Sex involving the vagina.

sexually transmitted infection (STI) Any of a group of bacterial, fungal, and viral infections and parasites that are transmitted during sexual activity.

sickle cell anemia, sickle cell disease Hereditary, chronic form of **anemia**. Blood cells take on an abnormal sickle or crescent shape when deprived of oxygen.

speculum A medical tool used to widen a body opening to better see inside. A speculum is inserted into the vagina to help see the cervix.

sperm The male sex cell. Sperm are produced in the **testes** of an adult male, mixed with **semen** in the **seminal vesicles**, and released during **ejaculation** (see Male Anatomy, p. 435).

spermatic cord A cord consisting of the **vas deferens,** arteries, veins, nerves, and lymphatic vessels that passes from the groin down to the back of each **testis** (see Male Anatomy, p. 435).

spontaneous abortion See **miscarriage**.

spotting See **vaginal bleeding**.

sterilize (medical equipment) To destroy all microorganisms, including spores that are not killed by **high-level disinfection**.

stroke See Stroke, Appendix B, p. 385.

superficial thrombophlebitis Inflammation of a vein just beneath the skin due to a blood clot.

syphilis A **sexually transmitted infection** caused by a bacterium. If untreated, may progress to systemic infection, causing general paralysis and dementia. May be transmitted to the fetus during pregnancy or childbirth.

tampon A plug of cotton or other absorbent material used to absorb fluids, such as a plug inserted in the vagina to absorb bloody flow during **monthly bleeding**.

testes, testicles The 2 male reproductive organs that produce **sperm** and the **hormone** testosterone. Located in the **scrotum**. (Testis if referring to one of the testes; see Male Anatomy, p. 435).

thalassemia An inherited type of **anemia**.

thromboembolic disorder (or disease) Abnormal clotting of blood in the blood vessels.

thrombogenic mutations Any of several genetic disorders that cause abnormal thickening or clotting of the blood.

thrombophlebitis Inflammation of a vein due to the presence of a blood clot (see **thrombosis**).

thrombosis Formation of a blood clot inside a blood vessel.

thrush See **candidiasis**.

thyroid disease Any disease of the thyroid (see **hyperthyroid, hypothyroid**).

toxic shock syndrome See Toxic shock syndrome, Appendix B, p. 385.

trichomoniasis A **sexually transmitted infection** caused by a protozoan.

trophoblast disease See **gestational trophoblastic disease**.

tuberculosis A contagious disease caused by a bacterium. Most commonly infects the respiratory system; also infects the organs in a woman's **pelvis**, and then known as **pelvic tuberculosis**.

urethra Tube through which urine is released from the body (see Female Anatomy, p. 432, and Male Anatomy, p. 435). In men **semen** also passes through the urethra.

uterine fibroid Noncancerous tumor that grows in the muscle of the **uterus**.

uterine perforation Puncturing of the wall of the **uterus**, which may occur during an induced abortion or with insertion of an intrauterine device.

uterine rupture A tear of the **uterus**, typically during labor or late pregnancy.

uterus The hollow, muscular organ that carries the **fetus** during pregnancy. Also called the womb (see Female Anatomy, p. 432).

vagina The passage joining the outer sexual organs with the **uterus** in females (see Female Anatomy, p. 432).

vaginal bleeding Any bloody vaginal discharge (pink, red, or brown) that requires the use of sanitary protection (pads, cloths, or tampons). Different vaginal bleeding patterns include:

> **amenorrhea** No bleeding at all at expected bleeding times.
>
> **breakthrough bleeding** Any bleeding outside of expected bleeding times (i.e., outside of regular monthly bleeding) that requires use of sanitary protection.
>
> **heavy bleeding (menorrhagia)** Bleeding that is twice as heavy as a woman's usual bleeding.
>
> **infrequent bleeding** Fewer than 2 bleeding episodes over 3 months.
>
> **irregular bleeding** Spotting and/or breakthrough bleeding that occurs outside of expected bleeding times (i.e., outside of regular monthly bleeding).
>
> **menstrual bleeding, monthly bleeding.** Bleeding that takes place, on average, for 3–7 days about every 28 days.
>
> **prolonged bleeding** Bleeding that lasts longer than 8 days.
>
> **spotting** Any bloody vaginal discharge outside of expected bleeding times that requires no sanitary protection.

vaginal mucus The fluid secreted by glands in the **vagina**.

vaginitis Inflammation of the **vagina**. May be due to infection by bacteria, viruses, or fungi, or to chemical irritation. Not a sexually transmitted infection.

valvular heart disease Health problems due to improperly functioning heart valves.

varicose veins Enlarged, twisted veins, most commonly seen in veins just beneath the skin of the legs.

vas deferens (vas, vasa) 2 muscular tubes that transport **sperm** from the **testes** to the **seminal vesicles**. These tubes are cut or blocked during a vasectomy (see Male Anatomy, p. 435).

vascular disease Any disease of the blood vessels.

vulva The exterior female genitals.

warts See **genital warts**.

withdrawal bleed See **monthly bleeding**.

womb See **uterus**.

yeast infection See **candidiasis**.

Index

D

Index

I

J

K

L

M

R

S

T

U

V

W

Y

Methodology

This handbook provides evidence-based guidance developed through worldwide collaboration. For the first edition of this handbook, the World Health Organization (WHO) Department of Reproductive Health and Research invited more than 30 organizations to participate. The INFO Project at the Johns Hopkins Bloomberg School of Public Health/Center for Communication Programs led the handbook development process. The INFO Project was the precursor to the Knowledge for Health Project, a publisher of this update to the Global Handbook along with WHO.

The Global Handbook is the successor to *The Essentials of Contraceptive Technology* (Johns Hopkins School of Public Health, Population Information Program, 1997).

Guidance in the first edition came from several similar consensus processes:

- The *Medical Eligibility Criteria for Contraceptive Use and the Selected Practice Recommendations for Contraceptive Use.* WHO expert Working Groups developed these guidelines.
- For additional questions specific to this handbook, WHO convened an expert Working Group that met in Geneva on 21–24 June 2005. To discuss topics needing special attention, several subgroups met between October 2004 and June 2005. At the June 2005 meeting the full expert Working Group reviewed and endorsed the subgroups' recommendations.
- Content not addressed in these consensus processes was developed through collaboration between researchers at the INFO Project and technical experts. Then, a group of experts and, finally, representatives of collaborating organizations had the opportunity to review the entire text.

The 2011 update of the handbook added guidance from the expert Working Group meeting in April 2008 for the Medical Eligibility Criteria and the Selected Practice Recommendations and 2 Technical Consultations related to these guidelines in October 2008 and January 2010. Further guidance came from an expert Working Group meeting on HIV and infant feeding in October 2009 and a Technical Consultation on community-based provision of injectable contraceptives in June 2009.

The current update (2018) also reflects the recommendations of the expert Working Group on the Medical Eligibility Criteria and the Selected Practice Recommendations that met in May 2013, March 2014, and September 2014. Other current WHO guidance forms the basis for updates throughout the book. For WHO guidance publications used in preparing this update, see the next page.

A group of experts reviewed the updates to this edition, made revisions, and contributed new content. Their names are listed in the Acknowledgements, p. viii.

Definitions used in this handbook

Effectiveness: Rates are largely the percentages of US women estimated to have unintended pregnancies during the first year of use, unless noted otherwise. See Appendix A, p. 383.

Side effects: Conditions reported by at least 5% of users in selected studies, regardless of evidence of causality or biological plausibility, listed in order of frequency with the most common at the top.

Terms describing health risks (percentage of users experiencing a risk):
Common: ≥15% and <45%
Uncommon: ≥1% and <15%
Rare: ≥0.1% and <1% (<1 per 100 and ≥1 per 1,000)
Very rare: ≥0.01% and <0.1% (<1 per 1,000 and ≥1 per 10,000)
Extremely rare: <0.01% (<1 per 10,000)

WHO Guidance Documents Used in Preparation of This Edition of the Handbook

Medical eligibility criteria for contraceptive use, 5th edition. 2015. http://www.who.int/reproductivehealth/publications/family_planning/MEC-5/en/

Selected practice recommendations for contraceptive use, 3rd edition. 2016. http://www.who.int/reproductivehealth/publications/family_planning/SPR-3/en/

Comprehensive cervical cancer control: a guide to essential practice, 2nd edition. 2014. http://apps.who.int/iris/bitstream/10665/144785/1/9789241548953_eng.pdf?ua=1

Consolidated guidelines on the use of antiretroviral drugs for treating and preventing HIV infection: recommendations for a public health approach – 2nd ed. 2016. http://apps.who.int/iris/bitstream/10665/208825/1/9789241549684_eng.pdf?ua=1

Eliminating forced, coercive and otherwise involuntary sterilization. An interagency statement by OHCHR, UN Women, UNAIDS, UNDP, UNFPA, UNICEF and WHO. 2014. http://www.who.int/reproductivehealth/publications/gender_rights/eliminating-forced-sterilization/en/

Ensuring human rights in the provision of contraceptive information and services. Guidance and recommendations. 2014. http://who.int/reproductive health/publications/family_planning/human-rights-contraception/en/

Ensuring human rights within contraceptive service delivery: Implementation guide. 2015. http://www.who.int/reproductivehealth/publications/family_planning/hr-contraceptive-service-delivery/en/

Health care for women subjected to intimate partner violence or sexual violence. A clinical handbook – field testing version. 2014. http://www.who.int/reproductivehealth/publications/violence/vaw-clinical-handbook/en/

Health worker roles in providing safe abortion care and post-abortion contraception. 2015. http://www.who.int/reproductivehealth/publications/unsafe_abortion/abortion-task-shifting/en/

Monitoring human rights in contraceptive services and programmes. 2017. http://www.who.int/reproductivehealth/publications/contraceptive-services-monitoring-hr/en/

Preventing HIV during pregnancy and breastfeeding in the context of PrEP. Technical brief. 2017. http://www.who.int/hiv/pub/toolkits/prep-preventing-hiv-during-pregnancy/en/

Programming strategies for postpartum family planning. 2013. http://www.who.int/reproductivehealth/publications/family_planning/ppfp_strategies/en/

Promoting sexual and reproductive health for persons with disabilities. WHO/UNFPA guidance note. 2009. http://www.who.int/reproductivehealth/publications/general/9789241598682/en/

Responding to intimate partner violence and sexual violence against women. WHO clinical and policy guidelines. 2013. http://www.who.int/reproductivehealth/publications/violence/9789241548595/en/

Technical consultation on the effects of hormonal contraception on bone health. Summary report. 2005. http://apps.who.int/iris/bitstream/10665/69845/1/WHO_RHR_07.08_eng.pdf

Use of antiretroviral drugs for treating pregnant women and preventing HIV infection in infants. Programmatic update. 2012. http://www.who.int/hiv/pub/mtct/programmatic_update2012/en/

WHO guidelines for screening and treatment of precancerous lesions for cervical cancer prevention. 2013. http://who.int/reproductivehealth/publications/cancers/screening_and_treatment_of_precancerous_lesions/en/

WHO implementation tool for pre-exposure prophylaxis (PrEP) of HIV infection. 2017. http://www.who.int/hiv/pub/prep/prep-implementation-tool/en/

WHO recommendations on antenatal care for a positive pregnancy experience. 2016. http://www.who.int/reproductivehealth/publications/maternal_perinatal_health/anc-positive-pregnancy-experience/en/

WHO recommendations on postnatal care of the mother and newborn. 2013. http://www.who.int/maternal_child_adolescent/documents/postnatal-care-recommendations/en/

WHO recommendations: optimizing health worker roles to improve access to key maternal and newborn health interventions through task shifting. 2012. http://apps.who.int/iris/bitstream/10665/77764/1/9789241504843_eng.pdf

Illustration and Photo Credits

Illustrations by Greg Dayman, Rita Meyer, and Rafael Avila, unless otherwise noted below. Adaptations by Rafael Avila.

Covers	Mark Beisser, CCP
p. 34	DELIVER
p. 38	Cheikh Fall, CCP, courtesy of Photoshare
p. 50	Francine Mueller, CCP
p. 66	David Alexander, CCP, courtesy of Photoshare
p. 70	PATH/Will Boase
pp. 81–82	PATH
pp. 84–85	PATH
p. 98	Schering AG
p. 120	Ortho-McNeil Pharmaceutical
p. 124	David Alexander, CCP, courtesy of Photoshare
p. 127	Population Council
p. 144	Jhpiego. Source: Bluestone B, Chase R, and Lu ER, editors. IUD guidelines for family planning service programs. 3rd ed. Baltimore: Jhpiego; 2006. (adapted)
p. 158	David Alexander, CCP, courtesy of Photoshare
p. 166	David Alexander, CCP, courtesy of Photoshare
pp. 168–169	Jhpiego. Source: Bluestone B, Chase R, and Lu ER, editors. IUD guidelines for family planning service programs. 3rd ed. Baltimore: Jhpiego; 2006. (adapted)
p. 189	David Alexander, CCP, courtesy of Photoshare
pp. 197–198	Jhpiego. Source: Bluestone B, Chase R, and Lu ER, editors. IUD guidelines for family planning service programs. 3rd ed. Baltimore: Jhpiego; 2006. (adapted)
p. 221	EngenderHealth (adapted)
p. 239	EngenderHealth (adapted)
p. 262	David Alexander, CCP, courtesy of Photoshare
p. 265	Female Health Foundation (adapted)
p. 272	David Alexander, CCP, courtesy of Photoshare
p. 290	Francine Mueller, CCP
p. 296	Institute for Reproductive Health, Georgetown University (adapted)

p. 302	Institute for Reproductive Health, Georgetown University (adapted)
p. 317	LINKAGES Project, Academy for Educational Development
p. 323	Bangladesh Center for Communication Programs
p. 346	Rick Maiman, David and Lucile Packard Foundation, courtesy of Photoshare
p. 348	CCP, courtesy of Photoshare
p. 376	Lamia Jaroudi, CCP, courtesy of Photoshare
p. 379	CCP, courtesy of Photoshare
pp. 439–440	FHI 360
Inside back cover	FHI 360

Design and composition by Prographics, Inc., Annapolis, Maryland, USA

Comparing Contraceptives

Comparing Combined Methods

Characteristic	Combined Oral Contraceptives	Monthly Injectables	Combined Patch	Combined Vaginal Ring
How it is used	Pill taken orally.	Intramuscular injection.	Patch worn on upper outer arm, back, abdomen or buttocks. Not on breasts.	Ring inserted in the vagina.
Frequency of use	Daily.	Monthly: Injection every 4 weeks.	Weekly: Patch is changed every week for 3 weeks. No patch worn 4th week.	Monthly: Ring kept in place for 3 weeks and taken out during 4th week.
Effectiveness	Depends on user's ability to take a pill every day.	Least dependent on the user. User must obtain injection every 4 weeks (plus or minus 7 days).	Requires user's attention once a week.	Depends on user keeping the ring in place, not leaving it out for more than 48 hours at a time.
Bleeding patterns	Typically, irregular bleeding for the first few months and then lighter and more regular bleeding.	Irregular bleeding or no monthly bleeding is more common than with COCs. Also, some have prolonged bleeding in the first few months.	Similar to COCs, but irregular bleeding is more common in the first few cycles than with COCs.	Similar to COCs, but irregular bleeding is less common than with COCs.
Privacy	No physical signs of use but others may find the pills.	No physical signs of use.	Patch may be seen by partner or others.	Partner may be able to feel the ring.

Comparing Injectables

Characteristic	DMPA	NET-EN	Monthly Injectables
Time between injections	3 months.	2 months.	1 month.
How early or late a client can have the next injection	2 weeks before or 4 weeks after scheduled injection date.	2 weeks before or after scheduled injection date.	7 days before or after scheduled injection date.
Injection technique	Deep intramuscular (IM) injection into the hip, upper arm, or buttock. Subcutaneous injection into back of upper arm, abdomen, or front of thigh.	Deep intramuscular injection into the hip, upper arm, or buttock. May be slightly more painful than DMPA-IM.	Deep intramuscular injection into the hip, upper arm, buttock, or outer thigh.
Typical bleeding patterns in first year	Irregular and prolonged bleeding at first, then no bleeding or infrequent bleeding. About 40% of users have no monthly bleeding after 1 year.	Irregular or prolonged bleeding in first 6 months but shorter bleeding episodes than with DMPA. After 6 months bleeding patterns are similar to those with DMPA. 30% of users have no monthly bleeding after 1 year.	Irregular, frequent, or prolonged bleeding in first 3 months. Mostly regular bleeding patterns by 1 year. About 2% of users have no monthly bleeding after 1 year.
Average weight gain	1–2 kg per year.	1–2 kg per year.	1 kg per year.
Pregnancy rate, as commonly used	About 4 pregnancies per 100 women in the first year.	Assumed to be similar to DMPA.	About 3 pregnancies per 100 women in the first year.
Average delay in time to pregnancy after stopping injections	4 months longer than for women who used other methods.	1 month longer than for women who used other methods.	1 month longer than for women who used other methods.

Comparing Implants

Characteristic	Jadelle	Implanon NXT	Levoplant
Type of progestin	Levonorgestrel	Etonogestrel	Levonorgestrel
Number	2 rods	1 rod	2 rods
Approved lifespan	5 years	3 years	4 years

Comparing Condoms

Characteristic	Male Condoms	Female Condoms
How to wear	Rolled onto man's penis. Fits the penis tightly.	Inserted into the woman's vagina. Loosely lines the vagina and does not constrict the penis.
When to put on	Put on erect penis right before sex.	Can be inserted up to 8 hours before sex.
Material	Most made of latex; some of synthetic materials or animal membranes.	Most made of a thin, synthetic film; a few are latex.
How they feel during sex	Change feeling of sex.	Fewer complaints of changed feeling of sex than with male condoms.
Noise during sex	May make a rubbing noise during sex.	May rustle or squeak during sex.
Lubricants to use	Users can add lubricants: • Water-based or silicone-based only. • Applied to outside of condom.	Users can add lubricants: • Water-based, silicone-based, or oil-based (but not with latex condoms). • Before insertion, applied to outside of condom. • After insertion, applied to inside of condom or to the penis.

Comparing Condoms (continued)

Characteristic	Male Condoms	Female Condoms
Breakage or slippage	Tend to break more often than female condoms.	Tend to slip more often than male condoms.
When to remove	Require withdrawing from the vagina before the erection softens.	Can remain in vagina after erection softens. Requires removal before woman stands.
What they protect	Cover and protect most of the penis, protect the woman's internal genitalia.	Cover both the woman's internal and external genitalia and the base of the penis.
How to store	Store away from heat, light, and dampness.	Plastic condoms are not harmed by heat, light or dampness.
Reuse	Cannot be reused.	Reuse not recommended (see Female Condoms, Question 5, p. 270).
Cost and availability	Generally low cost and widely available.	Usually more expensive and less widely available than male condoms.

Comparing IUDs

Characteristic	Copper-Bearing IUD	Levonorgestrel IUD
Effectiveness	Nearly equal. Both are among the most effective methods.	
Length of use	Approved for 10 years.	Approved for 3 to 5 years.
Bleeding patterns	Longer and heavier monthly bleeding, irregular bleeding, and more cramping or pain during monthly bleeding.	More irregular bleeding and spotting in the first few months. After 1 year no monthly bleeding is more common. Causes less bleeding than copper-bearing IUDs over time.
Anemia	May contribute to iron-deficiency anemia if a woman already has low iron blood stores before insertion.	May help prevent iron-deficiency anemia.
Main reasons for discontinuation	Increased bleeding and pain.	No monthly bleeding and hormonal side effects.
Noncontraceptive benefits	May help protect against endometrial cancer.	Effective treatment for long and heavy monthly bleeding (alternative to hysterectomy). May also help treat painful monthly bleeding. Can be used to provide the progestin in hormone replacement therapy.
Postpartum use	Can be inserted up to 48 hours postpartum. After 48 hours, delay until 4 weeks or more.	
Use as emergency contraception	Can be used within 5 days after unprotected sex.	Not recommended.
Insertion	Requires specific training.	
Cost	Less expensive.	More expensive.

If You Miss Pills

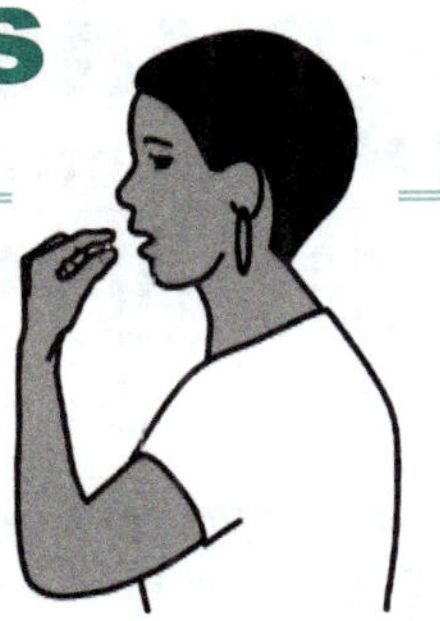

Always take a pill as soon as you remember, and continue taking pills, one each day.

Also...

If you miss pills 3 days or more in a row, or if you start a pack 3 days or more late:

Use condoms or avoid sex for the next 7 days

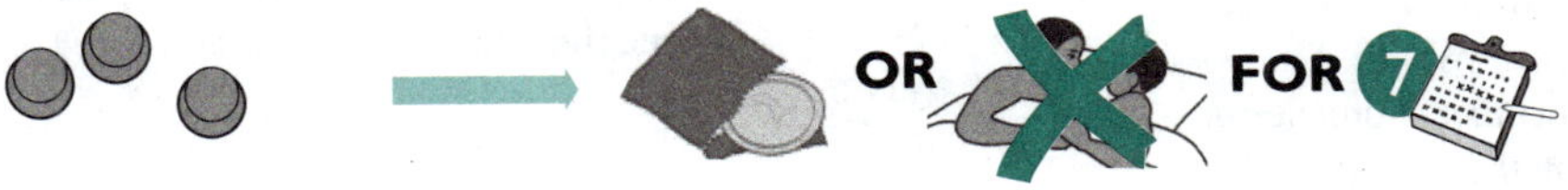

If you miss those 3 or more pills in a row in week 3:

Use condoms or avoid sex for the next 7 days

Also, skip the nonhormonal pills (or skip the pill-free week) and start taking pills at once from the next pack

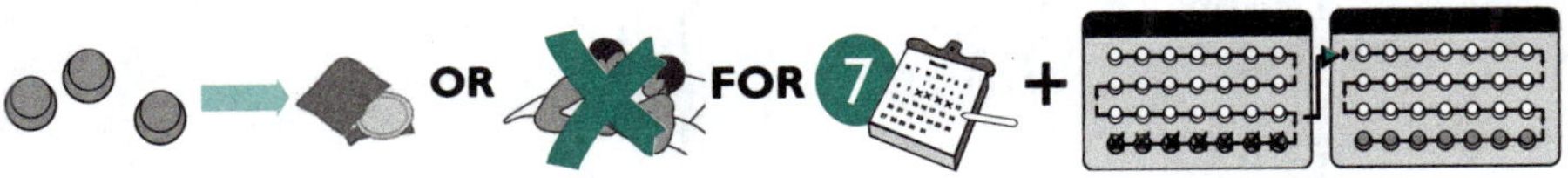

If you miss any nonhormonal pills (last 7 pills in 28-pill packs only):

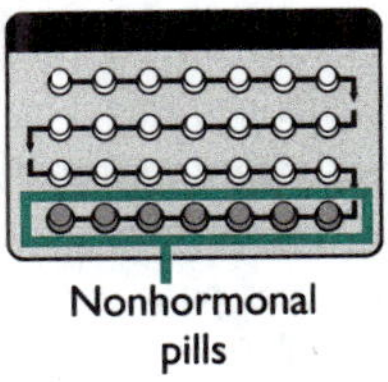

Discard the missed pills and continue taking pills, one each day

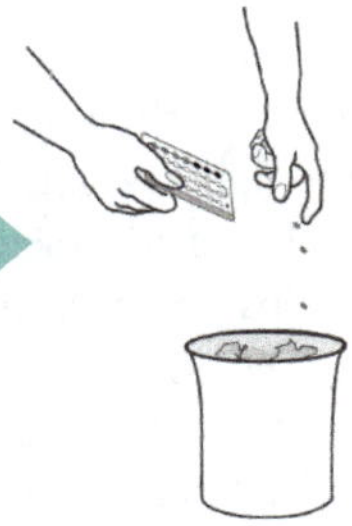

Job Aids/Tools

Female Anatomy

and How Contraceptives Work in Women

Internal Anatomy

Womb (uterus)
Where a fertilized egg grows and develops into a fetus. *IUDs* are placed in the uterus, but they prevent fertilization in the fallopian tubes. *Copper-bearing IUDs* also kill sperm as they move into the uterus.

Ovary
Where eggs develop and one is released each month. The *lactational amenorrhea method (LAM)* and *hormonal methods*, especially those with estrogen, prevent the release of eggs. *Fertility awareness methods* require avoiding unprotected sex around the time when an ovary releases an egg.

Uterine lining (endometrium)
Lining of the uterus, which gradually thickens and then is shed during monthly bleeding.

Fallopian tube
An egg travels along one of these tubes once a month, starting from the ovary. Fertilization of the egg (when sperm meets the egg) occurs in these tubes. *Female sterilization* involves cutting or clipping the fallopian tubes. This prevents sperm and egg from meeting. *IUDs* cause a chemical change that damages sperm before they can meet the egg in the fallopian tube.

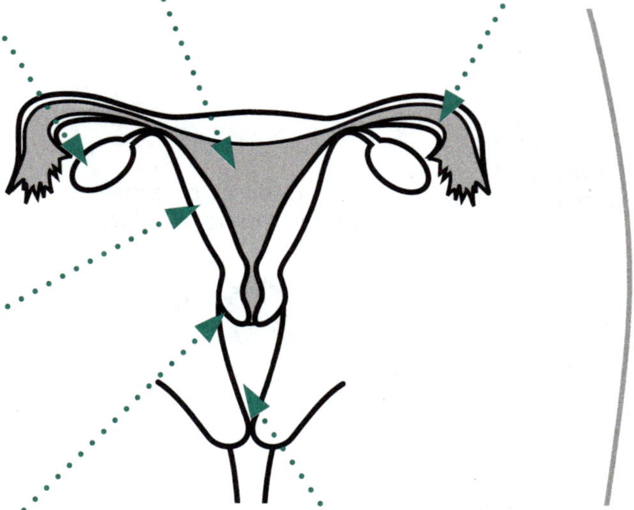

Cervix
The lower portion of the uterus, which extends into the upper vagina. It produces mucus. *Hormonal methods* thicken this mucus, which helps prevent sperm from passing through the cervix. Some *fertility awareness methods* require monitoring cervical mucus. The *diaphragm*, *cervical cap*, and *sponge* cover the cervix so that sperm cannot enter.

Vagina
Joins the outer sexual organs with the uterus. The *combined ring* and the *progesterone-releasing vaginal ring* are placed in the vagina, where they release hormones that pass through the vaginal walls. The *female condom* is placed in the vagina, creating a barrier to sperm. *Spermicides* inserted into the vagina kill sperm.

External Anatomy

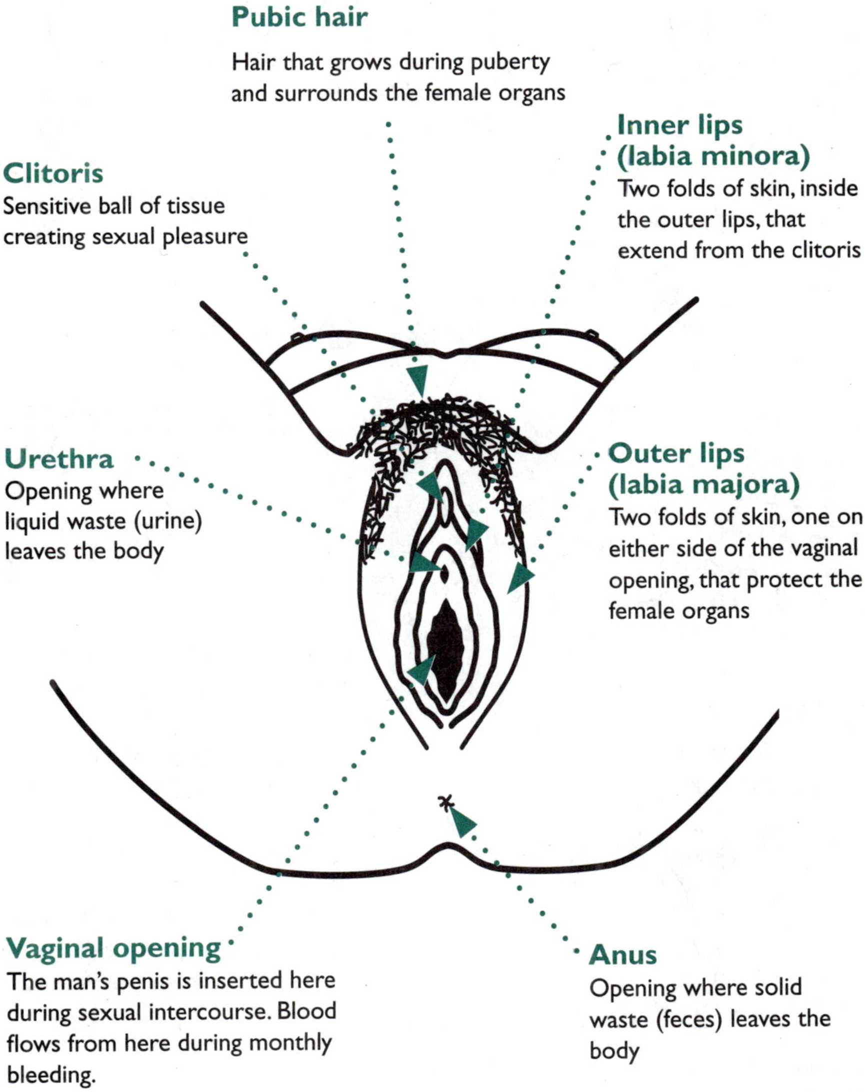

The Menstrual Cycle

1 *Days 1–5:* Monthly bleeding

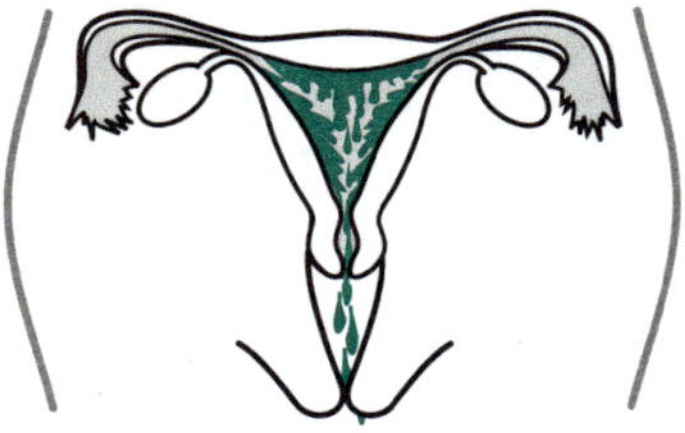

Usually lasts from 2–7 days, often about 5 days

If there is no pregnancy, the thickened lining of the womb is shed. It leaves the body through the vagina. This monthly bleeding is also called menstruation. Contractions of the womb at this time can cause cramps. Some women bleed for a short time (for example, 2 days), while others bleed for up to 8 days. Bleeding can be heavy or light. If the egg is fertilized by a man's sperm, the woman may become pregnant, and monthly bleeding stops.

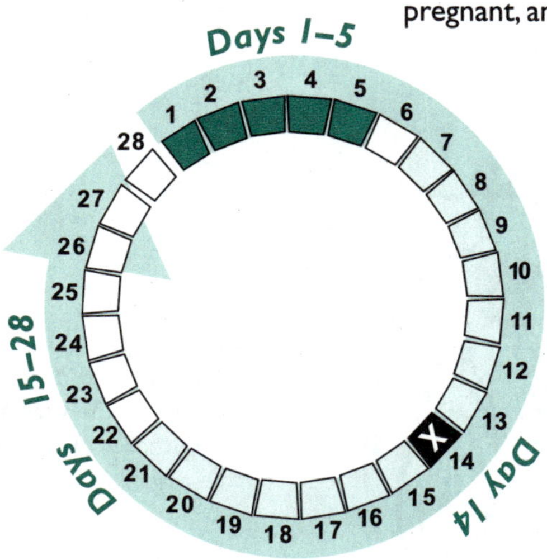

2 *Day 14:* Release of egg

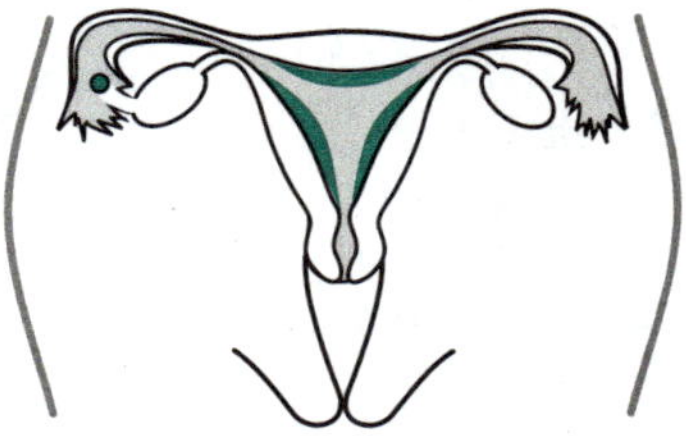

Usually occurs between days 7 and 21 of the cycle, often around day 14

Usually, one of the ovaries releases one egg in each cycle (usually once a month). The egg travels through a fallopian tube towards the womb. It may be fertilized in the tube at this time by a sperm cell that has travelled from the vagina.

3 *Days 15–28:* Thickening of the womb lining

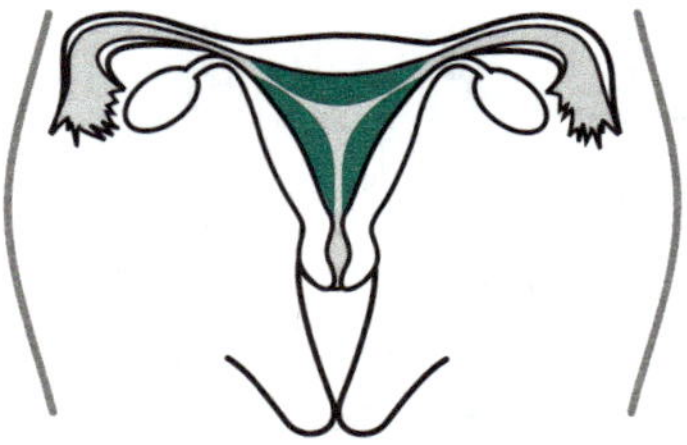

Usually about 14 days long, after ovulation

The lining of the uterus (endometrium) becomes thicker during this time to prepare for a fertilized egg. Usually there is no pregnancy, and the unfertilized egg cell dissolves in the reproductive tract.

Male Anatomy

and How Contraceptives Work in Men

Penis

Male sex organ made of spongy tissue. When a man becomes sexually excited, it grows larger and stiffens. Semen, containing sperm, is released from the penis (ejaculation) at the height of sexual excitement (orgasm). A *male condom* covers the erect penis, preventing sperm from entering the woman's vagina. *Withdrawal* of the penis from the vagina avoids the release of semen into the vagina.

Urethra

Tube through which semen is released from the body. Liquid waste (urine) is released through the same tube.

Seminal vesicles

Where sperm is mixed with semen.

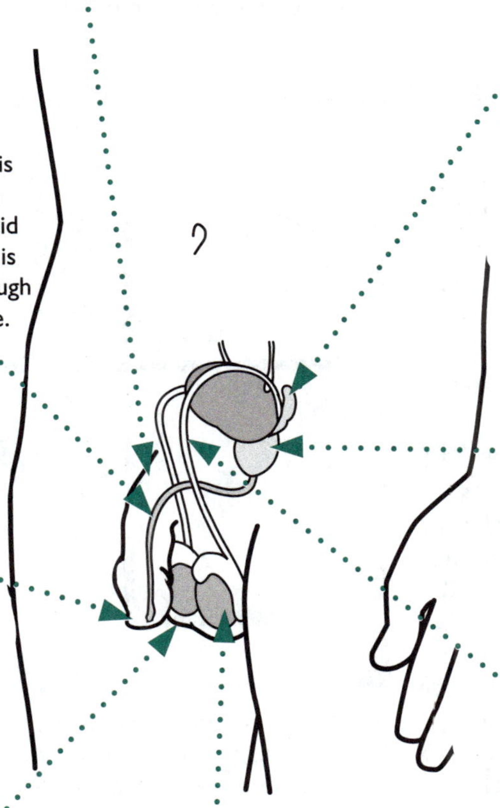

Foreskin

Hood of skin covering the end of the penis. Circumcision removes the foreskin.

Prostate

Organ that produces some of the fluid in semen.

Vas deferens

Each of the 2 thin tubes that carry sperm from the testicles to the seminal vesicles. *Vasectomy* involves cutting or blocking these tubes so that no sperm enters the semen.

Scrotum

Sack of thin loose skin containing the testicles.

Testicles

Organs that produce sperm.

Identifying Migraine Headaches and Auras

Identifying women who suffer from migraine headaches and/or auras is important because migraines, and aura in particular, are linked to higher risk of stroke. Some hormonal contraceptives can increase that risk further.

Migraine Headaches

- Recurring, throbbing, severe head pain, often on one side of the head, that can last from 4 to 72 hours.
- Moving about often makes the migraine headache worse.
- Nausea, vomiting, and sensitivity to light or noise may also occur.

Migraine Auras

- Nervous system disruptions that affect sight and sometimes touch and speech.
- Almost all auras include a bright area of lost vision in one eye that increases in size and turns into a crescent shape with zigzag edges.
- About 30% of auras also include a feeling of "pins and needles" in one hand that spreads up the arm and to one side of the face. Some auras also include trouble with speaking. Seeing spots or flashing lights, or having blurred vision, which often occurs during migraine headaches, is not aura.

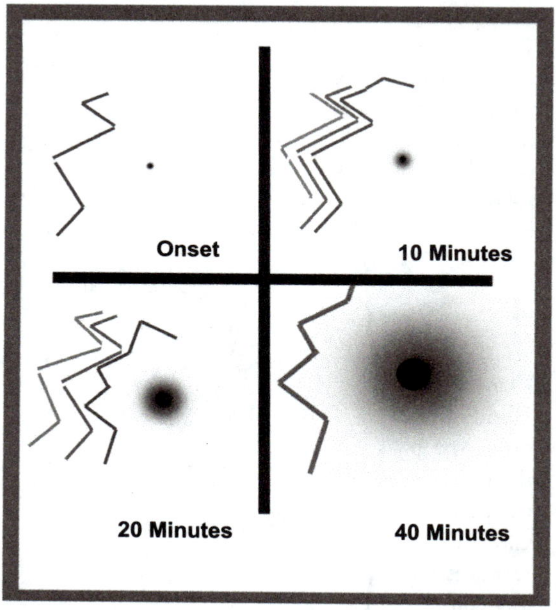

People describe visual auras as bright, shimmering lines or waves around a bright area of lost vision that increase in size and turn into a crescent shape with zigzag edges. The black spot represents how the area of lost vision increases in size over time.

- Auras develop slowly over several minutes and go away within an hour, typically before the headache starts. (In contrast, a sudden blackout in one eye, particularly with a feeling of "pins and needles" or weakness in the opposite arm or leg, may indicate a stroke.)

Identifying Migraine Headaches

For women who want a hormonal method‡,§ or are using one.

If a woman reports having very bad headaches, ask her these questions to tell the difference between a migraine headache and an ordinary headache. If she answers "yes" to any 2 of these questions, she probably suffers from migraine headaches. Continue to Identifying Migraine Auras, below.

1. **Do your headaches make you feel sick to your stomach?**
2. **When you have a headache, do light and noise bother you a lot more than when you do not have a headache?**
3. **Do you have headaches that stop you from working or carrying out your usual activities for one day or more?**

Identifying Migraine Auras

Ask this question to identify the most common migraine aura. If a woman answers "yes," she probably suffers from migraine auras.

1. **Have you ever had a bright light in your eyes lasting 5 to 60 minutes, loss of clear vision usually to one side, and then a headache?** (Women with such aura often bring one hand up beside their heads when describing the vision change. In some cases the bright light is not followed by a headache.)

If her headaches are not migraines and she does not have aura, she can start or continue hormonal methods if she is otherwise medically eligible. Any later changes in her headaches should be evaluated, however.

Can a Woman With Migraines and/or Aura Use a Hormonal Method?

In situations where clinical judgment is limited:

Yes = Yes, can use; No = No, do not use; I = Initiation; C = Continuation

	Combined methods†		Progestin-only methods§	
Migraine headaches	I	C	I	C
Without aura				
Age < 35	Yes	No	Yes	Yes
Age ≥ 35	No	No	Yes	Yes
With aura, at any age	No	No	Yes	No

† *Methods with estrogen and progestin: combined oral contraceptives, monthly injectables, combined patch, and combined vaginal ring*

§ *Methods with progestin only: progestin-only pills, progestin-only injectables, and implants*

Considering Progestin-Only Injectables Where HIV Risk Is High: Counseling Tips

Countries and programs where many family planning clients are at high risk of HIV infection may decide to tell all women interested in progestin-only injectables about research findings concerning HIV risk (see Progestin-Only Injectables, Question 2, p. 92). Women at high HIV risk can still choose to use a progestin-only injectable if they wish.

For providers in these programs, here are some counseling tips:

- **Tell the client interested in a progestin-only injectable these facts:**

  1. **Some research has found that women who use a progestin-only injectable and are exposed to HIV are slightly more likely than other women to get an HIV infection.**
  2. **The meaning of these findings is not clear.** We do not know whether or not this method causes this higher risk.
  3. **You can protect yourself from HIV.**
  4. **You can still choose this method,** but we want you to think about this information.
  5. **We have other long-acting and effective methods**, and we can discuss them if you would like.

- **Help the woman consider:**

  1. **Are you doing something to protect yourself from HIV infection?** [Discuss how she protects herself from HIV.] **If not, could you start protecting yourself now?** [Discuss HIV protection choices.]
  2. **Do you prefer a progestin-only injectable much more than any other method?** [If so, reassure her that she can choose a progestin-only injectable if she prefers it.] **Would you like to discuss and think about other methods, too?** [Mention and discuss especially other long-lasting, effective and convenient methods, such as implants and IUDs.]

Note: This counseling is for women who are *not now infected with HIV* but who face a high risk that they may become infected in the future. It is not relevant for women who already have HIV infection. Women who already have HIV infection also can safely use a progestin-only injectable.

Ruling Out Pregnancy

Ruling out pregnancy is recommended before starting a hormonal contraceptive and before IUD insertion. Family planning providers have 3 tools available for this routine task:

1. Medical history (often collected using the Pregnancy Checklist shown on the inside back cover)
2. Pregnancy tests
3. Delaying the start of the method until the client's next monthly bleeding.

Which tool should a provider use first, and when?

The job aid on the next page, How and When to Use the Pregnancy Checklist and Pregnancy Tests, offers guidance based on the client's chosen method and on whether she has been having bleeding each month or she is not having monthly bleedings due to recent childbirth or other reasons. This job aid also addresses the situation for a woman who has been having monthly bleedings but now has missed her expected monthly bleeding.

Important points to note

- Unless the client has missed her monthly bleeding, ruling out pregnancy **starts with the Pregnancy Checklist.** This checklist can provide reasonable certainty that a woman is not pregnant.
- **Pregnancy tests are not likely to work before the first day of missed monthly bleeding.** Using a test earlier is pointless and wasteful.
- **The only contraceptive method known to pose a health risk if started during pregnancy is the IUD (either copper or hormonal).** If the Pregnancy Checklist cannot rule out pregnancy, a provider should use another tool to rule out pregnancy before inserting an IUD.
- **All hormonal methods except the LNG-IUD can be provided without delay** even when uncertainty about pregnancy exists. Follow-up is required in some cases (see job aid on next page).
- **Delaying the start of the method is the worst choice** among the 3 tools for assessing pregnancy. She may become pregnant before her next monthly bleeding. The other tools should be used first whenever possible.
- Both the Pregnancy Checklist and a pregnancy test are highly accurate for ruling out pregnancy when used appropriately. **When the checklist can be used, there is no reason to prefer a test.**

How and When to Use the Pregnancy Checklist and Pregnancy Tests

Match your client's menstrual status and chosen contraceptive method with one of the options below and follow the instructions.

Client with amenorrhea (postpartum or other type)

Implants, pills, ring, injectables, or patch | **IUDs** Copper or LNG

Use Pregnancy Checklist.[1]
Pregnancy ruled out: Provide method.

Pregnancy not ruled out:
Use a pregnancy test.

Implants, pills, ring, injectables, or patch: Pregnancy test is negative (or test is not immediately available): Provide the method now.[2]

Schedule a follow-up pregnancy test in 3–4 weeks.

IUDs: Pregnancy test is negative (or test is not immediately available): Advise woman to use COCs, DMPA, or condoms or abstain for 3–4 weeks, then repeat the pregnancy test.

Second pregnancy test is negative: Provide the IUD.

Client between two regular menses (monthly bleeding)*

Implants, pills, ring, injectables, or patch | **IUDs** Copper or LNG

Use Pregnancy Checklist.[1]
Pregnancy ruled out: Provide method.
Do not use a pregnancy test (in most cases it is too early for the test to be effective).

Implants, pills, ring, injectables, or patch: Pregnancy not ruled out: Provide the method now.[2]

Return for a pregnancy test if next menses are delayed.

IUDs: Pregnancy not ruled out: Do not provide method.

Advise woman to return for LNG-IUD insertion within 7 days of onset of her next menses, or within 12 days for a copper IUD; but in the meantime, use COCs, DMPA, or condoms or abstain.

Return for a preganancy test if next menses are delayed.

[1] See inside back cover for Pregnancy Checklist.

[2] For implants, counsel about the need to remove the implant if pregnancy is confirmed and she wishes to continue the pregnancy.

In cases where pregnancy cannot be ruled out, offer emergency contraception if the woman had unprotected sex within the last 5 days.

Counsel all women to come back any time they have a reason to suspect pregnancy (for example, she misses a period).

* **If the client presents with a late/missed menses, use a pregnancy test to rule out pregnancy.** If using a highly sensitive pregnancy test (for example, 25 mIU/ml) and it is negative, provide her desired method.

If using a test with lower sensitivity (for example, 50 mIU/ml) and it is negative during the time of her missed period, wait until at least 10 days after expected date of menses and repeat the test. Advise the woman to use condoms or abstain in the meantime. If the test is still negative, provide her desired method.

If test sensitivity is not specified, assume lower sensitivity.